Handbook of Venous Thromboembolism

Handbook of Venous Thromboembolism

Edited by

Jecko Thachil, MBBS, MD, MRCP, FRCPath
Consultant Haematologist,
Department of Haematology, Manchester Royal Infirmary,
Manchester, UK

Catherine Bagot, BSc, MBBS, MD, MRCP, FRCPath
Consultant Haematologist,
Department of Haematology, Glasgow Royal Infirmary,
Glasgow, UK

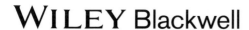

This edition first published 2018
© 2018 John Wiley & Sons Ltd

Registered Office
John Wiley & Sons Ltd, The Atrium, Southern Gate, Chichester, West Sussex, PO19 8SQ, UK

Editorial Offices
9600 Garsington Road, Oxford, OX4 2DQ, UK
The Atrium, Southern Gate, Chichester, West Sussex, PO19 8SQ, UK

For details of our global editorial offices, customer services, and more information about Wiley products visit us at www.wiley.com.

Wiley also publishes its books in a variety of electronic formats and by print-on-demand. Some content that appears in standard print versions of this book may not be available in other formats.

Limit of Liability/Disclaimer of Warranty
The publisher and the authors make no representations or warranties with respect to the accuracy or completeness of the contents of this work and specifically disclaim all warranties, including without limitation any implied warranties of fitness for a particular purpose. This work is sold with the understanding that the publisher is not engaged in rendering professional services. The advice and strategies contained herein may not be suitable for every situation. In view of ongoing research, equipment modifications, changes in governmental regulations, and the constant flow of information relating to the use of experimental reagents, equipment, and devices, the reader is urged to review and evaluate the information provided in the package insert or instructions for each chemical, piece of equipment, reagent, or device for, among other things, any changes in the instructions or indication of usage and for added warnings and precautions. The fact that an organization or website is referred to in this work as a citation and/or potential source of further information does not mean that the author or the publisher endorses the information the organization or website may provide or recommendations it may make. Further, readers should be aware that websites listed in this work may have changed or disappeared between when this works was written and when it is read. No warranty may be created or extended by any promotional statements for this work. Neither the publisher nor the author shall be liable for any damages arising here from.

Library of Congress Cataloging-in-Publication Data

Names: Thachil, Jecko, editor. | Bagot, Catherine, editor.
Title: Handbook of venous thromboembolism / edited by Jecko Thachil and Catherine Bagot.
Description: Chichester, West Sussex ; Hoboken : John Wiley & Sons, 2018. |
   Includes bibliographical references and index. |
Identifiers: LCCN 2017039383 (print) | LCCN 2017040998 (ebook) | ISBN 9781119095590 (pdf) |
   ISBN 9781119095583 (epub) | ISBN 9781119095576 (cloth)
Subjects: | MESH: Venous Thromboembolism
Classification: LCC RC697 (ebook) | LCC RC697 (print) | NLM WG 610 | DDC 616.1/45–dc23
LC record available at https://lccn.loc.gov/2017039383

Cover Design: Wiley
Cover Image: ©London_England/iStockphoto

Set in 10/12pt Warnock by SPi Global, Pondicherry, India

Printed in Singapore by C.O.S. Printers Pte Ltd

10 9 8 7 6 5 4 3 2 1

Contents

List of Contributors

William R. Auger, MD
University of California, San Diego, USA

Catherine Bagot, BSc, MBBS, MD, MRCP, FRCPath
Consultant Haematologist, Department of
Haematology, Glasgow Royal Infirmary,
Glasgow, UK

Rebecca Barton, MBBS, BBioMedSc
Department of Clinical Haematology, Royal
Children's Hospital, Melbourne, Australia

Enrico Bernardi, MD, PhD
Department of Emergency and Accident Medicine,
Hospital of Conegliano, Italy

Karen Breen, MD, MRCPI, FRCPath
Dept of Thrombosis, St.Thomas' Hospital, London

Andrew Busuttil, MD, MRCS
Academic Section of Vascular Surgery, Charing
Cross Hospital, Imperial College London, UK

Giuseppe Camporese, MD
Unit of Angiology, Department of Cardiac-
Thoracic-Vascular Sciences, University Hospital of
Padua, Italy

Lana A. Castellucci, MD, MSc
Department of Medicine, Ottawa Hospital Research
Institute, University of Ottawa, Ottawa, Canada

Yen-Lin Chee, MBChB, MRCP, PhD, MRCPath
Consultant Haematologist, Department of
Hematology-Oncology, National University Cancer
Institute, Singapore

Marco Das, MD, PhD, MBA
Department of Radiology and Nuclear Medicine,
Maastricht University Medical Center (MUMC+),
Maastricht, The Netherlands

Alun H. Davies, MA, DM, DSc, FRCS, FHEA, FEBVS, FACPh
Academic Section of Vascular Surgery, Charing
Cross Hospital, Imperial College London, UK

Kerstin de Wit, MBChB, BSc, MSc, MD
Department of Medicine, McMaster University,
Hamilton, Ontario, Canada

C.E.A. Dronkers, MD
Department of Thrombosis and Hemostasis, Leiden
University Medical Center, Leiden, The Netherlands

*Emmanuel J. Favaloro, BSc (Hons), MAIMS,
PhD, FFSc (RCPA)*
Department of Haematology, Institute of Clinical
Pathology and Medical Research (ICPMR),
Pathology West, NSW Health Pathology, Westmead
Hospital, Westmead, NSW, Australia

David Fitzmaurice, MBChB, MRCGP, MD, FRCGP
Professor of Cardiorespiratory Primary Care,
University of Warwick, Coventry, UK

Lauren Floyd, MBBS, MRCP
Core Trainee, Manchester Royal Infirmary,
Manchester, UK

Massimo Franchini, MD
Department of Hematology and Transfusion
Medicine, C. Poma Hospital, Mantova, Italy

Emma Gee, BSc
Nurse Consultant, Thrombosis and Anticoagulation, King's College Hospital NHS Foundation Trust, London, UK

Francesca Gianniello, MD
A. Bianchi Bonomi Hemophilia and Thrombosis Center, Fondazione IRCCS Ca' Granda - Ospedale Maggiore Policlinico, Milan, Italy

Carlos J. Guevara, MD
Interventional Radiology Section, Mallinckrodt Institute of Radiology, Washington University in St. Louis, USA

Paul Hahn, MD, PhD
Department of Ophthalmology, Duke University Medical Center, Durham

Dan Horner, BA, MBBS, MD, PgCert, MRCP (UK) FCEM FFICM
Consultant in Emergency Medicine and Intensive Care, Salford Royal NHS Foundation Trust, Manchester, UK

M.V. Huisman, MD
Department of Thrombosis and Hemostasis, Leiden University Medical Center, Leiden, The Netherlands

Francesca Jones, MBBS, MRCP, FRCPath
Haematology consultant
Department of Haematology, University Hospital Coventry and Warwick, NHS Foundation Trust, UK

David Keeling, BSc MD FRCP FRCPath
Consultant Haematologist, Oxford Haemophilia and Thrombosis Centre, Oxford University Hospitals, Oxford, UK

Dianne Patricia Kitchen
Point of Care, UK NEQAS for Blood Coagulation, Sheffield, UK

F.A. Klok, MD, PhD
Department of Thrombosis and Hemostasis, Leiden University Medical Center, Leiden, The Netherlands

Dawn Kyle, BSC, RGN
Team Leader, Glasgow and Clyde Anticoagulation Service, Glasgow, UK

Kathryn Lang, MBBS, MRCP(UK)
King's Thrombosis Centre, Department of Haematological Medicine, King's College Hospital Foundation NHS Trust, London

Will Lester, MBChB, BSc, FRCP, FRCPath, PhD
Haematology Consultant
Department of Haematology, University Hospital Birmingham NHS Foundation Trust

Giuseppe Lippi, MD
Section of Clinical Biochemistry, University of Verona, Verona, Italy

Molly W. Mandernach, MD, MPH, FACP
University of Florida College of Medicine, Gainesville, Florida, USA

Ida Martinelli, MD, PhD
A. Bianchi Bonomi Hemophilia and Thrombosis Center, Fondazione IRCCS Ca' Granda - Ospedale Maggiore Policlinico, Milan, Italy

Paul Monagle, MBBS, MD, MSc, FRACP, FRCPA, FCCP
Department of Clinical Haematology & Department of Paediatrics, University of Melbourne Royal Children's Hospital, Victoria, Australia

Kathy Macintosh, BSc
Team Leader, Glasgow and Clyde Anticoagulation Service, Glasgow, UK

Alison Moughton
Anticoagulant Nurse Specialist
Department of Haematology, University Hospital Birmingham NHS Foundation Trust

Simon Noble, MBBS, MD, FRCP
Division of Population Medicine, Cardiff University, Cardiff, Wales

Serena M. Passamonti, MD, PhD
A. Bianchi Bonomi Hemophilia and Thrombosis Center, Fondazione IRCCS Ca' Granda - Ospedale Maggiore Policlinico, Milan, Italy

Jignesh Patel, BSc(Hons), MSc, PhD
Institute of Pharmaceutical Science, Faculty of Life Sciences and Medicine, King's College, London & King's Thrombosis Centre, Department of Haematological Medicine, King's College Hospital Foundation NHS Trust, London, UK

Demosthenes G. Papamatheakis, MD
University of California, San Diego, USA

Catherine Nelson Piercy, PhD, FRCP, FRCOG
Professor of Obstetric Medicine, Women's Health Academic Centre, Guy's and St Thomas' Foundation Trust, London, UK

Anita Rajasekhar, MD, MS
University of Florida College of Medicine, Gainesville, Florida, USA

Gill Parmilan, MBBS, MRCP
Core Trainee, Manchester Royal Infirmary, Manchester, UK

Peter E. Rose, BSc(Hons), PhD
Consultant Haematologist, Warwick Hospital, South Warwickshire Foundation Trust, UK

Linda Smith, RGN/BSC
Team Leader, Glasgow and Clyde Anticoagulation Service, Glasgow, UK

Scott M. Stevens, MD
Department of Medicine, Intermountain Medical Center, Murray, Utah, and Department of Medicine, University of Utah School of Medicine, Salt Lake City, Utah, USA

R. Campbell Tait, MBChB, FRCPSG, FRCPath
Honorary Professor of Haemostasis and Thrombosis, Department of Haematology, Glasgow Royal Infirmary, Glasgow, UK

Jecko Thachil, MBBS, MD, MRCP, FRCPath
Department of Haematology, Manchester Royal Infirmary, Manchester, UK

Suresh Vedantham, MD
Interventional Radiology Section, Mallinckrodt Institute of Radiology, Washington University in St. Louis, USA

Henry G. Watson, MD, FRCP, FRCPath
Consultant Haematologist and Honorary Professor of Medicine, Aberdeen Royal Infirmary, Foresterhill Health Campus, Aberdeen, Scotland, UK

Christian Weimar, MD
Department of Neurology and Stroke Center, University Duisburg-Essen, Germany

Joachim E. Wildberger, MD, PhD
Department of Radiology and Nuclear Medicine, Maastricht University Medical Center (MUMC+), Maastricht, The Netherlands

Scott C. Woller, MD
Department of Medicine, Intermountain Medical Center, Murray, Utah, and Department of Medicine, University of Utah School of Medicine, Salt Lake City, Utah, USA

Wenlan Zhang, MD
Department of Ophthalmology, Duke University Medical Center, Durham

Foreword

Venous thromboembolism (VTE) is ubiquitous in both primary and secondary care, and therefore, having a clear understanding of the presentation, diagnosis and treatment of this condition is important. However, remaining up to date with this rapidly changing field is a challenge for the non-expert.

Over the last 20 years, the management of VTE has undergone a paradigm shift. Investigation and diagnosis of Deep Vein Thrombosis (DVT) and, in recent years, pulmonary embolism (PE), has moved from an in-patient setting into well-defined out-patient pathways. Warfarin, the mainstay of treatment for venous thrombosis for over 70 years, is rapidly being replaced by use of direct oral anticoagulants, a new class of drugs which have their own characteristics and challenges. Finally, when once all patients would have received six months of anticoagulation following a VTE, patients are now risk-stratified, using a combination of both laboratory and demographic markers, demonstrating that a single duration of anticoagulation cannot be universally applied.

In addition to changes in VTE management, the prevention of VTE in hospital inpatients has become paramount in recent years, with the realisation that a significant number of thromboses occur as a result of hospital admission. Prevention strategies have reached the top of national health agendas, and remain a significant focus of safe patient care. Implementing effective VTE prevention strategies can be a significant challenge for healthcare professionals who may not have a primary role in VTE.

The purpose of this book is to provide all healthcare professionals involved in VTE with an easy-to-use tool, written by experts in the field, which summarises the most effective strategies for VTE investigation, diagnosis, management and prevention. We hope it can also be a practical reference for all those involved in the care of patients with VTE, both in its treatment and prevention.

Dr Catherine Bagot, Consultant Haematologist, Glasgow, UK
Dr Jecko Thachil, Consultant Haematologist, Manchester, UK

Section I

Clinical Overview

1

Risk Factors for Venous Thromboembolism

Peter E. Rose

Consultant Haematologist, Warwick Hospital, South Warwickshire Foundation Trust, UK

Introduction

There are many risk factors reported to increase the risk of venous thromboembolism (VTE), as shown in Table 1.1.

Large national registries for VTE patients have helped to elucidate and quantify the relative risk of individual factors. The risk factors for deep vein thrombosis (DVT) and pulmonary embolism (PE) are largely similar, as DVT and PE represent a spectrum of the same disease process. There is also some overlap between venous and arterial thrombotic risk, with age, smoking and obesity common to both, although they are much more important factors in arterial disease. Part of this may be an indirect association – for example, smoking increases cancer risk, and hence VTE, while medical in-patients with heart failure have a marked increase in risk for pulmonary embolism. Figure 1.1 shows the increasing rate of VTE with age, from the UK VTE registry, VERITY. Overall, the risk for VTE is increasing, with an ever aging population, receiving multiple medications many of which increase thrombotic risk, particularly in the field of cancer medicine.

The most important risk factors for VTE are a history of previous VTE, recent surgery, hospital in-patient stay and cancer. While there is much comment around factors such as long-haul travel and inherited risk factors for VTE, these represent less common and less important factors. In general the more risk factors present, the greater will be the cumulative risk for VTE.

Previous VTE

For patients with a known history of VTE, it is important to identify if the previous event was provoked, in association with temporary risk factors, or unprovoked. The risk of recurrence is less than 3% if provoked, but is near 10% in unprovoked VTE within 12 months of discontinuing anticoagulant therapy. It can be difficult to determine what is and is not provoked; for example, a DVT post orthopaedic surgery is clearly provoked, while a female on the combined pill preparation for three years without previous thrombosis is not necessarily a provoked event. A VTE within three months of starting the pill however, would be provoked.

Provoking factors can be further divided into surgical, with a recurrence rate of 1% within 12 months of treatment, and non-surgical factors, with a 6% risk in this time period. For patients with unprovoked VTE, the risk persists with time, with 40% recurrence within ten years. For a cohort of young male patients presenting with unprovoked PE, there is a 20% risk of recurrence of PE within 12 months which persists, making recurrence almost inevitable.

Table 1.1 Risk factors for venous thromboembolic disease.

Patient Related	Additional factors
Increasing age	Surgery within 90 days
Previous history VTE	Lower limb cast
Family history 1st degree relative	Hospital stay > 3 days
Thrombophilia	Cancer in past six months/ongoing disease
Pregnancy	Medical comorbidities
Obesity > 30 kg/m^2	Extended travel
Smoking/alcohol/substance abuse	Medication related

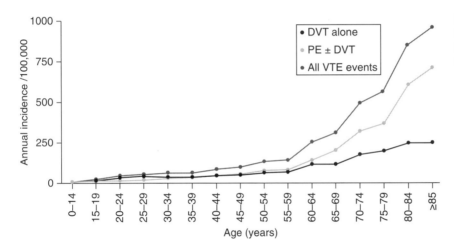

Figure 1.1 VTE risk increases with age. Taken from UK VERITY (Venous Thromboembolism registry).

Surgery

Pulmonary embolism remains the most widely reported preventable cause of death in patients undergoing surgery. It is the most common cause of death within 30 days of surgery, with 40% of VTE events occurring later than three weeks post operatively. Even for low-risk general gynaecological abdominal surgery for non-malignant disease, the risk for VTE extends up to at least 90 days post-surgery. Previous autopsy studies in surgical patients report VTE to be present in 5–10% of cases. Surgery, therefore, requiring general anaesthesia for over one hour, is a major risk factor for VTE. Surgical risk is compounded by many concomitant medical risk factors – for example, a further doubling of risk in cancer surgery. See Table 1.2.

Orthopaedic Surgery

Patients undergoing lower limb surgery are among the highest risk patients (odds ratio > 10), and this includes total hip and knee arthroplasty, hip/leg fractures, major orthopaedic trauma and spinal surgery. With improved surgical procedures and shorter time for anaesthesia, there is some recent risk reduction. The risk for VTE partly relates to prolonged stasis associated with immobility, and the release of tissue fragments of collagen and fat, which can directly activate coagulation factors. Furthermore, direct blood vessel damage during retraction of soft tissues can act as a nidus for thrombus formation.

Table 1.2 Surgical risk factors for VTE.

Personal	Surgical
Age > 60	Prolonged anaesthesia
Medical comorbidities	Major trauma
Previous VTE	Lower limb surgery
Thrombophilia	Major abdominal surgery
Obesity	Cancer surgery
	Post-operative admission to ITU
	Bariatric surgery

Lower limb immobilisation in casts, with or without surgery, increases the risk of VTE. The prevalence of lower limb injury-related DVT with cast immobilisation is reported to occur in 4–40% of cases. Further confirmation of the importance comes from studies using chemical thromboprophylaxis, which results in a 50% reduction in DVT rate. On this basis, NICE guidance recommends that all patients with lower limb immobilisation should be assessed for chemical thromboprophylaxis.

Other Surgeries

Other high-risk surgery includes major abdominal procedures, particularly in cancer patients. Evidence confirming the importance of general surgery as a major risk factor for VTE is provided from studies evaluating the efficacy of thromboprophylaxis. For example, a systematic review of cancer patients undergoing surgery showed a reduction in VTE events from 35% to 13% in patients receiving pharmacological thromboprophylaxis.

Additional risk factors for thrombus and surgery include the increasing use of indwelling venous catheters and filters for prolonged periods of time in the post-operative period. It is estimated that 14% of patients undergoing cardiac surgery without thromboprophylaxis develop VTE. As many of these patients are already on antiplatelet or anticoagulant therapy, the true risk associated with surgery is difficult to assess. Similarly, the risk with vascular surgery, while increased, is difficult to quantify in a largely elderly group with reduced mobility, on anti-platelet therapy and often with comorbidities. A careful VTE risk assessment is needed for all patients undergoing surgery, particularly where this involves general anaesthesia and prolonged hospital admission, evaluating the bleeding risk due to the procedure against the reduction in thrombotic events.

Hospitalised Medical Patients

Approximately 70–80% of fatal hospital acquired thrombosis (HAT) occurs in medical patients. Venous thrombosis is increased in most acute medical conditions, necessitating hospital admission. The risk of VTE is also increased in a number of chronic medical disorders (see Table 1.3). Medical inpatients are usually elderly, often with several conditions to compound VTE risk.

Stroke patients, whether due to ischaemic or haemorrhagic events, are at increased risk of VTE, with a wide range of estimates reported, namely, 15–60%. Prevention with chemical thromboprophylaxis is dependent on safety, with haemorrhagic risk often high. In the absence of haemorrhage, the presence of additional factors, such as severity of immobilisation and comorbidities, are important for risk assessment. Acute respiratory infection in hospitalised patients is a particularly high risk for VTE. Other medical conditions included in

Table 1.3 Medical conditions with increased risk of VTE.

Acute	Chronic
Congestive heart failure	Disorders of mobility (mechanical/ neurological)
Respiratory failure	Nephrotic syndrome
Severe infection/ sepsis	Sickle-cell disease
Rheumatological conditions	Paraproteinaemia
Inflammatory bowel disorders	Paroxysmal nocturnal haemoglobinuria
Stroke	Bechet's disease
Cancer	Porphyria

clinical trials for thromboprophylaxis in medical patients include congestive heart failure, respiratory failure, acute rheumatological and inflammatory bowel disorders.

Clinical studies have shown the risk of DVT to be between 4–5%, with mortality at 90 days 6–14%. Congestive heart failure patients commonly develop DVT in the absence of thromboprophylaxis, affecting 20–40% of patients, with a similar risk for medical intensive care patients. All hospitalised medical inpatients, therefore, require a risk assessment for VTE in order to reduce morbidity and mortality from HAT.

Several chronic medical conditions carry an increased life-time risk of VTE. Rheumatological disorders such as systemic lupus erythematosus, particularly associated with the anti-phospholipid syndrome, are pro-thrombotic conditions. Inflammatory bowel disease is associated with a 2–3 fold increased VTE risk. Less common medical conditions at high risk include Bechet's disease, nephrotic syndrome, sickle cell disease, and some porphyrias. Paroxysmal nocturnal haemoglobinuria, while rare, is complicated by thrombotic problems in over 50% of cases. Medical treatments may also be associated with VTE, with hormone therapies and erythropoietin being common examples. These medical conditions should evoke a high index of suspicion for VTE, particularly in those with a previous proven event.

Cancer Associated Thrombosis (CAT)

Twenty percent of all VTE cases occur in patients with cancer (those diagnosed within the previous six months or with ongoing disease or treatment for cancer). VTE is the second most common cause of death in cancer patients, and is associated with a very poor prognosis. Nearly 50% of cancer patients die within six months of developing VTE. CAT has a different pathogenesis, a different additional risk profile, and requires different management from non-cancer VTE. CAT is often undiagnosed, as it is found in 50% of cancer patients at autopsy. Important risk factors need to be considered for CAT, including the tumour site and the presence of metastatic disease. These risk factors are shown in Table 1.4 below.

Tumour sites with the highest thrombotic risk include pancreas, brain, stomach and lung. Rare tumours, such as head and neck plus endocrine, are also high risk for CAT – see Figures 1.2 and 1.3 from the UK VERITY registry.

While breast and prostatic cancer are the most commonly seen malignancies in patients presenting with CAT, this is due to their increased prevalence, with overall moderate to low risk, respectively, for these sites. The risk of VTE is greatly increased in the presence of metastatic disease, with increased tumour burden an important factor in promoting the pro-thrombotic state. This is illustrated in breast cancer, where the risk for localised Stage 1 disease not requiring adjuvant treatment for VTE is low, but increases 15 fold for those with Stage 4 disease requiring chemotherapy.

Table 1.4 Risk factors for cancer-associated VTE.

All cancer patients	Cancer patients receiving chemotherapy
Site of tumour high/intermediate/low risk	Platelets $> 350 \times 10^9$/l
Metastatic disease	Haemoglobin < 100 g/l
Surgery	White blood count $> 11 \times 10^9$/l
Chemotherapy	BMI > 35 kg/m^2
Radiotherapy	High D-dimer
Hormone treatment	High serum P-selectin
Anti-angiogenic therapy	
Indwelling venous catheter	

Figure 1.2 Risk factors for VTE. Taken from UK VERITY (Venous Thromboembolism registry).

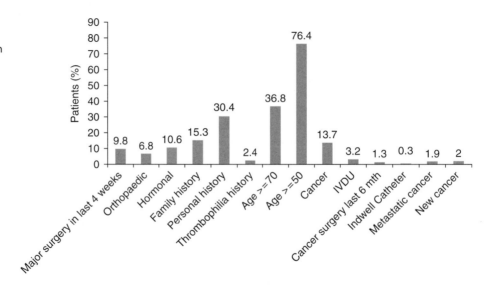

There is also a 28 fold increase in CAT patients with haematological malignancy, compared with population controls. This figure not only reflects the underlying pro-thrombotic state, but also the intensity and need for several modalities of treatment. Nearly all modalities of treatment increase the thrombotic risk in cancer patients. Many chemotherapeutic agents increase damage to the vascular endothelium, while radiotherapy also increases VTE. Many adjuvant treatments, such as hormone therapy, anti-angiogenic agents such as thalidomide, lenalidomide and anti- VEGF therapy, are associated with high risk for thrombosis. The use of indwelling lines for prolonged venous access, together with the additional risk where surgery is needed, all contribute to CAT. Supportive therapies, such as G-CSF, erythropoietin and even blood transfusion, have been reported to increase VTE risk.

The presence of malignancy appears such a significant risk factor for VTE that the risk profile is very different from non-cancer patients with VTE. In one large registry study, factors such as personal history of VTE, Thrombophilia, IV drug abuse and smoking were only significantly raised in non-cancer patients, with medical in-patient stay with immobilisation for more than three days in the last four weeks more common in CAT patients. In many, CAT is asymptomatic with increasing numbers of cases identified, due to improved imaging techniques. All cancer patients, as part of the multi-disciplinary treatment assessment at presentation, should have an appraisal of VTE risk in order to reduce the very high mortality with CAT. See Figure 1.4.

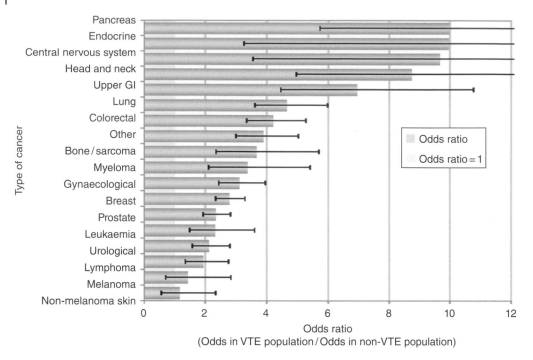

Figure 1.3 Rates of different cancers in the non-VTE and VTE population; odds ratios for different types of cancer. Taken from UK VERITY (Venous Thromboembolism registry).

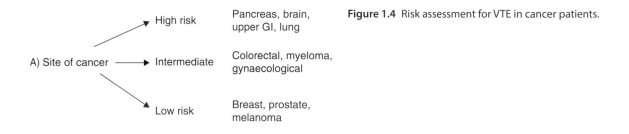

Figure 1.4 Risk assessment for VTE in cancer patients.

Pregnancy

Pregnancy is a pro-thrombotic state from the first trimester onwards, and is associated with a 4–5 fold increase in risk for VTE. The highest risk period is in the immediate eight weeks post-partum, with a 20 fold increased risk. The prevalence of all thrombotic events in pregnancy is two per 1000 deliveries, with 80% venous and 20% arterial. It is suggested that the pro-thrombotic state has evolved to reduce the haemorrhagic complications with childbirth. VTE accounts for approximately 10% of all maternal deaths, and is the most common cause in the western world. The risk of VTE increases with maternal age and multi-parity, and is higher in black females. The risk factors are shown in Table 1.5.

The clinical presentation is usually with an extensive clot in the proximal veins of the left leg. The predilection for the left leg is due to narrowing of the left common iliac vein, as it compresses between the lumbar vertebral body and right common iliac artery. There have also to be additional mechanical or hormonal factors in pregnancy to affect this change.

Table 1.5 Pregnancy and risk factors for VTE.

Patient-related	Additional factors
Increasing age > 35	Caesarean section
Previous VTE	Dehydration (hyperemesis)
Multi-parity	Pre-eclampsia
Varicose veins	Previous fertility treatment
Thrombophilia	Puerperal sepsis
Ethnicity (> Afro-Caribbean)	Ante-partum haemorrhage
Obesity	
Smoking	

Reduced venous flow in pregnancy is multi-factorial, with hormones mediating a reduction in venous tone and increased risk of varicosities. This is abetted by the expanding uterus and reduced mobility. The higher risk post-delivery is the result of increased tissue and vessel damage. A number of coagulation factors are significantly increased, including factors V, VIII, IX, XI and fibrinogen. There are changes in the natural anticoagulant free protein S, which reduces throughout pregnancy due to increased levels of binding protein C-4b, increasing thrombotic risk. Reduced fibrinolysis with increased levels of plasminogen activator inhibitors (PAI-1) and (PAI-2), is also seen in pregnancy. PAI-2 is produced in the placenta, and markedly increases in the third trimester. All of these changes contribute to the prothrombotic condition.

There are several additional risk factors to increase VTE in pregnancy. A personal history of VTE increases the risk by a further 3–4 fold. Dehydration and hyperemesis can be an important factor from early in pregnancy. Surgical intervention, with caesarean section, post-partum haemorrhage and puerperal sepsis, all increase thrombotic risk. While pregnancy can be considered an acquired form of thrombophilia, the risk for VTE increases further in the presence of a heritable thrombophilia. The risk varies dependent on the thrombophilia but, for those homozygous for Factor V Leiden or the Prothrombin mutation, there is a 30 fold increase in risk, while heterozygosity is associated with a 6–8 fold increase.

Patients with anti thrombin deficiency are high risk, with 50% risk for VTE in pregnancy. Protein C and S deficiency are reported to increase risk during pregnancy by 3–10% and 0–6%, respectively, with higher risk post-partum between 7–20%. Patients with thrombophilia, particularly with a proven history of VTE, would require specialist input to assess management.

Those who become pregnant as a result of fertility treatment have an added risk of VTE, sometimes presenting with thrombosis at unusual sites, resulting in subclavian and/or jugular vein thrombosis. A proper risk assessment for VTE in pregnancy is therefore essential, in order to avoid preventable morbidity and mortality. Combined assessment at an obstetric and haematology clinic is needed for patients at high risk, particularly those with a previous history of VTE.

Combined Oral Contraceptive Use

The highest risk period for VTE in users of the combined oral contraceptive (COC) is in the first few months of starting. The individual risk for VTE is very low but, as there are over 100 million users of reproductive age, it has an important impact on the incidence of VTE. The incidence in non-COC users is reported to be 0.16 per 1000 person years, while the relative risk in COC users compared to non-users is reported, in a Cochrane database study, to be 3.5. Similar to pregnancy, there are increased levels of several coagulation factors, and reduced levels of some natural anticoagulants in particular protein S. These changes have been reported to be more pronounced in some COC preparations than in others, most notably third generation COCs.

While all COC preparations increase VTE risk to some extent, studies have identified the dose of ethinyle-stradiol to be critical, with an important risk reduction in the dose from 150 to 30 micro grammes. The thrombotic risk is also dependent on the progestogen used in the preparation. Changes in the progestogen component have been made to try to reduce side-effects of COCs. Second-generation, from the 1970s, and third-generation COCs, together with further preparations, have had varying VTE risk outcomes. Overall, the most recent Cochrane review still reported the second-generation COC with 30 microgrammes of ethinylestradiol and levonorgestrel to have the lowest risk for VTE.

For all COC users of low-dose ethinylestradiol in combination with either gestodene, desogestrel, cyprop-terone acetate or drospinerone, the risk of VTE is 50–80% higher than with the second-generation COC. More recent studies, with the exception of norgestimate, also confirm the risk to be higher for the newer drug preparations. To date, there is limited information on the progestin-only contraceptive, although a recent meta-analysis concluded that VTE risk is not increased.

For postmenopausal women, increasing age is an important compounding factor and, for those taking hor-mone replacement therapy, there is a 2–5 fold increased risk for VTE. This risk is highest in the first 12 months of starting, when the risk is increased six-fold. The risk varies by preparation, but is higher in oestrogen-progestin preparations and increases with higher oestrogen dose. There is also a significant difference dependent on the mode of delivery, with transdermal patches safer. Overall, the risk, particularly when there are additional co-morbidities, needs to be assessed when considering optimal therapy.

Family History of VTE and Thrombophilia

A family history of an unprovoked VTE in a first-degree relative is associated with an additional risk for VTE. Screening for a significant heritable thrombophilia in patients with a proven history will, however, fail to identify an abnormality in nearly 50% of cases. The increased VTE risk remains, whether or not the screen is positive. For younger patients with an unprovoked PE, a thrombophilia screen should be considered if it is planned to stop anticoagulant treatment. This would also be the case where there is a known high-risk throm-bophilia in a first-degree relative and the patient is due to be exposed to additional risk factors.

Heterozygosity for Factor V Leiden can be identified in approximately 5% of people in the UK. It carries only a two-fold risk for VTE, and is the most commonly found abnormality in studies where thrombophilia screening has been undertaken in proven VTE patients, present in 30% of cases. For very rare cases homozygous for Factor V Leiden, the risk of VTE increases nearly 80 fold. The absolute risk for non-COC users heterozygous for Factor V Leiden is 35 per 100 000, rising to 285 per 100 000 for COC users. To put this in context, it compares to an absolute risk with fracture of femur of 6000 per 100 000. Overall, the risk of COC usage is not an absolute contraindication in carriers of Factor V Leiden, as the risk would be higher if pregnant. If known, it should, however, be part of the discussion around the most appropriate and safest form of contraception.

Overall, the risk of a first DVT in carriers of Factor V Leiden or Prothrombin gene mutation, and those with increased levels of FVIII, is under 0.5% per year, not high enough to warrant consideration for thrombo-prophylaxis.This is particularly the case as there is no difference in recurrence rate to patients with first DVT who have not had thrombophilia testing. Higher VTE risk is seen in deficiency of the natural anticoagulants protein C, protein S and antithrombin. The annual risk for VTE is reported as between 1.5 and 1.9%, with a recurrence risk at five years of 40%. The risk with deficiency of these factors in pregnancy, as previously discussed, is significantly higher and warrants expert input. While high levels of other coagulation factors, FIX, FXI and hyperhomocysteinaemia, have been reported to increase VTE risk, they are not independent risk factors and are usually seen in association with increased FVIII. The combination of two or more throm-bophilia factors would increase risk, and would require further expert input.

Obesity

A strong association between obesity and VTE has been reported. In a large population-based study, DVT risk increased with BMI, showing a hazard ratio of 1.3 in those overweight, 1.8 in moderate obesity, and 3.4 in severe obesity, compared with normal-weighted individuals. The risk is present for both males and females. Obese women using the COC, however have been reported to have a 24 fold increased VTE risk, compared with non-obese females not taking a COC.

Obesity risk for VTE is also increased in combination with a heritable thrombophilia – for example, it is associated with an eight- and seven-fold risk with heterozygosity for Factor V Leiden and Prothrombin 20210A mutations, respectively. For those with concomitant medical problems, the risk is high, as is the risk associated with bariatric surgery. Of the measures to quantify obesity, it is reported that waist circumference in males, and hip circumference in females, equate best with VTE. This contrasts with arterial and myocardial risk, in which waist-hip and waist to height are better measures. This emphasises differences in body fat distribution for venous and arterial disease and, perhaps, a different underling cause. Obesity has been suggested to correlate with increased thrombin generation in females with VTE, with increased fibrinogen and prothrombin associated with a pro-thrombotic state. Overall, the cause, independent of reduced mobility, still needs to be defined.

Travel

Extended travel is associated with an increased risk of venous thrombosis. The most compelling evidence relates to a study at Charles de Gaulle airport, where passengers diagnosed with acute pulmonary embolism were assessed in terms of distance travelled. For travellers of less than 5000 km, the event rate was 0.01 cases per million, compared with 4.8 cases per million for travel greater than 10 000 km. Overall there is a 2–4 fold increase in VTE events for air-travellers for flights greater than four hours, compared with non-travellers.

The absolute risk of a spontaneous VTE event within four weeks of flight is very low, at one per 4600 flights. The risk is increased with the frequency of flights within a short time frame, with a significant increase for two or more flights of over eight hours within six weeks. Additional risk factors are important, and can increase the event rate three-fold. These include increasing age, obesity, recent surgery, recent VTE off anti-coagulants, malignancy and pregnancy. The mechanism is likely to be multi-factorial, but prolonged immobilisation resulting in venous stasis, and changes in air pressure, are most important. While dehydration in flight has been suggested as a risk factor, there is currently no body of evidence to support this.

In conclusion, a VTE episode occurring within eight weeks of extended flight can be considered to have a role in causation. Risk associated with car travel, bus or train is highest in the week after travel. The greatest risk is reported in those with a BMI of more than 30kg/m^2, those over 1.9 m tall, or those with Factor V Leiden.

Substance Abuse

There is a marked increase in risk for DVT in users of opioid drugs. The prevalence of previous DVT in opioid users is reported to be 14%, with an annual incidence rate of 3%. The rate increases with age, female use, sex-worker status and intravenous administration. There is a high risk with iliac and femoral injection, often in combination with severe groin infection. High rates of venous leg ulceration (15%) are reported in young drug abusers which are usually chronic and recurring. Staphylococcus bacteraemia is a common problem with IV drug abuse and VTE; however, it is also a proven independent risk for VTE within 90 days of community acquired infection.

While moderate alcohol consumption has been suggested to reduce the risk of VTE, alcohol abuse and its associated medical complications increase the risk of DVT. The risk is increased, even in those without associated medical complications.

The magnitude of risk with smoking and VTE is much less than that seen with arterial disease. While VTE risk is small, smoking is very common, and is an additional risk factor for COC users and those with raised BMI. There is also a reported dose response relationship for smoking and VTE, with return to normal risk on discontinuation. The association is seen in patients with provoked and unprovoked VTE, and may be attributable to the reduced fibrinolysis, inflammation and raised viscosity seen in smokers.

Conclusion

VTE risk is multi-factorial, and requires a careful clinical appraisal in order to reduce the unacceptable high rates of morbidity and death currently seen in clinical practice. Early intervention in high risk patients is essential, and it is to be hoped that greater awareness of the important risk factors for VTE can reduce the incidence of a largely preventable problem.

Further Reading

NICE clinical guidance CG92. *Venous thromboembolism: reducing the risk of venous thromboembolism in patients admitted to hospitals.* www.nice.org.uk/guidance/ CG92.

Testroote M, Stiger WA, Janssen L, Janzing MN (2014). Low molecular weight heparin for prevention of venous thromboembolism in patients with lower limb immobilisation. *Cochrane Database of Systematic Reviews* **4**: CD00668.

Goldhaber SI, Turpie AG (2005). Prevention of venous thromboembolism among hospitalised medical patients. *Circulation* **111**: 1–3.

Rogers MA, Levine DA, Blumberg N *et al.* (2012). Triggers of hospitalisation for venous thromboembolism. *Circulation* **125**: 2092–99.

Watson HG, Keeling DM, Laffan M *et al.* (2015). Guideline on aspects of cancer-related venous thrombosis. *British Journal of Haematology* **170**(5): 640–8.

Klovaite J, Benn M, Nordestgaard BG (2015). Obesity as a causal risk factor for deep vein thrombosis; a Mendelian randomization study. *Journal of Internal Medicine* **277**: 573–84.

De Bastos m, Stegman BH, Rosendaal *et al.* (2014). Combined oral contraceptives: venous thrombosis. *Cochrane Database of Systematic Reviews* **3**(3): CD 010813.

Lijfering WM, Jan-Leendert P, Brouwer P *et al.* (2009). Selective testing for thrombophilia in patients with first venous thrombosis: results from a retrospective family cohort study in absolute thrombotic risk for currently known thrombophilic defects in 2479 relatives. *Blood* **113**: 5314–532.

Watson HG, Baglin T (2011). Guidelines on travel- related venous thrombosis. *British Journal of Haematology* **152**: 31–4.

VERITY (Venous thromboembolism Registry) (2007). *Fourth Annual Report.* www.e-dendrite verityonline.co.uk.

2

Management of Venous Thrombosis in the Lower Limbs

Dan Horner

Consultant in Emergency Medicine and Intensive Care, Salford Royal NHS Foundation Trust, Manchester, UK

Introduction

The annual incidence of deep vein thrombosis (DVT) throughout the developed world is approximately 1 : 1000 of the population. The condition carries significant morbidity in the form of embolisation, post-thrombotic venous insufficiency, pain, swelling and decreased mobility. Short-term mortality stands between 5% and 10% in most epidemiological studies. It is a condition that can range from a self-limiting minor nuisance to the presenting feature of disseminated malignancy. As such, all cases should be carefully managed, and considerable thought given to the what, the where and the why of each case.

Due to rising public and medical awareness of the condition (including caveats in clinical diagnosis) the pre-test probability continues to decline. Ten years ago, one in every four patients assessed would have disease confirmed by objective testing. This figure is now closer to one in ten. While this demonstrates an increase in our understanding of the need for objective testing, it is important to ensure that diagnostic workup is as evidence-based as possible. The focus must remain on improving patient outcomes, rather than providing invasive testing for those unlikely to have the condition, in an attempt to reassure.

Deep vein thrombosis is divided into proximal or distal disease, depending on the anatomical location of the thrombus. This is an important distinction for management, as will be discussed later. Superficial vein thrombosis in the lower limb refers to a clot outside the deep circulation, usually in the saphenous vein or superficial tributaries. This chapter is primarily concerned with disease of the deep veins.

Management of venous thrombosis focuses on two key areas: diagnosis and treatment.

Diagnosis

Clinical Diagnosis and Gestalt

While we will always have our clinical 'gut instinct', or Gestalt, regarding the likelihood of acute thrombotic disease in symptomatic patients, it has been proven time and again in the literature that this is neither sensitive nor specific. Vascular surgeons, thrombosis experts and emergency physicians have all been assessed for clinical reasoning in suspected DVT; even the most experienced clinicians are wrong approximately 40–50% of the time. This has been confirmed in systematic review and meta-analysis regarding the utility of individual signs and symptoms in suspected DVT. No single clinical sign or symptom generated a positive likelihood ratio greater than 2 or less than 0.5 in isolation, though it is notable that several *historical* features (such as malignancy or prior thrombosis) performed well. This paper, and many others, conclude that individual clinical features have limited use in assessment.

What does this mean for practising clinicians? Should we abandon clinical assessment? Absolutely not. Just because no single feature has sufficient discriminatory power to confirm or exclude disease, this does not mean we cannot build up a picture of clinical risk. In addition, this search for clinical signs and symptoms can often reveal a potential alternative diagnosis that may require a different diagnostic strategy. However, this information must be used as part of a patient centred discussion to explore the merits of further investigation, rather than wielded as confirmatory evidence of the absence or presence of DVT.

Scoring Systems

Several research teams have formalised this clinical assessment of risk, by combining historical and examination findings, together with Gestalt, as a quantitative clinical decision rule. The higher the score, the higher the risk of DVT. These tools aim to provide a more objective and reliable assessment of risk, such that further investigation can be based on clearly defined criteria, rather than Gestalt in isolation. The advantages of this approach are that it can be used cross-speciality, irrespective of seniority, and can streamline the decision-making process. As a point system, clear demarcation can be made to denote 'low' or 'high' risk and appropriate further management, tailored appropriately. Disadvantages include the accusation of 'check box' medicine, where clinicians focus more on the exclusion of a single disease than investigation of a differential diagnosis. Telling someone confidently that they are 'low risk' for DVT is of little use to them if, for example, the actual pathology is a tibial metastasis. An overview of clinical decision rules applicable to suspected DVT is provided at the end of this chapter.

Published and validated scoring systems for the assessment of risk in suspected DVT include the Hamilton score, the Khan score, the St Andre score, the Constans score and the Wells clinical decision rule. The latter of these has been most widely validated and, following modification from its original form, has now been adopted as a preferred two-level clinical scoring system for suspected DVT by the National Institute of Health and Care Excellence in the United Kingdom. It must be remembered that use of this score merely serves to estimate risk and direct further management – it cannot confirm or exclude disease in isolation. However, it is now considered to be a generalisable, reproducible and relatively accurate tool for the estimation of pre-test probability in patients presenting with suspected DVT.

Use of the D-dimer Assay

Why estimate pre-test probability? If we consider clinical assessment to be inaccurate, then why not simply proceed to definitive testing as soon as disease is suspected? This is certainly an option; some centres, with readily available seven-day/24-hour access to definitive imaging, will consider this as gold standard care. However, resource implications and cost prohibit this approach in most NHS hospitals and throughout Europe/North America. There is also a concern regarding overtreatment; definitive investigation may be inconclusive, or may suggest chronic incidental thrombus away from the symptomatic area in a patient deemed to be low-risk. There is little evidence that anticoagulation in this group will improve outcomes, although some clinicians will feel obliged to discuss therapeutic intervention.

More appropriate is a stratified approach to definitive imaging, based on the assessment of risk via a clinical decision rule. This can subsequently be followed by the appropriate measurement of fibrin degradation products within plasma. These products are best measured as D-dimer units, the final fragment of cross-linked fibrin degraded by the endogenous fibrinolytic system in the presence of thrombus. Assays to measure D-dimer units have been in clinical use since the 1980s, and are now widely available, quantitative, rapid and reliable. In the presence of low clinical risk, the test is highly sensitive, as such patients who are low-risk by a validated clinical decision rule, and who have a serum D-dimer value below a predetermined cut point, can be reassured that DVT has been excluded and that further investigation is unnecessary. This can avoid unnecessary medication, diagnostic delay and further hospital visits for definitive imaging. Several review articles are available discussing the adoption, utility and diagnostic test characteristics of the D-dimer assay.

Although sensitive, the test is well known for its relatively poor specificity. As such, it can never be used to 'rule in' disease; a positive result in a low risk patient simply mandates the need for further imaging. Likewise, sensitivity is limited in those patients deemed to be at high clinical risk and, as such, this cohort should proceed directly to further imaging, as stated in NICE guidance. However, the ability of a negative d-dimer to 'rule out' disease in patients deemed to be at low clinical risk is invaluable when one considers the low pre-test probability and the burden of unselected presentation.

It should be remembered that the D-dimer is a continuous variable. Although most labs will have a binary reference cut point between a positive and negative test, the value of this cut point is debated, which reflects previous research, standardisation between assays and pragmatic reasoning. An appropriate trade-off between sensitivity and specificity is given optimal balance; if the cut point is low, sensitivity will be excellent, but most patients will test positive, so specificity will be so low as to render the test useless. If the cut point is raised, specificity will improve, but some cases of DVT may be missed; sensitivity will reduce.

Most assays in common use reflect the cut point originally determined by Wells *et al.* during their validation of a strategy incorporating a clinical decision rule supplemented by D-dimer assay for exclusion of venous thromboembolism. However, the issue of cut points has received further attention within the last five years. Due to low specificity rates in the elderly, several authors have looked at the idea of an age-adjusted cut point for patients over 50 years old. Recent results have been encouraging, and suggest that use of an age-adjusted cut point may dramatically improve specificity without a proportionate decrease in sensitivity. Further research to clarify generalisability is warranted and ongoing in this area.

Definitive Testing: The Gold Standard?

Contrast venography is considered to be the gold standard test for evaluation of deep vein thrombosis, largely based on its long history and purported accuracy. This test involves cannulation of a pedal vessel, injection of radio-opaque contrast medium, and serial imaging of the leg to assess for the presence or absence of intraluminal filling defects. This direct pictorial evidence is taken as confirmation or exclusion of disease.

However, there are many issues with this technique that make it a less than ideal choice. Cannulation of a pedal vein can be challenging in those with gross swelling and oedema; inadequate studies, due to technical issues, can occur in up to 5% of cases; some veins fail to fill adequately with contrast routinely, such as the muscular branches of the calf veins or the profunda femoris; and contrast media extravasation or reactions can occur. Even with technical sufficiency, inter-observer agreement can be limited, with some studies showing varied conclusions between reporting radiologists in over 10% of cases.

Many alternatives to contrast venography have been described as a result of these concerns, with the most successful emerging as compression ultrasound (CUS). This test has now replaced contrast venography as the initial investigation of choice and the proxy gold standard. However, it is important to remember that, like any test, it comes with caveats.

Compression Ultrasound

Compression ultrasound refers to sonographic assessment of fluid filled structures, with compression to assess distension, flow and intraluminal masses. Duplex and triplex refer to use of two or more sonographic modalities, including standard B mode (assessment of architecture), Doppler (assessment of flow/velocity) and colour flow Doppler (direction of flow). CUS has been touted as the definitive investigation of choice for suspected thrombosis since the 1990s, as a result of its non-invasive nature, reproducibility and relatively low cost. It has also been extensively studied, and has been shown to be accurate for the diagnosis of proximal DVT when compared to a gold standard of contrast venography. A systematic review and diagnostic meta-analysis, pooling 100 cohorts, confirmed a sensitivity of 96.5% and a specificity of 94%. As such, it has proven to be reliable, generalisable and cost-effective.

The use of CUS to detect distal DVT is more debatable. The largest meta-analysis to date suggests the sensitivity to only reach the mid-70s when compared against contrast venography. However, the gold standard in this case is known to cause thrombi and to produce false positive results in up to 5% of cases. It is, perhaps, of more interest to study those patients with suspected DVT having anticoagulation withheld following a single whole leg negative ultrasound, and their rate of complications over a three-month period (implying missed disease). Johnson *et al* showed this to be < 0.5% in a recent systematic review. The implication from this data and other series/observational cohort studies is that whole-leg ultrasound is unlikely to miss significant disease. A further question yet to be answered is whether use of this modality leads to more diagnosed DVT without improving patient outcomes, as some have suggested.

Serial and Contralateral Imaging

Concern regarding the accuracy of whole-leg CUS has led to the use of serial proximal CUS as a recommended diagnostic strategy for the exclusion of DVT. Patients undergo CUS of the proximal veins and, if no thrombi are seen, further assessment is conducted. In the presence of an initial suspected high clinical risk, or a raised D-dimer level, patients return after one week for a further CUS of the proximal veins. It is suggested that any distal deep vein thrombosis not seen at the time of first scan will propagate during this week, and be detected at serial scan. Some facilities in North America will perform further imaging at 21 days even, to ensure no propagation. Concerns with this strategy include a lack of exploration for alternative diagnosis, a high rate of attrition (over 10% of patients will fail to return for follow-up imaging) and a low diagnostic yield (<2%). Despite these concerns, this is the approach currently recommended as first line by NICE and the American College of Chest Physicians (ACCP).

The idea of *contralateral* imaging stems from suggestion that, in patients with an acute lower limb thrombosis, almost a third will have evidence of bilateral disease. A high proportion of these patients will have multiple risk factors for thrombosis, or active malignancy. While knowledge of contralateral disease may not directly affect treatment, it can identify those patients in need of further investigation and record extent at the time of diagnosis. This can be very useful when the issue of recurrence arises. Many patients with treated DVT may re-present to the ED with pain and swelling in the affected or contralateral leg, both as a result of heightened awareness/knowledge, and as a pathological consequence of the original clot. Repeat imaging is most useful when a clear record exists of the location, extent and luminal defect associated with the original thrombi. Contralateral imaging is not currently routine practice in the UK.

When is Venography Still Useful?

Contrast venography has little role in the standard contemporary assessment of suspected DVT. However, it remains an available, and supposedly definitive, test in the presence of abnormal but non-specific ultrasound findings, or when a potentially false positive diagnosis carries significant risk. For example, in patients at high risk of bleeding, the consequences of anticoagulation must be carefully considered.

Other potential uses include assessment of cases where the accuracy of conventional ultrasound can be limited; assessment for suspected ipsilateral recurrence, or isolated iliac vein thrombosis, for example. The main caveat to use at present is lack of resource, experience and reliability. Some centres may perform no venograms for several years. As such, there are issues with requesting this test infrequently, and in the most complex of cases.

Alternative Diagnostic Strategies and When to Use Them

Several additional options exist to clarify diagnosis in suspected DVT. Study of leg venous capacitance, alterations in venous volume and assessment of blood flow have been investigated as plethysmography and rheography. Nearly all of these techniques have failed to demonstrate a sensitivity > 90% when compared to gold standard testing. Their use in practice, therefore, often requires additional levels of risk stratification to render them viable.

Computed tomography venography (CTV) is a further option, with a purported sensitivity of > 95% compared with proximal CUS. However, sensitivity for exclusion of distal disease is limited, and the test carries significant radiation exposure and cost implications.

Lastly, magnetic resonance venography (MRV) has also been investigated. Although sensitivity rates are poor, in particular for detection of distal disease, there seems to be an emerging role for MRV in the detection of isolated iliac vein thrombosis. This is a particular condition of pregnant patients, or those with pelvic trauma, and occurs principally due to obstructed flow at the pelvic inlet. Although Doppler CUS studies can suggest flow abnormalities, these thrombi are often too proximal to visualise. As such, MRV offers a non-invasive, radiation-free diagnostic method.

Treatment

Therapeutic Anticoagulation and Lower Limb Thrombosis

Proximal DVT

There is international agreement that the overwhelming majority of acute proximal lower limb thrombi should receive immediate and sustained therapeutic dose anticoagulation for at least three months. This is primarily based on evidence from the 1960s suggesting a sustained mortality reduction. Since this seminal work, ethical concerns have negated further large trials comparing any therapeutic intervention against an untreated control group. However, many studies since then have confirmed the benefit to anticoagulation. Work from the 1990s suggested a significant reduction in recurrence and extension when IV heparin was administered for five days concurrently with oral warfarin, compared to warfarin alone, for example. Another study, comparing six months of anticoagulation with just six weeks, confirmed a lower rate of recurrence in the group treated for six months.

What do we mean by therapeutic dose anticoagulation? This classically refers to immediate commencement of heparin, administered either as *unfractionated* heparin via intravenous infusion titrated to activated partial thromboplastin time, or given subcutaneously at treatment dose as a daily injection of *low molecular weight* heparin. Following this, patients are phased to oral anticoagulation with a vitamin K antagonist (usually warfarin), aiming for an international normalised prothrombin time ratio (INR) of 2.5 over the following five days. Once this INR is achieved, heparin can be discontinued. Other oral agents are now available, and these will be discussed separately below. It is recommended that, where clinically safe and practically feasible, early ambulation is encouraged and therapeutic anticoagulation facilitated in the home environment. This applies to all forms of acute DVT.

Distal DVT

A decision to anticoagulate patients with isolated distal DVT (IDDVT) is more complex. There are no large trials confirming a significant reduction in propagation, embolisation or mortality with therapeutic dose anticoagulation in this cohort. It is suggested by many that the risks of anticoagulation may not outweigh the benefits. Several small studies note a combined composite adverse outcome of approximately 12% in untreated IDDVT; approximately 3% of patients will go on to develop symptomatic pulmonary embolism, and 9–10% of cases will propagate above the level of the popliteal fossa.

Mortality is very rare in modern studies, but other risks also exist with untreated disease, such as ongoing pain/suffering, anxiety and the potential for post-thrombotic syndrome. These risks must be balanced against the risk of fatal bleeding (<0.5%) and major bleeding (2%) with therapeutic dose anticoagulation. Shared decision-making and patient-centred discussion are vital to direction on treatment strategy. Several authors have recently commented on the idea of stratified decision-making, and cases which are particularly symptomatic, unprovoked, or associated with a high level of risk (active malignancy) may benefit most from anticoagulation. Others can be followed with observation and serial CUS to assess for propagation. This strategy is supported by the most recent ACCP guidance.

Superficial Venous Thrombosis

Treatment of superficial venous thrombosis (SVT) is another area where the balance between risk and benefit is not clear-cut. Many practitioners believe this condition to be benign, and previous practice has been to treat with anti-inflammatory medication only. However, recent trial evidence suggests that complications, including extension to the saphenofemoral junction, recurrence, DVT and pulmonary embolism, can occur in up to 6% of untreated patients. In the 2013 prospective randomised CALISTO study, recruiting over 3000 patients, this was reduced to less than 1% with the use of prophylactic dose anticoagulation, with no increase in bleeding or adverse events. This translates to a number needed to treat of 1 : 20.

While this new data is convincing regarding clinical benefit, estimates of cost-effectiveness and additional trial data confirming generalisability are lacking. However, it seems prudent to consider location, provocation and symptoms in these patients; anyone with extensive or very symptomatic disease, without a clear provoking factor, or with multiple additional risk factors for thromboembolism, should be considered for imaging of the deep leg veins, prophylactic dose anticoagulation and definitive follow-up.

Novel and alternative agents

Direct Oral AntiCoagulants (DOAC)

The precedent of oral anticoagulation with vitamin K antagonists, while clinically effective, has always suffered from several drawbacks. Patients require regular monitoring of their INR to ensure that drug levels remain within a therapeutic window. This causes regular inconvenience, and requires large resource in the form of anticoagulation clinics or widely available point of care testing. Warfarin is notorious for interacting with many active drugs and other substances. Drug actions are also heavily affected by genetic polymorphisms, liver disease and inter-current illness.

Within the last decade, new oral agents have been developed that purport to provide similar efficacy of anticoagulation without the need for regular monitoring. These drugs principally consist of direct factor Xa inhibitors (rivaroXaban, edoXaban, apiXaban) or direct thrombin inhibtors (dabigaTran etexilate). They have a rapid onset over 1–2 hours, and are rapidly and efficiently excreted through the renal tract and biliary system, resulting in a half-life of between 7–12 hours. Routine monitoring of drug levels is not required.

Several large studies show these drugs to be non-inferior to standard phased anticoagulation, and suggest fewer bleeding complications than standard care. Cost-effectiveness has been reviewed, with the outcome that reduction in patient and clinician time in hospital, transport, monitoring and review combine to make the newer drugs cost-effective. As such, several of these agents are endorsed by national clinical bodies (such as NICE) as sole therapeutic anticoagulation options for patients with deep vein thrombosis.

At present, the main caveats to all new agents are accumulation in renal failure (unlike warfarin), a lack of real-world clinical experience, and the absence of a rapid available antidote. While information is currently being gathered as these drugs are utilised by practicing clinicians, the other concerns warrant careful review of each clinical scenario and patient-centred discussion. Some individuals with established renal impairment, or at high bleeding risk, may have viable concerns regarding side-effects and/or the lack of reversibility.

Alternative Treatment Options

Antiplatelet agents, such as aspirin, have been assessed for prophylaxis, treatment and prevention of recurrence in VTE. No large clinical trial has convincingly suggested benefit for these indications, although a recent study did suggest a significant reduction in pooled vascular adverse events.

Low molecular weight heparins are used in prophylactic and therapeutic dose for treatment of lower limb thrombosis. In particular, there is evidence that sustained treatment dose LMWH is of benefit to these patients with acute thrombosis and underlying active malignancy. There is no clear scientific explanation of this benefit.

Compression hosiery has been well studied in acute DVT for the prevention of post-thrombotic syndrome and the relief of symptoms. There is compelling evidence of benefit, and very little associated risk. As such, all patients should be offered stockings and verbal guidance regarding exercise/postural management.

Additional interventional options for the management of acute proximal DVT include catheter-directed thrombolysis, systemic thrombolysis and open surgical venous thrombectomy. While these options may be of benefit in specific clinical situations (acute iliofemoral DVT in patients with low risk of bleeding primarily), no robust trial data exists to support routine use. As such, they are not recommended over standard anticoagulation.

Provocation, Prognostication and Recurrence

Provocation and Malignancy Screening

The concept of provocation refers to a specific identifiable cause for development of an acute thrombosis. Several conditions have emerged within the literature as agreed 'provoking factors', such as recent surgery, pregnancy, flights of more than eight hours, immobilisation, lower limb fracture and hormone therapy. Other conditions (such as acute infective illness) remain more widely debated. Active cancer is a clear provocation, but this is often referred to separately. The others are segregated into surgical and non-surgical provoking factors. In the absence of these conditions, a thrombotic episode is referred to as 'unprovoked'. The risk of recurrence (without extended anticoagulation) at five years rises sequentially with initial surgical provocation (3%), non-surgical provocation (15%) and unprovoked disease (30%).

This risk mandates a careful exploration of provocation at the point of initial diagnosis, and a later discussion regarding the need for ongoing therapeutic anticoagulation at the end of the initial three-month treatment period. The exploration of provocation is essentially a focused history and examination, with ancillary investigation as warranted. NICE have suggested a formal malignancy screen in patients without clear evidence of provocation, for example through initial testing with urinalysis, sputum cytology, chest radiography and supplemental abdominopelvic CT imaging (and/or mammography in females) for patients over 40 years old.

Thrombophilia testing is also something to consider in those patients suffering an unprovoked thrombosis with a family history of disease. The decision to test is principally dependent on the decision to continue anticoagulation; testing is not recommended while drug therapy is continued, but may have a role if anticoagulation is to be withheld after three months.

Prognostication and Decisions Regarding Lifelong Anticoagulation

Following three months initial therapeutic anticoagulation for a proximal DVT, and a careful assessment of provocation, a patient-centred discussion must occur. This discussion must include a balanced assessment of the risk of further thrombosis, the risk of bleeding with anticoagulation, and patient preference. At present, extended anticoagulation is recommended for those patients with a first episode of unprovoked proximal DVT without a high bleeding risk, or those with DVT in the presence of active malignancy. Following this decision, a regular (annual) review should be undertaken to ascertain whether new events or changes have occurred which alter the risk benefit profile of current strategy.

Recurrence

In the event of a new episode of acute thrombus following cessation of anticoagulation, consideration should be given to immediate reintroduction and commencement of an extended course. This is recommended for patients with a second episode of unprovoked venous thrombosis in the absence of a high bleeding risk. If the recurrence is provoked, careful consideration is needed. Extended anticoagulation is not necessarily mandated.

Following this decision, regular (annual) review should be undertaken to ascertain whether new events or changes have occurred which alter the risk benefit profile of current strategy.

Further Reading

Goodacre S, Sutton AJ, Sampson FC (2005). Meta-analysis: The value of clinical assessment in the diagnosis of deep venous thrombosis. *Annals of Internal Medicine* **143**(2): 129–39.

Tamariz LJ, Eng J, Segal JB, *et al.* (2004). Usefulness of clinical prediction rules for the diagnosis of venous thromboembolism: a systematic review. *American Journal of Medicine* **117**(9): 676–84.

NICE (2012). *Venous throboembolic diseases: the management of venous thromboembolic diseases and the role of thrombophilia testing.* London: National Institute for Health and Clinical Excellence.

Rhigini M, Perrier A, Moerloose PD, Bounameaux H (2008). D-dimer for venous thromboembolism diagnosis: 20 years later. *Journal of Thrombosis and Haemostasis* **6**: 1059–71.

Wells P, Anderson D, Rodger M, *et al.* (2003). Evaluation of D-dimer in the Diagnosis of Suspected Deep Vein Thombosis. *The New England Journal of Medicine* **349**: 1227–35.

Goodacre S, Sampson F, Thomas S, van Beek E, Sutton A (2005). Systematic review and meta-analysis of the diagnostic accuracy of ultrasonography for deep vein thrombosis. *BMC Medical Imaging* **5**: 6.

Johnson SA, Stevens SM, Woller SC, *et al.* (2010). Risk of deep vein thrombosis following a single negative whole-leg compression ultrasound: a systematic review and meta-analysis. *JAMA* **303**(5): 438–45.

Guyatt GH, Akl EA, Crowther M, Gutterman DD, Schuunemann HJ (2012). Executive summary: Antithrombotic Therapy and Prevention of Thrombosis, 9th ed: American College of Chest Physicians Evidence-Based Clinical Practice Guidelines. *Chest* **141**(2 Suppl): 7S–47S.

Kearon C, Akl EA, Comerota AJ, *et al.* (2012). Antithrombotic therapy for VTE disease: Antithrombotic Therapy and Prevention of Thrombosis, 9th ed: American College of Chest Physicians Evidence-Based Clinical Practice Guidelines. *Chest* **141**(2 Suppl): e419S–94S.

Ageno W, Squizzato A, Dentali F (2012) Should the commonly accepted definition of 'unprovoked venous thrombembolism' be revisited? *Thrombosis and Haemostasis* **107**(5): 806–7.

3

Clinical Presentation of Acute Pulmonary Embolism

C.E.A. Dronkers, M.V. Huisman and F.A. Klok

Department of Thrombosis and Hemostasis, Leiden University Medical Center, Leiden, The Netherlands

Introduction

The diagnostic management of patients with suspected acute pulmonary embolism (PE) still remains a major challenge in current clinical practice, mainly because of its non-specific clinical presentation. For this reason, acute PE has been referred to as 'a wolf in sheep's clothing' since, if unrecognised and untreated, acute PE may be a lethal condition. In this chapter, the symptoms and signs associated with acute PE and the relevant differential diagnosis according to the different clinical presentations of PE, as well as the impact of presentation on the prognosis of the patient with PE, will be discussed.

Symptoms of Acute PE

In the vast majority of patients, a suspicion of PE is triggered by the symptoms of acute dyspnea, chest pain or coughing, with or without haemoptysis. One of the first and frequently cited studies on the clinical presentation of PE is a sub-study of the PIOPED (Prospective Investigation of Pulmonary Embolism Diagnosis), published in 1991. This sub-study focused on patients with no previous cardiac or pulmonary disease, in order to evaluate clinical characteristics that are specific for PE. A total of 117 patients with confirmed PE, and 248 patients in whom suspected PE was excluded, were studied.

The two largest and most recent cohort studies that focused on the clinical presentation of acute PE are the EMPEROR study (Multicentre Emergency Medicine Pulmonary Embolism in the Real World Registry) and the PIOPED II study. The EMPEROR study was a multicentre observational registry study, including 1880 patients with confirmed PE, and 528 patients with clinically suspected PE but negative imaging studies. The PIOPED II was a prospective multicentre investigation, primarily conducted to compare imaging techniques, that also evaluated the clinical characteristics of 192 patients with confirmed acute PE. The main observations from these three studies with regard to reported symptoms are summarised in Table 3.1, which shows the striking diversity of clinical presentations of acute PE.

The most common presenting symptom of pulmonary embolism is dyspnea and, especially, dyspnea at rest (50–61% of patients). Dyspnea on exertion can be observed in 16–27% of patients. In the PIOPED II study, orthopnoea (use of > 2 pillows) was described in 36% of patients with PE. The onset of dyspnea is often rapid, and occurs within seconds in 41% of the PE patients reporting dyspnea, within minutes in 26%, within hours in 14%, and within days in the remaining 19% of patients. The dyspnea in PE is predominantly

Table 3.1 Prevalence of clinical characteristics in patients with suspected PE.

Symptom	PE confirmed (%)	PE not confirmed (%)
Any dyspnea	73–79	72–73
Dyspnea at rest	50–61	51–54
Dyspnea with exertion	16–27	17–18
Pleuritic chest pain	39–66	28–59
Sub-sternal chest pain	15–17	17–21
Cough without haemoptysis	23–43	23–39
Cough with haemoptysis	8–13	5–8
Syncope	6	6
Fever	2–10	2–12
Symptoms suggestive of DVT	24–39	18–20

a consequence of ventilatory and haemodynamic disturbances, such as shunting and dead space ventilation, due to obstruction of the pulmonary artery by emboli and, in severe PE, of low cardiac output. In addition, congestive atelectasis, pulmonary infarction and regional pulmonary oedema may also contribute to hypoxemia and dyspnea.

Pleuritic chest pain is the second most common presenting symptom of acute PE (39–47% of patients). It is most often described as lateral or posterior thoracic pain between the costal margin and clavicles, and typically increases with breathing. The pleuritic pain is caused by infarction of a segment of the lung that is adjacent to the pleura. Sub-sternal chest pain, described as compressing and resembling that of acute myocardial infarction or angina pectoris, is less common (15–17% of patients), although it may occur more frequently in patients with 'massive PE' who present with hemodynamic instability due to a very high thrombus burden.

Cough without haemoptysis, present in approximately 23% of patients, is usually non-productive, but purulent sputum and clear sputum are both reported. Small distal emboli may create areas of alveolar haemorrhage known as 'pulmonary infarction'. These infarctions may result in cough with haemoptysis, characterised as blood streaked, blood-tinged or pure blood, which occurs in only 8% of all PE patients. Despite its relative infrequent occurrence, haemoptysis has been shown to be very specific for the presence of acute PE.

Syncope occurs in 6% of all PE patients. Massive PE is known to cause acute right ventricular failure, impaired left ventricular function and reduced cerebral perfusion, which may result in loss of consciousness and muscle strength. A second mechanism implicated in the pathogenesis of syncope is dysrhythmia due to enlargement of the right ventricle or hypotension, especially in patients with pre-existing left bundle branch block. Also, PE can trigger an increased vaso-vagal reflex associated with syncope on a neurogenic basis.

Fever has long been recognised as commonly accompanying PE. PE-related fever is usually low-grade, rarely exceeding 38.3 °C, and is short-lived. Its peak is reached on the same day on which the PE occurs, and it gradually disappears within one week. The pathogenesis of PE-related fever has not yet been fully clarified. It has been suggested that a variety of potential pyrogenic mechanisms may occur: infarction and tissue necrosis; haemorrhage; local vascular irritation or inflammation; atelectasis; or self-limited occult super-infections.

Lastly, symptoms of deep venous thrombosis (DVT), such as leg swelling or leg pain, are reported by approximately one-quarter of patients with proven acute PE. Of note, non-symptomatic DVT can be shown in 35–55% of all PE patients.

Non-specific Presentation of Acute PE

Remarkably, there is little to no difference in the prevalence of the above described symptoms in patients with proven PE versus those with suspected PE in whom this diagnosis was ruled out, as shown in table 3.1. This observation underlines the non-specific presentation of acute PE, and demonstrates the great challenge faced by clinicians in day-to-day clinical practice who manage patients with chest or respiratory symptoms. In addition, this observation also suggests that clinical symptoms alone are never sufficient to exclude or confirm the diagnosis.

Clinical Signs of Acute PE

Physical Examination

On physical examination, several clinical signs may point to acute PE. Tachypnea (respiratory rate ≥ 20 per min) is the most common sign, occurring in more than half of patients (57%). Tachycardia (heart rate > 100 per min) occurs in about one-quarter. Clinical evidence of pulmonary hypertension, such as accentuated pulmonary component of the second sound, right ventricular pressure overload or enlargement, or elevated right atrial pressure, is present in 22% of patients with PE. Abnormal lung examination is found in 29% of patients. Crackles and decreased breath sounds are the most frequent lung findings, while rhonchi and wheezes occur less commonly. Signs suggestive of DVT, such as unilateral swelling of calf and/or thigh swelling, red skin or pain, occur in 11% of patients.

Non-PE-specific Diagnostic Tests

In addition to physical examination, several diagnostic tests may also indicate the presence of PE. For instance, the majority of patients with proven PE have an abnormal chest X-ray (54–84%). Pleural effusion, elevated hemi diaphragm, wedge-shaped atelectasis and pulmonary consolidation are the most common radiographic abnormalities.

Electrocardiogram (ECG) abnormalities occur in about 70% of patients, and may show sinus tachycardia, right ventricular strain or repolarisation abnormalities. The classic PE ECG pattern is a prominent S wave in lead I, a prominent Q wave and inverted T wave in lead III, the so-called S1Q3T3 pattern.

Arterial blood gas analysis typically shows hypoxia ($PaO_2 < 80$ mm Hg) in combination with a normal or reduced $PaCO_2$, attributable to hyperventilation. Hypoxia mostly occurs in combination with a high Alveolar-Arterial Oxygen Gradient ($AaPO_2 > 20$ mm Hg). However, as with X-ray and ECG findings, blood gas analysis is of insufficient discriminant value to permit exclusion of the diagnosis of PE.

Differential Diagnosis

Most cardiopulmonary diseases, such as chronic obstructive pulmonary disease (COPD) and heart failure, share at least one symptom with acute PE. In unselected patients hospitalised after triaging at an emergency department because of acute dyspnea, chest pain, syncope or palpitations, PE is diagnosed in a small minority only (4%), since heart failure, pneumonia and COPD exacerbation are by far the most common acute disorders explaining acute cardiopulmonary symptoms. It remains of key importance to distinguish potentially life-threatening causes of respiratory or chest symptoms, such as acute PE, coronary artery disease and aortic dissection, from the more frequently occurring innocent conditions such as oesophagitis or muscular-skeletal problems. Table 3.2 shows an overview of the differential diagnoses in relation to the most common presenting symptoms of acute PE.

Table 3.2 Differential diagnosis of PE according to the key presenting symptom.

Clinical feature	Differential diagnosis
(Acute) dyspnea	Asthma, COPD, cardiac asthma, pneumonia, pleural fluid, bronchitis, pneumothorax, foreign body, hyperventilation syndrome, neuromuscular disease, direct pulmonary injury, pulmonary haemorrhage
Chest pain	Coronary artery disease, pericarditis, aortic dissection, pleuritis, pneumonia, bronchitis, pneumothorax, tumour, musculoskeletal chest pain syndromes (costochondritis, Tietze syndrome), rheumatic diseases, gastrointestinal (reflux, oesophageal spasm), pancreatobiliary (pancreatitis, cholecystitis), herpes zoster
Cough	Infectious disease, corpus alienum, bronchitis, asthma, COPD, smoking
Haemoptysis	Nasopharyngeal bleeding, neoplasm, bronchitis, bronchiectasis, foreign body, lung abscess, pneumonia, tuberculosis, Granulomatosis with Polyangiitis and other vasculitides, Goodpasture's syndrome, lung contusion, pulmonary arteriovenous malformation, heart failure.
Symptoms or signs suggestive of DVT	Cellulitis, erysipelas, trauma, ruptured Baker's cyst, haematoma, lymphangitis, post-thrombotic syndrome
Syncope	Myocardial infarction, cardiac arrhythmia, bleeding, ruptured aortic aneurysm, pericardial tamponade, tension pneumothorax, aortic dissection, sepsis, anaphylaxis, intoxication, vasovagal collapse.

Clinical Presentation in Specific Patient Subgroups

Elderly

The incidence of PE increases with age, and its clinical presentation is often even less discriminative in the elderly than in younger patients. The most common explanation for this is that the elderly more frequently suffer from concomitant cardiopulmonary conditions that may mimic acute PE. The different clinical presentations between elderly and younger patients have been observed in several studies. These studies suggest that, in patients aged over 75 years, symptoms and signs of DVT, tachycardia, pleural effusion and hemi-diaphragmatic elevation at chest X-ray are no longer predictive of PE. Also, older people may present less often with pleuritic chest pain and haemoptysis, compared with younger patients. Conversely, syncope may present more frequently in older patients with PE than in younger ones.

Men and Women

In contrast to other cardiopulmonary diseases such as myocardial infarction, only slight differences have been described in the clinical presentation of PE in men versus women. It has been reported that haemoptysis may occur more frequently in men than in women (29% versus 13%), as does leg swelling as evidence of concurrent DVT (49% versus 30%). On the other hand, women have a higher mean heart rate than men (98/min versus 93/min). The presence of dyspnea, chest pains and cough are comparable between the sexes.

Patients With COPD and/or Congestive Heart Failure (CHF)

As described above, the symptoms of both COPD and CHF overlap with those of PE and, consequently, a PE diagnosis has been shown to be frequently ignored or delayed in these patients. In the majority of patients with known cardiopulmonary disease who present with new symptoms of acute onset, it proves impossible to distinguish between patients with and without PE by clinical assessment alone.

Patients with COPD and PE may present more often with dyspnea and cough than patients with PE, but without COPD (89% versus 82%). Chest X-rays of PE patients with COPD are more often abnormal than in PE patients without COPD (66% versus 54%). As for patients with CHF, PE presents more often with dyspnea

(90% versus 82%) and cough (23% versus 17%) than in PE patients without CHF, but less often with chest pain (43% versus 54%). Also, ECG and chest radiograph abnormalities are more commonly found in patients with concomitant CHF and PE than in patients without CHF, as are hypoxemia and hypercapnia on blood gas analysis. Lastly, syncope occurs less commonly in PE patients with COPD or CHF than in PE patients without COPD or CHF (10% versus 15%).

To aid in the identification of COPD patients with concurrent acute PE, Lippmann and Fein suggested that the diagnosis of PE in patients with COPD should be suspected when worsening of dyspnea is unresponsive to bronchodilator therapy. This recommendation was stronger when accompanied by a reduction of $PaCO_2$ in a previously hypercapnic patient. In the PIOPED study, however, this latter recommendation could not be confirmed, since no difference in alveolar-arterial oxygen gradients in either group could be demonstrated – nor was there evidence of a reduction in $PaCO_2$ in patients with PE who had prior hypercapnia.

Clinical Presentation and Associated Prognosis

The prognosis of patients with acute PE is highly variable, and greatly depends on the initial clinical presentation. For example, patients presenting with shock or arterial hypotension are at very high risk of in-hospital or 30-day mortality (30–100%). Acute right ventricle dysfunction, due to pressure overload caused by massive PE, is the critical determinant of hemodynamic compromise and outcome in acute PE. In short, pulmonary artery pressure starts to increase after more than 30–50% of the pulmonary arterial bed is occluded by thromboemboli. This increase is further fuelled by local vasoactive substances released by platelets and the endothelium in response to the PE. The resulting right ventricular dilatation triggers a cascade of increase in right ventricular wall tension, myocyte stretch and increased oxygen demand of the right ventricle.

After all physiological compensatory mechanisms are depleted, this cascade continues with ventricular desynchronisation, decrease of cardiac output and myocardial ischemia. This latter feature contributes to systemic hypotension, haemodynamic instability and, eventually, death. The absence of syncope or persistent hypotension at presentation, on the other hand, predicts a quite favourable outcome, with a reported mortality rate of 3–15%. Still, some of the initially normotensive patients with acute PE may suffer hemodynamic deterioration, which occurs most often in the first 24–48 hours following the PE diagnosis and initiation of anticoagulant treatment.

Delay in Clinical Presentation and Diagnosis of PE

The non-specific clinical presentation of PE frequently results in a delayed diagnosis. Interestingly, studies have shown that patients with delayed presentation, defined as a diagnosis after at least seven days from symptom onset, are of older age, and more frequently have cardiopulmonary comorbidity than patients without delayed presentation, again indicating the even more non-specific clinical presentation of acute PE in patients with known cardiopulmonary disease or of older age.

It has been postulated that this diagnostic delay may be associated with poor clinical outcome, due to the risk of higher thrombus load caused by ongoing thrombosis. One prospective cohort study indeed suggested that a more central PE localisation was more frequently present in patients after diagnostic delay (41% versus 26%), although a second study could not confirm this observation. Even so, longer delay has never been shown to be predictive of three-month recurrent PE, hospital readmission or mortality. These discrepancies could be explained by the lack of a clear association between thrombus load and PE-related mortality in general, as well as the fact that the most severe cases of PE with haemodynamic instability may be likely to present to the emergency ward without any delay.

Of note, these findings do not challenge the recommendation to initiate anticoagulant treatment as soon as a possible PE diagnosis is considered, even before radiological examinations are performed, because withholding anticoagulant treatment before radiological examinations is the so-called 'doctor's delay' or 'treatment delay', which is different from 'diagnostic delay', and has a more pronounced impact on prognosis.

Summary

In summary, PE presents with a wide variation of symptoms and signs, from no or mild symptoms to shock or sudden death. Symptoms and findings at physical examination do not differentiate between PE and the wide range of other acute or chronic cardiopulmonary conditions that may mimic the presentation of PE, but are more common. This is especially true in elderly patients with COPD and/or CHF. As such, acute PE remains a wolf in sheep's clothing. Therefore, physicians should consider this diagnosis in every patient with new or sudden worsening cardiopulmonary symptoms, in particular when no evident alternative diagnosis is present, to allow for early diagnostic assessment and, if PE is confirmed, prompt initiation of adequate treatment in order to prevent clinical deterioration and death.

Key Points

1) The clinical presentation of PE ranges from no or mild symptoms to shock or sudden death.
2) Symptoms and findings on physical examination do not differentiate between PE and the wide range of other acute or chronic cardiopulmonary conditions that mimic its presentation.
3) The most frequently reported symptoms of PE are dyspnea, chest pain and cough. The most frequent signs of PE at physical examination include tachypnea, tachycardia and signs of DVT.
4) PE often is accompanied by abnormal ECG, chest X-ray and blood gas analysis, although the diagnosis cannot be ruled out nor confirmed on the basis of these diagnostic tests.
5) The presentation of PE is different in younger healthier patients than in elderly patients with known cardiopulmonary comorbidity.
6) The clinical presentation of PE – and especially hemodynamic instability – is highly predictive of its clinical outcome.

Further Reading

Konstantinides SV, Torbicki A, Agnelli G *et al.* (2014). 2014 ESC guidelines on the diagnosis and management of acute pulmonary embolism. *European Heart Journal* **35**: 3033–3069k.

Stein PD, Terrin ML, Hales CA *et al.* (1991). Clinical, laboratory, roentgenographic, and electrocardiographic findings in patients with acute pulmonary embolism and no pre-existing cardiac or pulmonary disease. *Chest* **100**: 598–603.

Stein PD, Beemath A, Matta F *et al.* (2007). Clinical characteristics of patients with acute pulmonary embolism: data from PIOPED II. *American Journal of Medicine* **120**: 871–879.

Pollack CV, Schreiber D, Goldhaber SZ *et al.* (2011). Clinical characteristics, management, and outcomes of patients diagnosed with acute pulmonary embolism in the emergency department: initial report of EMPEROR (Multicenter Emergency Medicine Pulmonary Embolism in the Real World Registry). *Journal of the American College of Cardiology* **57**: 700–706.

Squizzato A, Luciani D, Rubboli A *et al.* (2013). Differential diagnosis of pulmonary embolism in outpatients with non-specific cardiopulmonary symptoms. *Internal and Emergency Medicine* **8**: 695–702.

Lesser BA, Leeper KV, Jr., Stein PD *et al.* (1992). The diagnosis of acute pulmonary embolism in patients with chronic obstructive pulmonary disease. *Chest* **102**: 17–22.

Section II

Diagnosis

4

Clinical Prediction Scores

Kerstin de Wit[1] and Lana A. Castellucci[2]

[1] Department of Medicine, McMaster University, Hamilton, Ontario, Canada
[2] Department of Medicine, Ottawa Hospital Research Institute, University of Ottawa, Ottawa, Canada

The evaluation of risk for pulmonary embolism and deep vein thrombosis always includes an assessment of clinical probability using clinical prediction scores or rules. The tools are designed to simplify and standardise need for diagnostic imaging to confirm or refute the diagnosis. Clinical prediction scores provide accurate and reproducible estimates of venous thrombosis outcomes. We describe several clinical prediction rules for the diagnosis of pulmonary embolism and deep vein thrombosis.

Pulmonary Embolism

Pulmonary Embolism in the Emergency Department

For clinicians in the emergency department, it can be challenging to determine whether pulmonary embolism should be part of the differential diagnosis for common presentations of dyspnea or chest pain. On one hand, failure to consider the diagnosis could lead to untreated and potentially fatal pulmonary embolic disease. On the other, evaluation for pulmonary embolism is a time-consuming, multi-step and complex process, which can prolong emergency department stay or, in some cases, necessitate hospital admission for an otherwise healthy individual. A good example is the young patient who presents with isolated pleuritic chest pain. We now know that around 5% of these patients will have pulmonary embolism. The vast majority will have no diagnosis after extensive workup. Physicians have wrestled with this controversy for many years.

This is where the Pulmonary Embolism Rule-out Criteria (PERC rule) is helpful. The rule was created to help emergency clinicians to determine whether pulmonary embolism should be part of the differential diagnosis when the clinician is really not sure whether testing is even merited. The PERC rule (Table 4.1) allocates a patient into one of two categories:

1) PE so unlikely that testing for the condition is not required; and
2) Testing for PE is necessary to rule out the condition.

The PERC rule has a negative likelihood ratio of 0.2. When applied to a population with pre-test probability of 7% or less, the post-test probability following a negative PERC test is 1.5% or less. No test excludes PE in 100% of patients (including negative diagnostic imaging) so, when the PERC rule is used to exclude PE, the patient should be informed that PE has been excluded to the best of our ability. There will be a very slim chance that they have PE and, when discharged home, they should return if their symptoms worsen.

Handbook of Venous Thromboembolism, First Edition. Edited by Jecko Thachil and Catherine Bagot.
© 2018 John Wiley & Sons Ltd. Published 2018 by John Wiley & Sons Ltd.

Table 4.1 PERC score.

Age ≥ 50	Any component positive = positive test
Prior venous thromboembolism	All components negative = negative test
Trauma or surgery < 4 weeks	
Exogenous Oestrogen	
Haemoptysis	
Unilateral Leg Swelling	
O2 Sat on Room Air < 95%	
HR ≥ 100	

Table 4.2 Wells score for pulmonary embolism.

Clinical signs and symptoms of DVT	Minimum swelling and tenderness along distribution of deep veins	3.0
An alternative diagnosis is less likely than PE		3.0
Heart rate > 100		1.5
Immobilisation or surgery	Bedbound for minimum three days, walking to bathroom only. Surgery < 4 weeks ago.	1.5
Prior venous thrombosis	Objectively diagnosed PE or DVT	1.5
Haemoptysis		1.0
Malignancy	Malignancy treated or palliated within the last six months	1.0
PE unlikely ≤4.0		
PE likely ≥5.0		

When it is clear that objective testing for PE is necessary, clinical probability estimation guides the choice of subsequent testing. Those with a low risk of disease are appropriate for D-dimer testing, and those at high risk require diagnostic imaging.

Prior to the advent of clinical probability rules, all patients underwent diagnostic imaging. This led to longer hospital stays, higher costs and greater radiation exposure. Clinical probability scores are particularly useful in the emergency department, where the majority of patients assessed for VTE are low-risk for PE. Applying the bedside clinical probability estimate enables subsequent exclusion of thrombosis with D-dimer in a large proportion of patients.

Clinical prediction scores do not require extensive medical experience to use, and therefore have an advantage over Gestalt estimates. Although experienced clinicians may find Gestalt estimation simpler and more discriminatory, it can take many years to build up the necessary experience to identify high- and low-risk patients. Evidence tells us that new clinicians are less able to identify correctly the probability of PE using a Gestalt estimate, and use of a clinical prediction rule improves the accuracy of clinical probability classification. Furthermore, it standardises the approach to PE diagnosis.

Many clinical probability scores have been developed for PE over the past two decades however, the Wells score (Table 4.2) is the most widely used and validated. The Wells score has also been simplified for ease of use over the years. The original Wells score for PE placed each patient into a low, intermediate or high probability category. Subsequently, the score has been dichotomised into 'PE unlikely' and 'PE likely' groups. More than 10 000 patients have been studied with the likely/unlikely version of the model (including randomised studies and outcomes studies). Moderate to good inter-rater agreement and reproducibility has been demonstrated. The dichotomised score has been sufficiently validated in conjunction with D-dimer testing; patients who score 4.0 or fewer points are suitable for D-dimer testing. The combination of a normal D-dimer level in a 'PE unlikely' patient reliably excludes PE in up to 30% of outpatients.

Pulmonary Embolism in Hospitalised Patients

Hospitalised patients differ from outpatients in the presence of comorbidity (such as cancer and recent surgery). They are also more likely to be tachycardic and to have leg swelling. The PERC rule should not be applied to hospitalised patients. Patients investigated for PE in a hospital ward are more likely to have a higher Wells score for PE, and a smaller proportion will score 'PE unlikely'. Two studies reported post-test prevalence of PE in the 'PE unlikely' group to be 8% and 20%. Both studies reported no false negative PE exclusion on the bases of 'PE unlikely' and a negative D-dimer. There has been little overall research on the use of the Wells rule for inpatients. We recommend cautious use of the Wells score in inpatients, and consideration of diagnostic imaging in all cases.

Pulmonary Embolism in Primary Care

One study showed that the Wells score, in combination with D-dimer, can safely exclude PE in general practice. Given the urgency for diagnosis, the Wells score could be combined with a point of care D-dimer.

Deep Vein Thrombosis

Deep Vein Thrombosis in the Emergency Department

The original Wells score, derived from data collection on 529 outpatients, identified patients as low pre-test probability of DVT (around 3–8% prevalence of DVT), intermediate (15–25% prevalence) or high probability (40–50% prevalence). Gestalt estimation is effective in centres that have previously used risk prediction tools (possibly due to experience with validated prediction tools), but the Wells score may be a safer exclusion tool in combination with D-dimer testing. The derivation study excluded patients with a history of previous DVT, and these patients make up around 15% of investigated patients.

To obviate the need to perform ultrasound on all patients with prior history of DVT, the Wells score was modified in 2003 to include past history of DVT, and then dichotomised into 'DVT likely' and 'DVT unlikely' (Table 4.3), clarifying which patients require ultrasound and who to test for D-dimer. The original and modified Wells scores have a similar ability to discriminate clinical probability of DVT. The score is less sensitive for calf DVT but, when combined with D-dimer, it is safe to exclude both proximal and distal DVT.

Deep Vein Thrombosis in Hospitalised Patients

The Wells score for DVT does not discriminate well between inpatients with and without DVT. One study found that the prevalence of DVT in patients with a high Wells score was only 16%. Leg oedema and skin colour changes are common among hospitalised patients, contributing to the lack of specificity of the Wells rule. Given that leg ultrasound carries no radiation exposure, and is readily available in all hospital settings, we recommend that all patients who are suspected of having developed DVT in hospital should undergo leg ultrasound.

Deep Vein Thrombosis in Primary Care

In 2005, a study from the Netherlands found an unusually high prevalence of DVT among the low Wells score patient group (12%). This is the sole study to have examined the use of the Wells score by general practitioners. The authors analysed the same cohort to derive a new DVT rule for primary care general practitioners, which uses the D-dimer result within the score and determines which patients to refer for ultrasound. The Oudega rule (Table 4.4) excludes DVT without ultrasound in around half of the cohort, which could represent considerable savings in cost and time. However, the rule is less discriminatory in the elderly, and has only been evaluated in the Netherlands.

Table 4.3 Wells score for deep vein thrombosis.

Prior DVT	Objectively diagnosed DVT.	1.0
Paralysis, paresis, or recent plaster immobilisation of the lower extremity	Paralysis of one or more limbs or rigid immobilisation of a leg.	1.0
Immobilisation or surgery	Bedbound for minimum three days, walking to bathroom only. Surgery < 4 weeks ago.	1.0
Calf swelling > 3 cm compared to the other leg	Measured 10 cm below tibial tuberosity.	1.0
Entire leg swollen	Swelling visualised from groin to foot.	1.0
Dilated superficial veins present	New appearance of small veins beneath skin, compared to unaffected leg. These have become larger, as they are carrying blood past the deep vein obstruction.	1.0
Localised tenderness along the deep venous system	Tenderness over the proximal calf or the medial aspect of the thigh.	1.0
Unilateral pitting oedema	No oedema of the contralateral leg.	1.0
Alternative diagnosis to DVT is likely	Findings such as cellulitis, hematoma of the calf, history compatible with gastrocnemius rupture.	−2.0

DVT unlikely ≤ 1.0

DVT likely ≥ 2.0

Table 4.4 Oudega rule.

Male sex	1.0
Oestrogen use	1.0
Malignancy	1.0
Recent surgery	1.0
Absence of trauma	1.0
Dilated collateral veins	1.0
Calf circumference ≥ 3 cm difference compared to contralateral leg	2.0
Elevated D-dimer	6.0

Ultrasound required if ≥ 4.0

Potential Pitfalls

There are many unforeseen challenges associated with using clinical probability scoring systems, and these challenges are all the more exaggerated in the emergency department and internal medicine wards. Rule application relies on accurate recall of the individual components, a detailed understanding of each component definition, the conversion of positive and negative findings into points, and tallying of the total score. The clinician then has to convert the final score into a dichotomous category. There is room for error at every step, and only a meticulous evaluation will give accurate patient allocation. This is challenging when evaluation is conducted in a pressurised, noisy, overcrowded emergency department.

Some of this error can be minimised by the use of cell phone 'apps' or online scoring sites. At the very minimum, there should be simple access to an *aide memoire*.

Specific areas for improvement in rule application include a clear understanding of each component definition. For example, a long-distance flight or two days in bed do not qualify as 'immobility' for the Wells score. Chronic lymphocytic leukaemia which is under yearly review and no active treatment does not qualify as 'cancer'. To correctly evaluate for DVT, the clinician has to measure calf circumference, rather than estimate whether there is 3 cm difference.

The Wells rule for PE includes 1.5 points for tachycardia. In our experience, many patients in emergency triage are tachycardic. However, when assessed at the bedside, a proportion who were tachycardic at triage have a normal heart rate. Heart rate is influenced by anxiety, pain and emotion, and the triage vital signs may not give an accurate evaluation of the patient in question. We recommend recording the heart rate at the time of bedside evaluation and, ideally, in a quiet environment, following analgesia for those in pain.

The Wells rules ask whether there is another diagnosis more likely than PE/DVT. This component has remained a contentious issue for PE. The evaluation for DVT is simpler, since other diagnoses are generally quite obvious (such as cellulitis or muscular tear). However, this is not the case for PE. The most frequent diagnosis in a young person with pleuritic chest pain is no diagnosis at all (sometimes interpreted as anxiety, viral pleurisy, costochondritis or atypical chest pain). This is often apparent to the clinician at the time of evaluation, and it has become our practice not to allocate the 3.0 points for such patients. Furthermore, some studies have modified the wording to read 'PE is the most likely diagnosis', without affecting score performance.

The PERC rule is safe to exclude PE as a differential diagnosis of patients with a pre-test probability of 7% or less. However the PERC rule is not safe to apply to patients with a Wells score of 2.0 or more (the conventional cut-off for moderate probability), or a patient whom you feel is at high risk of PE.

The Wells scores are most studied in the outpatient, emergency department population. There is evidence that these scores perform less well in the inpatient population and in primary care centres. Clinicians should have a low threshold for diagnostic imaging in hospitalised patients, and for referring to the emergency department in primary care.

Finally, a prospective study from France demonstrated that deviation from standardised diagnostic PE protocols (including clinical probability estimation) resulted in a 6% increase in mortality when compared to those who had appropriate protocol driven investigation. Failure to evaluate clinical probability results in inferior medical care.

Key Points

- The PERC rule can exclude pulmonary embolism in emergency department patients when the physician is not clear whether pulmonary embolism is on the list of differential diagnoses.
- Diagnosis of pulmonary embolism or deep vein thrombosis in the emergency department starts with a structured clinical probability estimate.
- Clinical decision rules are the preferred method to estimate clinical probability, especially for inexperienced clinicians.
- The Wells scores are the most widely studied and validated clinical probability rules.
- The Wells rules should be used with caution in hospitalised inpatients, where there should be a low threshold for diagnostic imaging.
- Meticulous attention should be used when performing and calculating clinical probability scores in order to avoid allocation of patients to the wrong group.
- Deviation from predetermined clinical probability scores is associated with worse patient outcome.

Key Reading

Ceriani E, Combescure C, Le Gal G, Nendaz M, Perneger T, Bounameaux H *et al.* (2010). Clinical prediction rules for pulmonary embolism: a systematic review and meta-analysis. *Journal of Thrombosis and Haemostasis* **8**(5): 957–970.

Geersing GJ, Erkens PM, Lucassen WA, Buller HR, Cate HT, Hoes AW *et al.* (2012). Safe exclusion of pulmonary embolism using the Wells rule and qualitative D-dimer testing in primary care: prospective cohort study. *BMJ* **345**: e6564.

Geersing GJ, Zuithoff NP, Kearon C, Anderson DR, Ten Cate-Hoek AJ, Elf JL *et al.* (2014). Exclusion of deep vein thrombosis using the Wells rule in clinically important subgroups: individual patient data meta-analysis. *BMJ* **348**: g1340.

Goodacre S, Sutton AJ, Sampson FC (2005). Meta-Analysis: The Value of Clinical Assessment in the Diagnosis of Deep Venous Thrombosis. *Annals of Internal Medicine* **143**(2): 129–139.

Kline JA, Kabrhel C (2015). Emergency Evaluation for Pulmonary Embolism, Part 2: Diagnostic Approach. *The Journal of Emergency Medicine* **49**(1): 104–117.

Silveira PC, Ip IK, Goldhaber SZ, Piazza G, Benson CB, Khorasani R (2015). Performance of Wells score for deep vein thrombosis in the inpatient setting. *JAMA Internal Medicine* **175**(7): 1112–7.

van der Velde EF, Toll DB, ten Cate-Hoek AJ, Oudega R, Stoffers HEJH, Bossuyt PM *et al.* (2011). Comparing the Diagnostic Performance of 2 Clinical Decision Rules to Rule Out Deep Vein Thrombosis in Primary Care Patients. *The Annals of Family Medicine* **9**(1): 31–36.

5

Laboratory Aspects in Diagnosis and Management of Venous Thromboembolism

Giuseppe Lippi[1] *and Emmanuel J. Favaloro*[2]

[1] *Section of Clinical Biochemistry, University of Verona, Verona, Italy*
[2] *Department of Haematology, Institute of Clinical Pathology and Medical Research (ICPMR), Pathology West, NSW Health Pathology, Westmead Hospital, Westmead, NSW, Australia*

Introduction

Venous thromboembolism (VTE), which is conventionally defined as the occurrence of deep venous thrombosis (DVT), pulmonary embolism (PE), or both, is a severe, often life-threatening disorder, characterised by the onset of venous thrombi in peripheral veins (i.e. DVT), most frequently in the lower limbs, and by their possible detachment and embolisation in the pulmonary artery circulation (i.e. PE).

Although the precise epidemiology of VTE is difficult to estimate, recent statistics report that its frequency can be as high as 1–2 : 1000 per year in the general population, gradually increasing up to 1 : 100 per year in the elderly (Beckman *et al.*, 2010). The prevalence is also higher in Blacks and in the male gender (Montagnana *et al.*, 2010). The overall mortality is considerable, being between 10–30% within one month of diagnosis. Even more importantly, sudden death is the first 'symptom' to appear in approximately 25% of those affected. In individuals who survive, nearly 50% will experience long-term complications, principally the post-thrombotic syndrome (i.e. swelling, pain, discoloration and scaling in the affected limb), and approximately 33% will have a recurrence of VTE within ten years (Beckman *et al.*, 2010).

Due to the prevalence and severity of disease, a timely diagnosis and subsequent appropriate therapeutic management are essential aspects of managed care, for preventing both adverse outcomes and recurrence. As with other frequent human disorders, laboratory diagnostics plays a crucial role in several aspects of the natural history of VTE, including prevention, diagnosis, prognostication and therapeutic monitoring.

Laboratory Diagnostics of Venous Thromboembolism

After several decades of research, it is now widely acknowledged that an effective diagnosis of VTE can only be based on a multifaceted approach, encompassing the integration of clinical judgment, laboratory testing and diagnostic imaging to overcome the inherent shortcomings of each individual branch of clinical science.

Indeed, clinical judgment is a mainstay of clinical decision-making, and should guide the appropriate prescription of subsequent diagnostic investigations. The clinical expressions of DVT and PE encompass a wide range of signs and symptoms that are each not sufficiently sensitive or specific to achieve a final diagnosis. In brief, the onset of DVT is often associated with oedema, swelling, pain or tenderness of the affected limb (nearly 95% of DVTs are located in the lower or uppers arms), warmth or erythema of the skin over the area of thrombosis, Homans' sign (i.e. calf pain on dorsiflexion of the foot), and presence of palpable, indurated, cordlike, tender subcutaneous venous segment (Bates *et al.*, 2012). Patients with PE may instead present with tachycardia, shortness of breath, pain with deep breathing and cough, leading to haemoptysis and syncope in the most severe forms (Tapson, 2008).

According to the evidence-based clinical practice guidelines of the American College of Chest Physicians (ACCP) (Bates *et al.*, 2012), the investigation of a patient with suspected DVT should start with clinical assessment of pre-test probability, rather than with indiscriminate performance of diagnostic testing (recommendation of Grade 2B). The preferred recommended scoring system is that originally proposed by Wells, which incorporates signs, symptoms and risk factors for DVT, and enables the categorisation of patients as having low (i.e. ≈ 5%), moderate (i.e. ≈ 15%) or high (i.e. ≈ 50%) probability of DVT (Wells *et al.*, 1997).

A more recent and simplified version of the score was published in 2003 (Wells *et al.*, 2003), enabling the categorisation of patients as being likely (≈30% prevalence of DVT) or unlikely (≈6% prevalence of DVT) of having DVT (Table 5.1). The ACCP then recommends initial testing with D-dimer or ultrasound (US) in patients with low pre-test probability of DVT (Grade 1B recommendation), initial testing with a high sensitivity (HS) D-dimer, proximal compression US, whole-leg US or venography (Grade 1B recommendation) in

Table 5.1 Wells' score for the diagnosis of venous thromboembolism (Wells *et al.*, 1997, 2003).

Sign or symptom	Score
Deep Vein Thrombosis (DVT)	
• Active cancer	1
• Immobilisation of lower limbs	1
• Recently bedridden (three days or more), or major surgery (within 12 weeks) requiring anaesthesia	1
• Localised tenderness	1
• Leg swollen	1
• Calf swelling (≥3 cm than the asymptomatic side)	1
• Pitting oedema	1
• Collateral superficial veins	1
• Previous diagnosis of DVT	1
• Alternative diagnosis	−2
Pulmonary embolism (PE)	
• Clinical signs and symptoms of DVT	3
• Alternative diagnosis less likely than PE	3
• Tachycardia (i.e. heart rate >100 per min)	1.5
• Recently bedridden (three days or more), or major surgery (within 12 weeks) requiring anaesthesia	1.5
• Previous diagnosis of PE or DVT	1.5
• Haemoptysis	1
• Active cancer	1

DVT score:
≥2 likely of having DVT
PE score:
<2 low probability of PE
2–6 modest probability of PE
>6 high probability of PE
≤4 likely of not having PE.
>4 likely of having PE.

Figure 5.1 Diagnostic algorithm for deep vein thrombosis. DVT – deep vein thrombosis; HS – high sensitivity; US – ultrasonography.

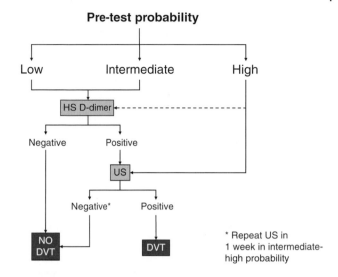

Figure 5.2 Diagnostic algorithm for pulmonary embolism. HS – high sensitivity; PA – pulmonary angiography; PE – pulmonary embolism; US – ultrasonography; V/Q scan – pulmonary ventilation/perfusion scan.

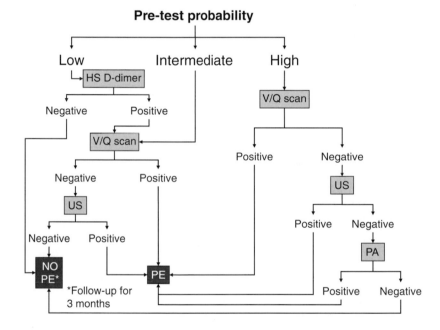

patients with moderate pre-test probability of DVT, and proximal compression, whole-leg US or venography (Grade 1B) in patients with high pre-test probability of DVT. The derived diagnostic algorithm is shown in Figure 5.1.

Another version of the Wells' scoring system was subsequently proposed for the diagnostic approach to patients with suspected PE (Wells *et al.*, 2000), which enables the categorisation of patients as having low (i.e. ≈ 2%), moderate (i.e. ≈ 20%) or high (i.e. ≈ 50%) probability of PE (Table 5.1). As for DVT, the use of a simplified version of the scoring system also enables the categorisation of patients as being likely (≈40% prevalence of PE) or unlikely (≈5% prevalence of PE) of having PE (Table 5.1). The resulting diagnostic algorithm is shown in Figure 5.2.

Interestingly, a key aspect in both algorithms for the diagnosis of DVT or PE is the presence of one laboratory biomarker measurement (i.e. D-dimer) in patients with low and intermediate pre-test probability of DVT, as well as in those with low pre-test probability of PE. Indeed, the introduction of this sensitive marker of VTE revolutionised the diagnostic approach to VTE nearly 20 years ago (Lippi *et al.*, 1998), in that VTE may now be safely ruled out in the vast majority of patients with low pre-test probability and negative D-dimer test results.

The selection of D-dimer as the preferred test has not been an easy task, however (Lippi *et al.*, 2010a). Several potential biomarkers have been proposed over past decades for diagnosing VTE. These have conventionally included prothrombin fragment 1 + 2 (PF1 + 2), fibrinopeptide A (FPA) and fibrinopeptide B (FPB), thrombin-antithrombin complex (TAT), plasmin-antiplasmin complex (PAP), thrombus precursor protein (TpP), activated protein C-protein C inhibitor complex (APC-PCI), soluble fibrin monomers (SFMs), fibrin/fibrinogen degradation products (FDPs) and, perceptibly, D-dimer (Lippi *et al.*, 2015a).

Among these, widespread consensus has now been reached that D-dimer exhibits the best compromise between analytical and clinical characteristics, and should therefore be regarded as the biochemical gold standard for the diagnosis of VTE. The elevated sensitivity (up to 1.00), combined with the availability of fast, accurate and relatively inexpensive techniques (i.e. latex-enhanced immunoassays or enzyme-linked immunoassays) for its measurement, has contributed to considerably enhancing its diffusion in clinical laboratories in recent times (Lippi *et al.*, 2014a, 2015b).

D-dimer is an end product of plasmin-catalysed degradation of stabilised fibrin. Unlike FDPs, D-dimer is generated by the covalent cross-linking of two adjacent D fibrin subunits, when both blood coagulation (and, thus, thrombin) and fibrinolysis (and, thus, plasmin) are activated (Figure 5.3).

Intuitively appealing to this biological pathway, the clinical value (and, most precisely, the diagnostic specificity) of D-dimer is several orders of magnitudes higher than that of FDPs, since an increased blood concentration of this biomarker specifically mirrors the presence of a recent clot and its subsequent fibrinolysis. Unfortunately, there are several potential sources of misunderstanding regarding the clinical interpretation of D-dimer concentration in blood. First, D-dimer is not a single molecule, but a mixture of many molecular products of fibrin degradation that are all characterised by the presence of a covalent cross-linking between adjacent D fibrin subunits (Figure 5.3; Lippi *et al.*, 2008a). The identification of a universal standard material for calibrating and harmonising the different immunoassays is, therefore, challenged by this inherent structural characteristic.

Another frequent misinterpretation occurs when physicians attempt to relate increased values of D-dimer with *only* VTE or disseminated intravascular coagulation (DIC), thus ignoring the fact that D-dimer can be generated in a variety of physiological and pathological conditions, such as pregnancy, cancer, localised or

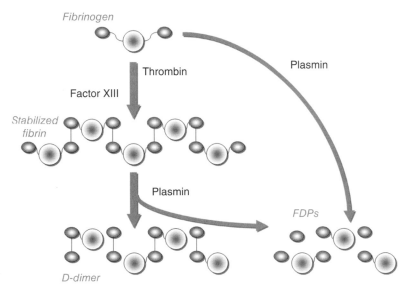

Figure 5.3 Generation of fibrin/fibrinogen degradation products (FDPs) and D-dimer.

systemic infections (i.e. sepsis) and atrial fibrillation, among others (Lippi *et al.*, 2014b, Danese *et al.*, 2014). As such, although displaying a comparable sensitivity for the diagnosis of VTE, the diagnostic *specificity* of D-dimer, while greater than that of FDPs, remains overall modest, approximating 0.50.

Additional aspects that should be considered when interpreting D-dimer results include the fact that its concentration depends on the time of occurrence and extension of the thrombotic process, so that negative results may be frequently encountered when D-dimer is measured too early or too late after development of thrombosis, especially in patients with small and distal DVT, as well as in those undergoing anticoagulant therapy (Lippi *et al.*, 2009a). Physiological ageing is an additional drawback to interpretation, in that the development of age-related changes has been documented for a number of procoagulant and anticoagulant proteins, including D-dimer (Favaloro *et al.*, 2014). Finally, analytical artefacts such as spurious haemolysis (Lippi *et al.*, 2006) and the presence of heterophile antibodies in the plasma sample (Lippi *et al.*, 2014c) may decrease the diagnostic accuracy of D-dimer. Taken together, these drawbacks explain why the measurement of D-dimer is now preferable to that of other biomarkers, but its use as a rule-out test is only indicated in patients with low (or intermediate) pre-test probability of VTE (Figures 5.1 and 5.2).

Laboratory Prediction of Recurrent Venous Thromboembolism

VTE is currently regarded as a chronic disease, which exhibits a considerably high recurrence rate. Basically, the risk of recurrence after a first episode of VTE is influenced by a number of factors, including the type of first event and the presence of (additional) prothrombotic conditions (Poli and Palareti, 2013). In a recent systematic review including prospective cohort studies and randomised trials in patients with a first episode of symptomatic VTE (Iorio *et al.*, 2010), Iorio *et al.* estimated a 3.3% recurrence rate at 24 months per patient-year in subjects with a transient risk factor, 0.7% per patient-year in those with a surgical factor, 4.2% per patient-year in those with non-surgical factors, and 7.4% per patient-year in those with unprovoked VTE. Overall, patients with unprovoked VTE exhibited a recurrence rate that was nearly double than that of patients with non-surgical factors. Due to such a high recurrence rate, several studies have attempted to stratify the risk of patients with unprovoked VTE according to clinical risk factors (e.g. sex, gender, comorbidities), or using laboratory biomarkers.

Rodger *et al.* performed a multicentre prospective cohort study including 646 participants with a first, unprovoked major VTE who completed a mean 18-month follow-up (Rodger *et al.*, 2008). Information on as many as 69 potential predictors of recurrent VTE was collected, but no combination could accurately satisfy the criteria for identifying a low-risk subgroup of patients in men. Nonetheless, in women, the presence of two or more factors, including hyper-pigmentation, oedema or redness of either leg, D-dimer $\geq 250\,\mu g/L$, body mass index $\geq 30\,kg/m^2$ and age ≥ 65 years, was associated with a 14.1% greater annual risk of VTE.

Eichinger *et al.* also performed a prospective cohort study including 929 patients with a first unprovoked VTE, who were followed up from three weeks after the end of anticoagulation, up to a median period of 43.3 months (Eichinger *et al.*, 2010). Interestingly, a number of factors were associated with a higher recurrent risk, including male sex (hazard ratio (HR) versus female sex 1.9), proximal DVT (HR versus distal DVT, 2.1), diagnosis of PE (HR versus distal thrombosis, 2.6), and elevated D-dimer values (HR per doubling D-dimer concentration, 1.3).

An algorithm was therefore developed using these variables (60 points for male sex and 0 for females sex; 90 points for PE, 70 for proximal DVT and 0 for distal DVT; 100 points for D-dimer $2000\,\mu g/L$ down to 0 points for D-dimer $100\,\mu g/L$ or lower), which was applied to estimate risk scores and cumulative probability of VTE recurrence. The recurrence risk at 60 months was 50% (or higher) in patients with a score of 300 or higher, compared with 10% in patients with a score of 100 or lower. Similarly, the recurrence risk at 12 months was 15% (or higher) in patients with a score of 300 or higher, compared with 3% (or lower) in patients with a score of 100 or lower. This normogram was then validated in a further study for estimating the 60-month cumulative recurrence rate, from three weeks to 15 months after end of anticoagulation (Eichinger *et al.*, 2014).

Tosetto *et al.* studied 1818 patients with unprovoked VTE treated for at least three months with a vitamin K antagonist (Tosetto *et al.*, 2012). A number of parameters (i.e. increased D-dimer value after anticoagulation was stopped, age < 50 years, male sex and VTE not associated with hormonal therapy in women) were then used to generate a prognostic recurrence score (DASH score; D-dimer, Age, Sex, Hormonal therapy), which exhibited good accuracy to predict VTE recurrence (area under the curve, 0.71).

As specifically regards D-dimer, a meta-analysis published by Schouten *et al.* (2013) including 13 cohorts and totalling 12 497 patients, concluded that the specificity of the conventional D-dimer threshold value decreases with increasing age, from 0.58 in patients aged 51–60 years to 0.15 in those aged > 80. Conversely, the use of age-adjusted threshold values was associated with a much higher specificity across all age categories, from 0.62 in patients aged 51–60 years, to 0.35 in those aged > 80. The diagnostic sensitivity remained unvaried using conventional or age-adjusted thresholds (i.e. always equal to or greater than 0.97).

Palareti has also recently demonstrated that serial D-dimer measurement represents a reliable approach for identifying VTE patients in whom anticoagulation can be safely discontinued (Palareti *et al.*, 2014). Briefly, 1010 patients with a first VTE were followed for up to two years, during which serial D-dimer measurements with predefined age/sex-specific threshold were performed. In patients with persistently negative D-dimer ($n = 528$), anticoagulation was stopped whereas, in the remaining, anticoagulation was continued ($n = 373$) or refused ($n = 109$). A diagnosis of recurrent VTE was made in 0.7% of patients with persistently negative D-dimer in whom anticoagulation was stopped, compared with 8.8% in those with abnormal D-dimer who refused anticoagulation (HR, 2.9; 95% CI, 1.9–9.7). Interestingly, in patients with negative D-dimer, the events were significantly more frequent in those aged 70 years or older, and in those with idiopathic VTE.

According to these evidences it can, hence, be concluded that D-dimer exhibits a high predictive value for VTE recurrence, and can be used in the clinical decision-making process, more specifically for establishing the optimal type and duration of anticoagulation (Palareti, 2015). This is in agreement with the current recommendations of the ACCP, concluding that in patients at risk of recurrent lower extremity DVT, initial evaluation with highly sensitive D-dimer testing (all Grade 1B), eventually followed by proximal CUS in patients with diagnostic D-dimer values (Bates *et al.*, 2012). In patients with a negative value of HS D-dimer, consideration should be made that anticoagulation be suspended after the conventional therapeutic period (3–12 months) whereas, in those with a positive D-dimer value, long-term or indeterminate anticoagulation should be advisable (Figure 5.4). In analogy with the diagnosis of VTE, recent evidence also suggests that the use of age-dependent D-dimer cut-offs is advisable for enhancing the diagnostic effectiveness of this biomarker with increasing age (Lippi *et al.*, 2014d).

Laboratory Monitoring of Anticoagulant Therapy

The foremost reason underlying the establishment of anti-coagulant or anti-thrombotic therapy in patients with (or at high risk of) VTE is based on the fact that anticoagulant drugs are relatively effective for inhibiting blood coagulation and reducing fibrin formation, thus representing the mainstay for prevention and treatment of venous thrombosis (Ko and Hylek, 2014). The current armamentarium of anti-coagulant or anti-thrombotic drugs mainly entails three types of agents: heparins; vitamin K antagonists (VKAs); and the more recently developed direct oral anticoagulants (DOACs) (Table 5.2; Figure 5.5).

Heparin is a highly sulphated glycosaminoglycan, which is commercially available as unfractionated heparin (UFH) or low molecular weight heparin (LMWH). LMWH, which principally acts by inhibiting activated factor X (FXa) and, to a lower extent, thrombin, can only be parentally administered (e.g. by subcutaneous injection), has a relatively short half-life (i.e. 3–6 hours), and its anticoagulant effect can be conventionally reversed by administration of protamine sulphate.

The VKAs, mainly represented by warfarin and acenocumarol, act through inhibiting the synthesis of functional vitamin K-dependent factors (i.e. FII, FVII, FIX, FX, protein S and C), are orally administered (usually once daily), have a relatively longer half-life (10–60 hours), and their anticoagulant effect can be typically

Figure 5.4 Diagnostic algorithm for recurrent deep vein thrombosis. DVT – deep vein thrombosis; HS – high sensitivity; US – ultrasonography.

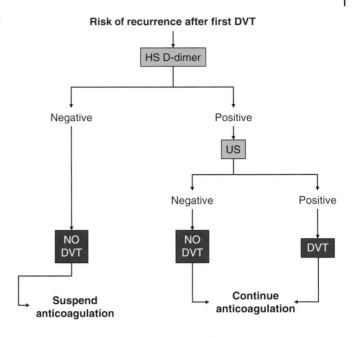

Table 5.2 Characteristics of current anticoagulant drugs and their laboratory monitoring.

	LMWH	VKAs	Dabigatran	Rivaroxaban	Apixaban	Edoxaban
Action	Inhibition of FXa	Inactivation of vitamin K-dependent factors	Thrombin inhibition	Inhibition of FXa	Inhibition of FXa	Inhibition of FXa
Administration	Parenteral (i.e., subcutaneous)	Oral	Oral	Oral	Oral	Oral
Half-life	3–6 hours	10–60 hours	12–17 hours	5–9 hours	6–12 hours	6–8 hours
Laboratory test (reference)	Anti-FXa chromogenic assay	PT-INR	dTT (or ECT)	Anti-FXa chromogenic assay	Anti-FXa chromogenic assay	Anti-FXa chromogenic assay
Urgent screening	APTT	PT-INR	APTT (ratio) or dRVVT	PT (ratio) or dRVVT	PT (ratio) or dRVVT	Not established

APTT – activated partial thromboplastin time; dRVVT – dilute Russell viper venom time; dTT – dilute thrombin time; ECT – ecarin clotting time; FXa – activated factor X; LMWH – low molecular weight heparin; PT – prothrombin time; VKAs – vitamin K antagonists.

reversed by administration of vitamin K or factor replacement therapy (i.e. administration of plasma, prothrombin complex concentrate and similar agents).

The DOACs act through selective inhibition of either thrombin (dabigatran) or FXa (i.e. rivaroxaban, apixaban and edoxaban), can be orally administered (once or twice daily), have a half-life of usually between 5–20 hours, and the neutralisation of their anticoagulant effect can only be achieved with replacement therapy (e.g. prothrombin complex concentrate) or by-passing agents in urgent conditions (Lippi *et al.*, 2014e), although potentially more effective antidotes are in development. Unlike heparin, the administration of DOACs does not carry a risk of developing heparin-induced thrombocytopenia (Cuker, 2014).

So far, the US Food and Drug Administration (FDA) and the European Commission (EC) have licensed dabigratan, rivaroxaban and apixaban for treatment and reducing the risk of recurrence of VTE, whereas the use of edoxaban for these indications is currently licensed in Japan and the USA, but not in other countries.

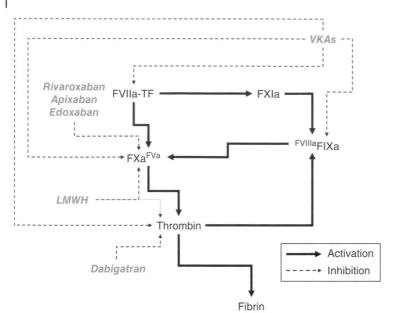

Figure 5.5 Mechanism of action of the leading anticoagulant drugs. F – factor; LMWH – low molecular weight heparin; VKAs – vitamin K antagonists.

Although the comprehensive description of anticoagulant therapy is beyond the scope of this chapter, according to the most recent guidelines of the ACCP for treatment of acute DVT or PE, the initial therapy should be based on administration of parenteral anticoagulant therapy with LMWH (or fondaparinux), or anticoagulation with the DOACs for three months. For unprovoked VTE, or that associated with active cancer, extended therapy (i.e. >3 months) is instead recommended when the bleeding risk is low to moderate (Kearon *et al.*, 2012). Pharmacological prophylaxis with antithrombotic agents is also recommended in acutely ill hospitalised medical patients at increased risk of thrombosis throughout (but not beyond) the period of patient immobilisation or acute hospital stay, and in non-orthopaedic surgical patients at moderate or high risk (i.e. (3–6%) of VTE who are not at high risk for major bleeding, as well as in all orthopaedic surgery patients.

Whatever the anticoagulant drug used in the specific patient setting, the role of the hemostasis laboratory is always crucial.

Heparin Monitoring

Compared with UFH, LMWHs have a number of advantages, including a higher inhibitory activity against FXa than thrombin, more predictable pharmacokinetic and pharmacodynamic profiles and longer half-life. They therefore carry a much lower risk of bleeding, and have now almost completely replaced the former compound for management of VTE in clinical practice. The laboratory monitoring of UFH has been based for decades on the conventional activated partial thromboplastin time (APTT), with a therapeutic range typically being a ratio of patient test result to 'normal' (usually a reference pool of normal plasmas) of between 1.5 and 2.5.

The APTT is a first-line, clot-based hemostasis assay, based on exposure of citrated plasma to substances (e.g. silica, ellagic acid, kaolin or celite) capable of activating the intrinsic coagulation pathway in the presence of calcium and phospholipids (Lippi and Favaloro, 2008b). Therefore, this test is prevalently sensitive to perturbation of the intrinsic and common pathway (i.e. FXII, FXI, FIX, FVIII, FX, FV, thrombin and fibrinogen; Lippi *et al.*, 2010b). Interestingly, owing to the fact that LMWHs have a much greater inhibitory activity against FXa than thrombin, the APTT is almost insensitive to these compounds when present in therapeutic doses, and therefore cannot be used for therapeutic monitoring of LMWH treatment.

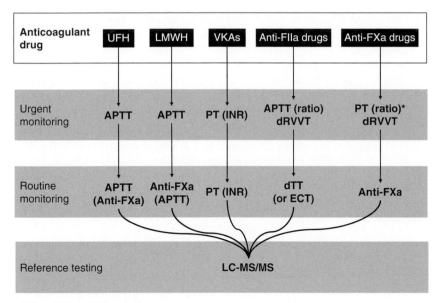

* Not validated for edoxaban

Figure 5.6 Laboratory assessment of the leading anticoagulant drugs. APTT – activated partial thromboplastin time; dRVVT – dilute Russell viper venom time; dTT – dilute thrombin time; ECT – ecarin clotting time; FXa – activated factor X; LC-MS/MS – liquid chromatography tandem mass spectrometry; LMWH – low molecular weight heparin; PT – prothrombin time; UFH – unfractionated heparin; VKAs – vitamin K antagonists.

Conventionally, LMWHs are administered at a fixed dose and display predictable pharmacokinetics, so that laboratory monitoring is usually unnecessary. Nevertheless, since a perturbation of the pharmacodynamic profile may occur in some clinical conditions (i.e. obesity, extreme low weight, impaired renal function and pregnancy), the anti-FXa functional assay is recommended when monitoring may be advisable or required (Garcia *et al.*, 2012; Figure 5.6).

Monitoring of Vitamin K Antagonists

The laboratory monitoring of VKAs is traditionally based on a simple and inexpensive test, the prothrombin time (PT), which was originally described by Quick (1935). The test, although originally being developed for the assessment of prothrombin, from which its name originates, is mostly sensitive to abnormalities of clotting factors of the extrinsic and common coagulation pathways (i.e. FVII, FX, FV, thrombin and fibrinogen). In brief, the PT is a one-stage clotting assay based on the time required for fibrin generation after addition of tissue factor (TF), phospholipid and calcium to decalcified, platelet poor plasma (Hood and Eby, 2008).

Although the results of this test can be conventionally expressed in seconds or ratio (i.e. the ratio between the clotting time of a patient sample and that of a reference pool of plasmas), the extreme variability among the different types of thromboplastin used for activating FVII have led the way to the development of a major degree of inter-laboratory harmonisation for monitoring VKAs, with introduction of the International Normalized Ratio (INR) (Favaloro and Adcock, 2008).

The INR is a mathematical algorithm, in which the ratio is elevated at a reagent- and often instrument-specific coefficient called ISI (International Sensitivity Index), as follows: $INR = PT\ ratio^{ISI}$. In general, the INR value in patients on anticoagulant therapy for an episode VTE should be maintained between 2.0 and 3.0.

Due to this narrow therapeutic range, and to the fact that the metabolism of VKAs may be impaired by a number of comorbidities (i.e. decreased liver or renal function, intestinal disorders), dietary habits (i.e. vitamin K ingestion with foods) or interfering drugs (e.g. antibiotics), laboratory monitoring of INR should be planned on a regular basis, which can vary between days and weeks according to the specific patient. This is an obvious source of inconvenience for patients, wherein blood has to be drawn on regular basis and VKAs dosage systematically adjusted according to the actual derived INR value.

Although regular monitoring of INR can also be based on point of care testing (Testa *et al.*, 2015), this approach is inherently more expensive, and also requires a specific and challenging quality control system (Tange *et al.*, 2014; Kitchen *et al.*, 2015; Bonar *et al.*, 2015). Interestingly, although more than 50% of the pharmacological response to VKAs is influenced by polymorphisms in the genes encoding for vitamin K epoxide reductase (*VKOR*) and cytochrome P450 CYP2C9 (Lippi *et al.*, 2009b), ACCP advise against the routine use of pharmacogenetic testing for guiding the initial dosage and maintenance of VKAs therapy (Holbrook *et al.*, 2012).

Monitoring of Direct Oral Anticoagulants

The leading theoretical aspects driving the development and introduction of DOACs into clinical practice is the fact that laboratory monitoring may be unnecessary under most clinical circumstances. The only exceptions may be represented by: the onset of thrombotic or hemorrhagic events in patients under regular therapy; perioperative screening in patients who have recently taken the drug; suspicion of over-dosage or intoxication; or impaired kidney and liver function. The assessment may also be indicated in patients with extremes of body weight, in women suspected to be pregnant and taking these drugs, or in subjects taking potentially interfering drugs, such as certain classes of antibiotics (Lippi *et al.*, 2014f).

As with therapeutic monitoring of other drugs, the reference approach for measuring DOACs is obviously based on direct concentration assessment in serum, plasma (Favaloro *et al.*, 2011, 2012; Harenberg *et al.*, 2014a; Favaloro and Lippi, 2015; Harenberg *et al.*, 2015) or even urine (Harenberg *et al.*, 2013). Indeed, although liquid chromatography tandem mass spectrometry (LC-MS/MS) remains the gold standard for accurately estimating the concentration of DOACs (Gous *et al.*, 2014), this approach is impractical in most clinical laboratories. It is generally not available, or would require dedicated instrumentation and personnel, is more expensive than conventional hemostasis testing, and is also plagued by a longer turnaround time, which ultimately makes it inadequate for stat testing in patients requiring urgent clinical management (i.e. those needing an invasive procedure or experiencing severe bleeding). Accordingly, alternative and more convenient testing would be needed to be performed for routine or urgent assessment of these drugs in clinical laboratories.

According to recent evidence, routine monitoring of dabigatran may be performed using a modified thrombin time (TT), called diluted TT (dTT), in which one volume of patient plasma is mixed with three volumes of pooled reference plasma to overcome the extreme sensitivity of the conventional test. An alternative approach entails the performance of the ecarin clotting time (ECT) (or alternatively a chromogenic assay), in which prothrombin is activated by the highly purified metalloprotease ecarin isolated from the viper *Echis carinatus*'s venom (Nowak, 2003). The available data gathered so far suggest that the dTT assay is very sensitive, accurate and reproducible, so that it should be preferred over the ECT test (Lippi and Favaloro, 2015c).

As regards the DOACs targeting FXa, current evidence suggests that the anti-FXa functional (chromogenic) assays should be used when monitoring is required. More specifically, the different assays should be calibrated by spiking pooled normal plasma samples with known and increasing concentrations of the single drugs, and results should be reported by interpolation of clotting times from the local calibration curves (Lippi and Favaloro, 2015c).

Due to high costs and specific technical requirements, the use of dTT, ECT and anti-FXa assays for urgent monitoring of DOACs has also been debated, since it may impose serious challenges to most clinical laboratories, especially those which cannot afford to have specialised personnel dedicated to hemostasis testing (Lippi *et al.*, 2014g). As such, an alternative approach, by use of more conventional (screening) tests, has recently been proposed by several national and international organisations.

In brief, the recommended screening assay for anti-FIIa drugs (only dabigatran, so far) is the APTT (results expressed as ratio) or the dilute Russell Viper Venom Time (dRVVT), whereas the PT (results expressed as ratio) may be used for screening the anticoagulant effect of some anti-FXa drugs (i.e. rivaroxaban and apixaban) (Figure 5.6; Harenberg *et al.*, 2014b). Incidentally, clear indications about the potential usefulness of PT or dRVVT for edoxaban are currently lacking, so that the screening of anticoagulant effect of this drug should be more cautiously based on anti-FXa assays.

Indeed, the PT, APTT and dRVVT assays are primarily intended for screening the anticoagulant effect, rather than for establishing the actual concentration of the drug. This is due to the fact that normal results will provide reliable evidence that significant anticoagulant effects of DOACs are absent in the patient sample (provided that the sensitivity of the assays to the different agents has been validated), whereas abnormal results would be suggestive of over-dosage, thus reserving the more accurate estimation of the drug concentration by means of more sensitive techniques (Figure 5.6).

Key Points

- Laboratory diagnostics plays a crucial role in several aspects of the natural history of venous thromboembolism, including prevention, diagnosis, prognostication and therapeutic monitoring.
- D-dimer assessment within a diagnostic algorithm integrating pre-test probability and diagnostic imaging represents the biochemical gold standard for diagnosing venous thromboembolism.
- The measurement of D-dimer may help predict the risk of recurrent venous thromboembolism.
- D-dimer values should be preferably compared against age-specific cut-offs.
- The therapy with vitamin K antagonists is routinely monitored with the prothrombin time (expressed as an INR (International Normalised Ratio)).
- The therapy with low molecular weight heparin can be routinely monitored with an anti-activated factor X assay.
- The therapy with direct thrombin inhibitors can be monitored with dilute thrombin time and activated partial thromboplastin time (ratio) in routine and urgent condition, respectively.
- The therapy with direct activated factor X inhibitors can be monitored with an anti-activated factor X assay and occasionally with prothrombin time (ratio) in routine and urgent condition, respectively.

References

Bates SM, Jaeschke R, Stevens SM, Goodacre S, Wells PS, Stevenson MD, Kearon C, Schunemann HJ, Crowther M, Pauker SG, Makdissi R, Guyatt GH; American College of Chest Physicians (2012). Diagnosis of DVT: Antithrombotic Therapy and Prevention of Thrombosis, 9th ed: American College of Chest Physicians Evidence-Based Clinical Practice Guidelines. *Chest* **141**(2 Suppl): e351S–418S.

Beckman MG, Hooper WC, Critchley SE, Ortel TL (2010). Venous thromboembolism: a public health concern. *American Journal of Preventive Medicine* **38**(4 Suppl): S495–501.

Bonar R, Mohammed S, Favaloro EJ (2015). International normalized ratio monitoring of vitamin K antagonist therapy: comparative performance of point-of-care and laboratory-derived testing. *Seminars in Thrombosis and Hemostasis* **41**: 279–86.

Cuker A (2014). Clinical and laboratory diagnosis of heparin-induced thrombocytopenia: an integrated approach. *Seminars in Thrombosis and Hemostasis* **40**: 106–14.

Danese E, Montagnana M, Cervellin G, Lippi G (2014). Hypercoagulability, D-dimer and atrial fibrillation: an overview of biological and clinical evidence. *Annals of Medicine* **46**: 364–71.

Eichinger S, Heinze G, Jandeck LM, Kyrle PA (2010). Risk assessment of recurrence in patients with unprovoked deep vein thrombosis or pulmonary embolism: the Vienna prediction model. *Circulation* **121**: 1630–1636.

Eichinger S, Heinze G, Kyrle PA (2014). D-dimer levels over time and the risk of recurrent venous thromboembolism: an update of the Vienna prediction model. *Journal of the American Heart Association* **3**: e000467.

Favaloro EJ, Adcock DM (2008). Standardization of the INR: how good is your laboratory's INR and can it be improved? *Seminars in Thrombosis and Hemostasis* **34**: 593–603.

Favaloro EJ, Lippi G, Koutts J (2011). Laboratory testing of anticoagulants: the present and the future. *Pathology* **43**: 682–92.

Favaloro EJ, Lippi G (2012). The new oral anticoagulants and the future of haemostasis laboratory testing. *Biochemia Medica* (Zagreb) **22**: 329–41.

Favaloro EJ, Franchini M, Lippi G (2014). Aging hemostasis: changes to laboratory markers of hemostasis as we age – a narrative review. *Seminars in Thrombosis and Hemostasis* **40**: 621–33.

Favaloro EJ, Lippi G (2015). Laboratory Testing in the Era of Direct or Non-Vitamin K Antagonist Oral Anticoagulants: A Practical Guide to Measuring Their Activity and Avoiding Diagnostic Errors. *Seminars in Thrombosis and Hemostasis* **41**: 208–27.

Garcia DA, Baglin TP, Weitz JI, Samama MM; American College of Chest Physicians (2012). Parenteral anticoagulants: Antithrombotic Therapy and Prevention of Thrombosis, 9th ed: American College of Chest Physicians Evidence-Based Clinical Practice Guidelines. *Chest* **141**(2 Suppl): e24S–43S.

Gous T, Couchman L, Patel JP, Paradzai C, Arya R, Flanagan RJ (2014). Measurement of the Direct Oral Anticoagulants Apixaban, Dabigatran, Edoxaban, and Rivaroxaban in Human Plasma Using Turbulent Flow Liquid Chromatography With High-Resolution Mass Spectrometry. *Therapeutic Drug Monitoring* **36**: 597–605.

Harenberg J, Krämer S, Du S, Weiss C, Krämer R (2013). Concept of a point of care test to detect new oral anticoagulants in urine samples. *Thrombosis Journal* **11**: 15.

Harenberg J, Kraemer S, Du S, Giese C, Schulze A, Kraemer R, Weiss C (2014a). Determination of direct oral anticoagulants from human serum samples. *Seminars in Thrombosis and Hemostasis* **40**: 129–34.

Harenberg J, Du S, Weiss C, Krämer R, Hoppensteadt D, Walenga J; working party: methods to determine apixaban of the Subcommittee on Control of Anticoagulation of the International Society of Thrombosis and Haemostasis (2014b). Report of the Subcommittee on Control of Anticoagulation on the determination of the anticoagulant effects of apixaban: communication from the SSC of the ISTH. *Journal of Thrombosis and Haemostasis* **12**: 801–4.

Harenberg J, Du S, Krämer S, Weiss C, Krämer R, Wehling M (2015). Patients' Serum and Urine as Easily Accessible Samples for the Measurement of Non-Vitamin K Antagonist Oral Anticoagulants. *Seminars in Thrombosis and Hemostasis* **41**: 228–36.

Holbrook A, Schulman S, Witt DM, Vandvik PO, Fish J, Kovacs MJ, Svensson PJ, Veenstra DL, Crowther M, Guyatt GH; American College of Chest Physicians (2012). Evidence-based management of anticoagulant therapy: Antithrombotic Therapy and Prevention of Thrombosis, 9th ed: American College of Chest Physicians Evidence-Based Clinical Practice Guidelines. *Chest* **141**(2 Suppl): e152S–84S.

Hood JL, Eby CS (2008). Evaluation of a prolonged prothrombin time. *Clinical Chemistry* **54**: 765–9.

Iorio A, Kearon C, Filippucci E, Marcucci M, Macura A, Pengo V, Siragusa S, Palareti G (2010). Risk of recurrence after a first episode of symptomatic venous thromboembolism provoked by a transient risk factor: a systematic review. *Archives of Internal Medicine* **170**: 1710–6.

Kearon C, Akl EA, Comerota AJ, Prandoni P, Bounameaux H, Goldhaber SZ, Nelson ME, Wells PS, Gould MK, Dentali F, Crowther M, Kahn SR; American College of Chest Physicians (2012). Antithrombotic therapy for VTE disease: Antithrombotic Therapy and Prevention of Thrombosis, 9th ed: American College of Chest Physicians Evidence-Based Clinical Practice Guidelines. *Chest* **141**(2 Suppl): e419S–94S.

Kitchen DP, Jennings I, Kitchen S, Woods TAL, Walker ID (2015). Bridging the gap between point-of-care testing and laboratory testing in hemostasis. *Seminars in Thrombosis and Hemostasis* **41**: 272–8.

Ko D, Hylek EM (2014). Anticoagulation in the older adult: optimizing benefit and reducing risk. *Seminars in Thrombosis and Hemostasis* **40**: 688–94.

Lippi G, Mengoni A, Manzato F (1998). Plasma D-dimer in the diagnosis of deep vein thrombosis. *JAMA* **280**: 1828–9.

Lippi G, Montagnana M, Salvagno GL, Guidi GC (2006). Interference of blood cell lysis on routine coagulation testing. *Archives of Pathology & Laboratory Medicine* **130**: 181–4.

Lippi G, Franchini M, Targher G, Favaloro EJ (2008a). Help me, Doctor! My D-dimer is raised. *Annals of Medicine* **40**: 594–605.

Lippi G, Favaloro EJ (2008b). Activated partial thromboplastin time: new tricks for an old dogma. *Seminars in Thrombosis and Hemostasis* **34**: 604–11.

Lippi G, Favaloro EJ (2009a). D-dimer measurement and laboratory feedback. *Journal of Emergency Medicine* **37**: 82–3.

Lippi G, Franchini M, Favaloro EJ (2009b). Pharmacogenetics of vitamin K antagonists: useful or hype? *Clinical Chemistry and Laboratory Medicine* **47**: 503–15.

Lippi G, Cervellin G, Franchini M, Favaloro EJ (2010a). Biochemical markers for the diagnosis of venous thromboembolism: the past, present and future. *Journal of Thrombosis and Thrombolysis* **30**: 459–71.

Lippi G, Salvagno GL, Ippolito L, Franchini M, Favaloro EJ (2010b). Shortened activated partial thromboplastin time: causes and management. *Blood Coagulation & Fibrinolysis* **21**: 459–463.

Lippi G, Cervellin G, Casagranda I, Morelli B, Testa S, Tripodi A (2014a). D-dimer testing for suspected venous thromboembolism in the emergency department. Consensus document of AcEMC, CISMEL, SIBioC, and SIMeL. *Clinical Chemistry and Laboratory Medicine* **52**: 621–8.

Lippi G, Bonfanti L, Saccenti C, Cervellin G (2014b). Causes of elevated D-dimer in patients admitted to a large urban emergency department. *European Journal of Internal Medicine* **25**: 45–8.

Lippi G, Ippolito L, Tondelli MT, Favaloro EJ (2014c). Interference from heterophilic antibodies in D-dimer assessment. A case report. *Blood Coagulation & Fibrinolysis* **25**: 277–9.

Lippi G, Favaloro EJ, Cervellin G (2014d). A review of the value of D-dimer testing for prediction of recurrent venous thromboembolism with increasing age. *Seminars in Thrombosis and Hemostasis* **40**: 634–9.

Lippi G, Favaloro EJ, Mattiuzzi C (2014e). Combined administration of antibiotics and direct oral anticoagulants: a renewed indication for laboratory monitoring? *Seminars in Thrombosis and Hemostasis* **40**: 756–65.

Lippi G, Ardissino D, Quintavalla R, Cervellin G (2014g). Urgent monitoring of direct oral anticoagulants in patients with atrial fibrillation: a tentative approach based on routine laboratory tests. *Journal of Thrombosis and Thrombolysis* **38**: 269–74.

Lippi G, Danese E, Favaloro EJ, Montagnana M, Franchini M (2015a). Diagnostics in venous thromboembolism: from origin to future prospects. *Seminars in Thrombosis and Hemostasis* **41**: 374–381.

Lippi G, Tripodi A, Simundic AM, Favaloro EJ (2015b). International Survey on D-Dimer Test Reporting: A Call for Standardization. *Seminars in Thrombosis and Hemostasis* **41**: 287–93.

Lippi G, Favaloro EJ (2015c). Recent guidelines and recommendations for laboratory assessment of the direct oral anticoagulants (DOACs): is there consensus? *Clinical Chemistry and Laboratory Medicine* **53**: 185–97.

Montagnana M, Favaloro EJ, Franchini M, Guidi GC, Lippi G (2010). The role of ethnicity, age and gender in venous thromboembolism. *Journal of Thrombosis and Thrombolysis* **29**: 489–96.

Nowak G (2003). The ecarin clotting time, a universal method to quantify direct thrombin inhibitors. *Pathophysiology of Haemostasis and Thrombosis* **33**: 173–83.

Palareti G, Cosmi B, Legnani C, Antonucci E, De Micheli V, Ghirarduzzi A, Poli D, Testa S, Tosetto A, Pengo V, Prandoni P; DULCIS (D-dimer and ULtrasonography in Combination Italian Study) Investigators (2014). D-dimer to guide the duration of anticoagulation in patients with venous thromboembolism: a management study. *Blood* **124**: 196–203.

Palareti G (2015). How D-dimer assay can be useful in deciding the duration of anticoagulation after venous thromboembolism: a review. *Expert Review of Hematology* **8**: 79–88.

Poli D, Palareti G (2013). Assessing recurrence risk following acute venous thromboembolism: use of algorithms. *Current Opinion in Pulmonary Medicine* **19**: 407–12.

Quick AJ (1940). The Thromboplastin Reagent for the Determination of Prothrombin. *Science* **92**: 113–4.

Rodger MA, Kahn SR, Wells PS, Anderson DA, Chagnon I, Le Gal G, Solymoss S, Crowther M, Perrier A, White R, Vickars L, Ramsay T, Betancourt MT, Kovacs MJ (2008). Identifying unprovoked thromboembolism patients at low risk for recurrence who can discontinue anticoagulant therapy. *CMAJ* **179**: 417–26.

Schouten HJ, Geersing GJ, Koek HL, Zuithoff NP, Janssen KJ, Douma RA, van Delden JJ, Moons KG, Reitsma JB (2013). Diagnostic accuracy of conventional or age adjusted D-dimer cut-off values in older patients with suspected venous thromboembolism: systematic review and meta-analysis. *BMJ* **346**: f2492.

Tange JI, Grill D, Koch CD, Ybabez RJ, Krekelberg BJ, Fylling KA, Wiese CR, Baumann NA, Block DR, Karon BS, Chen D, Pruthi RK (2014). Local verification and assignment of mean normal prothrombin time and International Sensitivity Index values across various instruments: recent experience and outcome from North America. *Seminars in Thrombosis and Hemostasis* **40**: 115–20.

Tapson VF (2008). Acute pulmonary embolism. *New England Journal of Medicine* **358**: 1037–52.

Testa S, Paoletti O, Bassi L, Dellanoce C, Morandini R, Lippi G (2015). A global quality control system to check PT-INR portable monitor for Antivitamin K antagonists. *International Journal of Laboratory Hematology* **37**: 71–8.

Tosetto A, Iorio A, Marcucci M, *et al.* (2012). Predicting disease recurrence in patients with previous unprovoked venous thromboembolism: a proposed prediction score (DASH). *Journal of Thrombosis and Haemostasis* **10**: 1019–25.

Wells PS, Anderson DR, Bormanis J, Guy F, Mitchell M, Gray L, Clement C, Robinson KS, Lewandowski B (1997). Value of assessment of pretest probability of deep-vein thrombosis in clinical management. *Lancet* **350**: 1795–8.

Wells PS, Anderson DR, Rodger M, Ginsberg JS, Kearon C, Gent M, Turpie AG, Bormanis J, Weitz J, Chamberlain M, Bowie D, Barnes D, Hirsh J (2000). Derivation of a simple clinical model to categorize patients probability of pulmonary embolism: increasing the models utility with the SimpliRED D-dimer. *Thrombosis and Haemostasis* **83**: 416–20.

Wells PS, Anderson DR, Rodger M, Forgie M, Kearon C, Dreyer J, Kovacs G, Mitchell M, Lewandowski B, Kovacs MJ (2003). Evaluation of D-dimer in the diagnosis of suspected deep-vein thrombosis. *New England Journal of Medicine* **349**: 1227–35.

6

Thrombophilia Testing

Massimo Franchini

Department of Hematology and Transfusion Medicine, C. Poma Hospital, Mantova, Italy

Introduction

Thrombophilia is defined as a hypercoagulable state leading to a thrombotic tendency. In 1856, the German physician Rudolf Virchow conceived the theory of the triad i.e. endothelial injury, stasis of blood flow and hypercoagulability, to explain the aetiology of thrombosis. This concept was prophetic, in that it has now been shown that all three components of the triad play active roles in the development of venous thromboembolism (VTE). Thrombophilic abnormalities can be inherited, acquired, or mixed (both congenital and acquired) and the risk of VTE is different according to each abnormality (Table 6.1).

Inherited thrombophilias include deficiencies of the natural anticoagulant proteins antithrombin, protein C and protein S, as well as gain-of-function mutations in the factor V gene (factor V G1691A Leiden) and prothrombin gene (prothrombin G20210A). Acquired thrombophilia is mainly represented by the presence of antiphospholipid antibodies, while the most frequently investigated mixed abnormality is mild to moderate hyperhomocysteinemia. This chapter will discuss the role of the main thrombophilia markers in the management of VTE.

Inherited Risk Factors

Antithrombin Deficiency

Antithrombin is a single chain glycoprotein synthesised in the liver, belonging to the serine protease inhibitor (serpin) superfamily, which functions as a natural anticoagulant by binding to, and inactivating, thrombin and other serine proteases, such as activated FX. The result of this activity is a reduction in both the generation and the half-life of thrombin. In addition to the active site responsible for coagulation factor inactivation, the antithrombin molecule contains a heparin-binding site. When exogenous heparin or endogenous heparan sulphate binds to this site, the ability of antithrombin to inactivate the abovementioned activated factors is greatly enhanced. As expected, any type of mutation that leads to a reduction of plasma antithrombin levels, or to a decreased ability of antithrombin to interact with either activated coagulation factors or heparin, will result in an increased risk of thrombosis.

Antithrombin deficiency is mainly inherited as an autosomal dominant trait, and more than 250 gene variations have been identified so far, including missense and nonsense point mutations, insertions and deletions. Antithrombin deficiency is probably the most severe of the inherited thrombophilias, causing more than a 50 fold increased risk for VTE, compared with that of individuals not carrying this defect (Table 6.2). Its penetrance is very high, since most affected family members experience a thrombotic event by the age of 45.

Handbook of Venous Thromboembolism, First Edition. Edited by Jecko Thachil and Catherine Bagot.
© 2018 John Wiley & Sons Ltd. Published 2018 by John Wiley & Sons Ltd.

Table 6.1 Inherited, acquired and mixed coagulation-related risk factors for thrombosis.

Inherited	Acquired	Mixed
Antithrombin deficiency	Antiphospholipid antibodies	Hyperhomocysteinemia
Protein C deficiency		Increased levels of coagulation factors (fibrinogen, factor VIII, factor IX, factor XI)
Protein S deficiency		
Factor V Leiden		
Prothrombin G20210A		

Table 6.2 Prevalence of thrombophilia abnormalities and relative risk of thrombosis.

	Prevalence (%)		Relative risk	
Thrombophilia abnormality	General population	Patients with VTE	First VTE	Recurrent VTE
Antithrombin deficiency	0.02–0.17	1.1	50	2.5
Protein C deficiency	0.2–0.4	3.2	15	2.5
Protein S deficiency	0.03–0.1	2.2	6–10	2.5
Factor V Leiden heterozygous	5	20–50	7	1.4
Factor V Leiden homozygous	0.02	1.5	80	N/A
Prothrombin G20210A heterozygous	2	6	3–4	1.4
Prothrombin G20210A homozygous	0.02	<1	40–80	N/A
Factor V Leiden + prothrombin G20210A	0.01	2.2	20–60	2–5
Antiphospholipid antibodies	1–2	5–15	1–10	2–6
Hyperhomocysteinemia	5	10–15	1.5	0.9–2.7

VTE – venous thromboembolism; N/A – Data not available.

Two types of antithrombin deficiency can be distinguished. In type I, antithrombin activity and antigen level are both reduced in plasma, owing to a lack of protein production or secretion by the mutant allele. In type II, low antithrombin activity contrasts with normal antigen levels, indicating functional defects in the molecule. The only individuals homozygous for antithrombin deficiency described to date carry heparin-binding site defects, suggesting that the other subtypes are associated with embryonic lethality.

Protein C Deficiency

Protein C is a vitamin K-dependent glycoprotein synthesised in the liver in an inactive form. Under physiological conditions, once activated by the thrombin-thrombomodulin complex, protein C acts as an anticoagulant by means of the proteolytic degradation of activated coagulant factors Va and VIIIa. As for other physiological inhibitors of coagulation, any mutation leading to a reduction of protein C activity increases the risk of VTE.

Inherited protein C deficiency is transmitted as an autosomal dominant trait, and more than 200 loss-of-function gene mutations have been reported to date. Heterozygous individuals, who have an approximately 15 fold increased risk for thrombosis compared to the general population (Table 6.2), often experience recurrent episodes of VTE before the age of 45. Homozygous individuals have a more severe clinical picture, not infrequently leading to neonatal purpura fulminans, a potentially fatal condition characterised by multiple thromboses in small vessels leading to skin necrosis.

Similar to antithrombin deficiency, protein C deficiency can be divided in two subtypes. Type I, which is the most common, is characterised by a parallel reduction in plasma antigen level and activity, reflecting a reduced synthesis of the functional protein. The less common type II is characterised by a normal antigen level with reduced functional activity, reflecting normal synthesis of a dysfunctional protein.

Protein S Deficiency

Protein S is a vitamin K-dependent protein synthesised in the liver, which circulates in plasma in both a free, functionally active, form (approximately 40%) and an inactive form bound to the acute phase C4b-binding protein (approximately 60%). Protein S functions as a cofactor of activated protein C (APC), which is responsible for the degradation of activated factors Va and VIIIa. In addition, protein S acts as a cofactor of tissue factor pathway inhibitor (TFPI), which inhibits factor Xa.

Inherited as an autosomal dominant trait (to date more than 130 loss-of-function mutations have been identified), familial protein S deficiency has a clinical presentation very similar to that observed for protein C deficiency. Thus, heterozygotes experience early recurrent VTE episodes and sometimes warfarin-induced skin necrosis, while rare homozygotes exhibit a very severe clinical picture with neonatal purpura fulminans. The penetrance of the disease is also similar to that of protein C deficiency, causing a nearly ten-fold increased VTE risk in affected individuals compared with the normal population (Table 6.2). Three types of protein S defects have been described: type I (low total and free antigen levels, reduced activity); type II (normal total and free antigen levels, reduced activity); and type III (normal total antigen level, reduced free antigen level and activity).

Factor V Leiden

In 1993, a poor anticoagulant response to APC was noted to be associated with an increased risk of VTE. The following year, a missense mutation (Arg506Gln) in the *F5* gene was first described in the city of Leiden, and was found to be responsible for the majority of cases of APC resistance. Factor V Leiden is inactivated by APC more slowly than wild type FVa, thus promoting a hypercoagulable state and an increased susceptibility to VTE. The FV Leiden gain-of-function mutation has a dominant autosomal transmission and, in its heterozygous form, is the most common prothrombotic gene mutation in the Caucasian population, with a prevalence of around 5%. The risk of VTE is increased approximately seven-fold in heterozygous carriers, and 80 fold in homozygous carriers, compared with non-carriers (Table 6.2).

Prothrombin G20210A

A heterozygous guanine to adenine nucleotide substitution at position 20210 in the 3'-untranslated region of the prothrombin gene causes increased basal plasma levels of functionally normal prothrombin. Similar to factor V Leiden, the prothrombin G20210A mutation has an autosomal dominant transmission, and is the second most common coagulation abnormality, with a prevalence of heterozygotes in the Caucasian population of approximately 2%, increasing to 6% in patients with VTE. Heterozygosity for the prothrombin G20210A mutation confers an approximately three- to four-fold increased risk of developing VTE. Thus, these individuals exhibit a relatively low thrombotic risk, and most will not develop a thrombotic episode by age 45–50 years. In contrast, homozygosity for the prothrombin gene mutation is much rarer, and causes a higher thrombotic risk (Table 6.2).

Acquired Risk Factors

Antiphospholipid Antibodies

Antiphospholipid antibodies represent one of the most important acquired risk factors for thrombosis. The corresponding syndrome is characterised by the presence of circulating antiphospholipid antibodies in plasma and either arterial and/or venous thrombosis, or pregnancy complications – particularly foetal loss.

The clinically relevant antiphospholipid antibodies include lupus anticoagulant, anticardiolipin and anti-β_2-glycoprotein I antibodies. These autoantibodies are directed against a wide variety of protein co-factors localised upon phospholipid membrane surfaces, including β_2-glycoprotein I, prothrombin, protein C, protein S, annexin V and coagulation factor XII. The resulting complexes interact with several cell types, including endothelial cells, monocytes and platelets, all of which play important roles in haemostasis and thrombosis. Antiphospholipid antibodies can be idiopathic, drug-related or associated with autoimmune disease (e.g. systemic lupus erythematosus, rheumatoid arthritis, lymphoproliferative or inflammatory diseases).

Mixed Risk Factors

Hyperhomocysteinemia

The amino acid homocysteine is formed from the demethylation of dietary methionine, and its plasma levels are controlled by two metabolic pathways. The first involves the enzyme cystathionine β-synthase (CBS) and requires vitamin B_6, while the second involves the enzyme methionine synthase and requires both vitamin B_{12} and N^5-methyltetrahydrofolate reductase (MTHFR). Both genetic (e.g. mutations in *MTHFR* and *CBS* genes) and acquired factors (e.g. deficiencies of folate, vitamin B12 or vitamin B6, advanced age, chronic renal failure and the use of anti-folate drugs) interact to determine plasma homocysteine concentrations. As a consequence, hyperhomocysteinemia is considered a mixed thrombophilia (i.e. genetic and/or acquired) that affects thrombosis risk.

Moderately increased plasma levels of homocysteine have been associated with a modest (1.5 fold) increased thrombotic risk and approximately five percent of the general population has higher than normal levels of homocysteine, while the prevalence of modest hyperhomocysteinemia among VTE patients is approximately 10–15% (Table 6.2).

High Levels of Coagulation Factors

An association between elevated levels of FVIII and an increased risk of VTE has been demonstrated in several studies. A similar association has also been shown with increased levels of factors IX and XI, and fibrinogen. The plasma levels of these factors are influenced by age and inflammation, and are also under genetic control. However, although a heritable component has been described to account for elevated levels of these clotting factors, no discrete genetic variations have been identified to date. Hence, few laboratories include measurement of these factors in the thrombophilia test panel.

Indications for Thrombophilia Testing

Table 6.1 reports the main thrombophilia abnormalities that should be investigated in individuals with suspected thrombophilia. However, a major issue is deciding when testing for thrombophilia is appropriate. It is, nowadays, well established that VTE is a multifactorial event, being the result of multiple gene-gene and/or gene-environment interactions. In keeping with this model, inherited thrombophilia does interact with several other well-established acquired predisposing factors for VTE, such as malignancy, inflammatory states, antiphospholipid antibodies, surgery, trauma, immobility, pregnancy/puerperium and the use of oral contraceptives or hormone replacement therapy. Moreover, age plays a key role in modulating thrombotic risk.

Overall, this model provides a dynamic concept of thromboembolic risk, encompassing a genetic predisposition (one or more co-inherited thrombophilic abnormalities) plus a variable contribution of environmental factors (potentially modifiable or preventable) during different stages of life. Therefore, thrombophilia markers cannot be interpreted in isolation, because interactions with other genetic and acquired risk factors are

Table 6.3 Current indications for which thrombophilia testing can be considered.

Clinical condition
Idiopathic thrombosis and/or age < 50 years at the time of first venous thrombosis
Unusual sites of venous thrombosis (hepatic, mesenteric, splenic, portal, cerebral)
History of recurrent venous thrombosis
Asymptomatic relatives of patients with severe thrombophilia
Venous thrombosis during pregnancy or in women taking oral contraceptives or under hormone replacement therapy

important determinants of the overall risk of VTE. It therefore appears evident that an indiscriminate search for thrombophilia carriers is of little use, and that a targeted screening strategy is potentially more useful. Thus, screening for thrombophilia should be performed only in selected conditions – namely, when it is expected to influence the management of affected individuals.

The current indications, reported in Table 6.3, include: unprovoked thrombosis and/or thrombosis at an age less than 50 years; VTE at unusual sites (such as hepatic, mesenteric and cerebral veins), recurrent VTE, asymptomatic relatives of patients with severe thrombophilia (i.e. natural anticoagulant deficiencies, homozygous defects and multiple abnormalities); and VTE during pregnancy or in women taking oral contraceptives or hormone replacement therapy. Notably, testing for thrombophilia in patients during the acute phase of a thromboembolic episode or whilst taking anticoagulation is usually uninformative, as there is frequently interference with functional laboratory assays.

In spite of these indications, there is no universal agreement on the clinical utility of thrombophilia screening in certain high-risk conditions. For instance, whether the presence of thrombophilia is able to predict VTE recurrence is still a matter of debate, with conflicting results, in various studies, that have compared the prevalence of thrombophilia in patients with recurrent VTE with that in patients without recurrence. Meta-analyses of prospective studies have revealed only a modest increased risk (approximately 1.5 fold) of VTE recurrence for mild thrombophilias such as heterozygous factor V Leiden or prothrombin G20210A mutation. A higher risk (approximately 2.5 fold) has been observed, however, in patients with severe thrombophilia, although the data available are limited, because of the rarity of these inherited disorders.

Another potential advantage of testing patients with VTE for thrombophilia could be the screening of asymptomatic relatives of patients with inherited thrombophilia. The rationale for this approach is the possibility of identifying those individuals carrying a thrombophilic trait who may benefit from targeted thromboprophylaxis in high-risk situations (pregnancy, puerperium, surgery, immobilisation and trauma).

A number of prospective and retrospective studies have specifically investigated the VTE risk among relatives of individuals with inherited thrombophilia. Collectively, these studies have reported that the VTE incidence among relatives is higher in carriers of antithrombin, protein C or protein S deficiency (with a range of 0.36–4.0% per individual-year) than in carriers of FV Leiden (0.19–0.58% per individual-year) and prothrombin G20210A (0.11–0.37% per individual-year). Considering these data globally, while screening asymptomatic relatives of patients with severe thrombophilia may be warranted, more uncertainty exists regarding the usefulness of familial screening among the relatives of probands with mild thrombophilia.

As regards the gender-related risk factors for VTE, universal screening for thrombophilia before exposure to environmental risks, such as oral contraceptives or pregnancy, has been demonstrated not to be cost-effective, but it can be considered in well-selected cases. For instance, the use of third-generation combined oral contraceptives is associated with a two-fold increased risk of VTE, and a supra-additive effect is observed (up to five-fold) when an inherited thrombophilic risk factor is also present.

However, although the increased risk of VTE in women with thrombophilia taking combined oral contraceptives suggests that there may be utility in screening women prior to prescribing oestrogen-progestogen therapy, the relatively low incidence (1–6 events per 1000 women-years) of VTE among unselected carriers indicates that such screening has a limited role. By contrast, testing for inherited thrombophilia before the prescription of oral contraceptives may be beneficial for women who are relatives of symptomatic carriers of severe thrombophilia because, in this category, the absolute incidence of VTE is much higher (4–10 events per 100 women-years).

The absolute incidence of VTE among post-menopausal women on hormone replacement therapy is higher than among oral contraceptive users, due to their older age. Accordingly, unrestricted or family-driven screening before prescribing hormone replacement therapy has been proposed by a number of investigators, because this medication is associated with a relatively high VTE risk in thrombophilic carriers. Finally, pregnant women with an asymptomatic inherited thrombophilia are considered at high VTE risk if they have a severe thrombophilia, and are thus eligible for prophylaxis with low molecular weight heparin (LMWH) during the antenatal period and for six weeks post-partum. The same LMWH prophylaxis is also recommended in pregnant women with mild thrombophilia, but only in the presence of multiple risk factors, such as family history of VTE, immobility, obesity, age over 35 years, or gross varicose veins.

Key Points

- Thrombophilia is defined as a hypercoagulable state leading to a thrombotic tendency.
- Thrombophilic abnormalities can be inherited, acquired or mixed (both congenital and acquired).
- Thrombophilic abnormalities cause blood hypercoagulability through the impairment of an anticoagulant or the potentiation of procoagulant pathways.
- Both inherited and acquired risk factors should be taken into account when assessing an individual's risk of thrombosis.
- Universal screening for inherited thrombophilia is unjustified.
- Screening asymptomatic relatives of carriers of severe thrombophilia should be considered.

Further Reading

Baglin T, Gray E, Greaves M *et al.* (2010). British Committee for Standards in Haematology. Clinical guidelines for testing for heritable thrombophilia. *British Journal of Haematology* **149**(2): 209–220.

Bertina RM, Koeleman BP, Koster T *et al.* (1994). Mutation in blood coagulation factor V associated with resistance to activated protein C. *Nature* **369**(6475): 64–67.

Brouwer JL, Veeger NJ, Kluin-Nelemans HC, van der Meer J (2006). The pathogenesis of venous thromboembolism: evidence for multiple interrelated causes. *Annals of Internal Medicine* **145**(1): 807–815.

Franchini M, Veneri D, Salvagno GL, Manzato F, Lippi G (2006). Inherited thrombophilia. *Critical Reviews in Clinical Laboratory Sciences* **43**(3): 249–290.

Franco RF, Reitsma PH (2001). Genetic risk factors of venous thrombosis. *Human Genetics* **109**(4): 369–384.

Kyrle PA, Rosendaal FR, Eichinger S (2010). Risk assessment for recurrent venous thrombosis. *Lancet* **376**(9757): 2032–2039.

Lussana F, Dentali F, Abbate R, *et al.* (2009). Italian Society for Haemostasis and Thrombosis. Screening for thrombophilia and antithrombotic prophylaxis in pregnancy: guidelines of the Italian Society for Haemostasis and Thrombosis (SISET). *Thrombosis Research* **124**(5): e19–e25.

Martinelli I, De Stefano V, Mannucci PM (2014). Inherited risk factors for venous thromboembolism. *Nature Reviews Cardiology* **11**(3): 140–156.

Miyakis S, Lockshin MD, Atsumi T, *et al.* (2006). International consensus statement on an update of the classification criteria for definite antiphospholipid syndrome (APS). *Journal of Thrombosis and Haemostasis* **4**(2): 295–306.

Simioni P (1999). The molecular genetics of familial venous thrombosis. *Baillière's Clinical Haematology* **12**(3): 479–503.

7

Radiological Diagnosis of Pulmonary Embolism

Joachim E. Wildberger and Marco Das

Department of Radiology and Nuclear Medicine, Maastricht University Medical Center (MUMC+), Maastricht, The Netherlands

Introduction

Pulmonary embolism (PE) is often referred to as the great masquerader, and remains a diagnostic challenge in daily practice due to its mostly unspecific clinical presentation. Diagnostic algorithms are needed to assist clinical assessment and optimise the use of investigations, especially under emergency conditions. A comprehensive survey on the evolution on imaging techniques for the assessment of venous thromboembolism has been published recently (Goodman, 2013).

Ventilation-perfusion Scanning (V/Q Scintigraphy)

Nuclear medicine V/Q scintigraphy has long been the imaging mainstay for the diagnosis of PE. This traditional imaging technique, using radioactive isotopes, is non-invasive and relatively inexpensive. It has a high sensitivity, which is why it remains a primary PE screening technique. However, the high sensitivity of perfusion scanning is associated with a moderate specificity, as it provides only indirect evidence for PE ('probability assessment'). Venous thromboembolism is not directly visualised but, rather, its effects on perfusion and ventilation. This necessitates the need for probability criteria, categorised as high, intermediate, low or very low probability, and normal. In daily practice, logistical considerations also have to be taken into account, including limited availability in many hospitals (especially state-of-the-art systems, such as V/Q scanning in SPECT technique) and 24-hour accessibility. However, V/Q scintigraphy remains the first imaging modality for patients with contraindications for iodinated contrast media, such as previous contrast-associated anaphylaxis and renal failure, as well as in pregnant patients.

Spiral Computed Tomography Pulmonary Angiography (CTPA)

Spiral computed tomography pulmonary angiography (CTPA) emerged in the 1990s as a new diagnostic technique. The basis of PE assessment on CTPA is the direct visualisation of clot material in the pulmonary arteries and frequent secondary findings, such as wedge-shaped opacities within the adjacent lung parenchyma. The first CTPA protocols allowed for visualisation of the central (and segmental) pulmonary arteries (based on 5 mm thick sections). However, it is now known that 5 mm thick sections lack precision when assessing for PE, and thin collimation data acquisition is mandatory if peripheral PE is to be confidently excluded.

Table 7.1 Recommendations for the use of CTPA for suspected PE.

Compared with V/Q scanning, CTPA:

a) is quicker to perform

b) rarely needs to be followed by other imaging

c) may provide the correct diagnosis when PE has been excluded

d) is now available in most hospitals

e) is easier to arrange urgently out of hours

(adapted and modified from British Thoracic Society (2003)).

The introduction of multi-slice spiral CT (MSCT) was a milestone in CTPA technology (Lell *et al.*, 2015). Using thin sections (≤1 mm) significantly decreases the number of arteries classified as indeterminate, and improves inter-observer agreement in detection of PE. Thin collimation CTPA of the entire chest can now be done within a single breath-hold, even in critically ill patients.

In daily clinical practice, standard MSCT with thin collimation is recommended as the method of choice for imaging of the pulmonary circulation in patients suspected of having non-massive PE (Remy-Jardin *et al.*, 2007). Furthermore, based on the guidelines of the British Thoracic Society from as early as 2003, no further examination or treatment is needed for patients with a high-quality negative MSCT PA (British Thoracic Society, 2003). Moreover, ancillary findings suggesting alternate diagnoses are clinically extremely beneficial, and all MSCT platforms are technically sufficient to detect most pathologies, in addition to PE, if used appropriately (see Table 7.1).

The Issue of Subsegmental PE

There is a recent trend to analyse the overall clinical accuracy of diagnostic tests, and the clinical outcome of patients with negative PE diagnoses has been highlighted in numerous studies. The risk of PE after an initial negative CTPA is approximately 1%, at a minimum follow-up of three months, allowing patients with a negative CTPA to be safely discharged. Conversely, the incidence of pulmonary embolism is increasing, with a lower severity of illness and lower mortality, suggesting that the increase may be due to more frequent diagnoses of minor thrombotic events, resulting from the greater sensitivity of current CTPA techniques (DeMonaco *et al.*, 2008).

In particular, the management of isolated sub-segmental PE remains a matter of controversy. On the one hand, small emboli may indicate a risk for recurrent, more significant emboli, with patients with underlying cardiorespiratory disease possibly at risk of respiratory compromise from these more minor events. On the other hand, otherwise healthy patients with isolated sub-segmental PE may not be at any increased risk of significant morbidity and mortality. The combination of a large increase in incidence and reduced case fatality may be resulting in inappropriate overdiagnosis, as stated in the 'too much medicine' campaign (Wiener *et al.*, 2013).

The clinical impact of these findings is part of an ongoing debate, especially in patients where small emboli are detected following CT scans undertaken for different reasons, such as in cancer patients. Therefore, additional functional information is desirable. Quantitative CT scores for PE, such as the Qanadli and Mastora score, are based on the overall amount of clot burden within the pulmonary vasculature and were adapted from angiographic indices. However, they are rarely applied routinely.

Haemodynamic Assessment of Patients with PE

The diameter of the central pulmonary artery and the right ventricle : left ventricle ratio are straightforward methods to assess the hemodynamic severity of PE. CT can identify characteristic cardiac changes, including acute dilatation of the right heart and interventricular septal shift, the latter resulting from reversal of the

Figure 7.1 Flowchart in patients with suspected PE, classified as high-risk patients (modified from Konstantinides *et al.*, 2014). CTPA – computed tomography pulmonary angiography; RV – right ventricle; PE – pulmonary embolism.

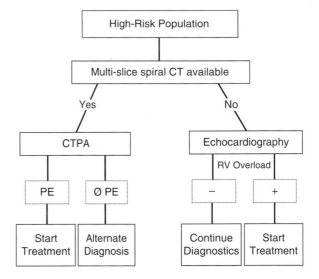

transseptal pressure gradient and convex bulging of the septum towards the left ventricle. In particular, the right ventricle : left ventricle ratio (as measured by the diameter at the mid-myocardial level in the right and left ventricle) is an easy assessable secondary sign for the severity of PE in everyday practice, with a right ventricle : left ventricle ratio greater than 1 being a well defined functional parameter for a haemodynamically relevant PE.

Depiction of cardiac and pulmonary function, in combination with the quantification of pulmonary obstruction, helps to grade the severity of PE for further risk stratification, and to monitor the effect of thrombolytic therapy. Assessment of haemodynamic stability of the patient and clinical probability of pulmonary embolism (PE) is the basis of all diagnostic strategies (Konstantinides, 2014).

CTPA is an appropriate initial test in patients with high-clinical suspicion of PE under emergency conditions, such as in patients with shock or hypotension (Figure 7.1). Although logistical and clinical aspects have to be considered, if a CTPA scan can be performed under these conditions, a fast assessment of the pulmonary situation, including a right heart assessment, is possible. If appropriate, treatment can then be started immediately thereafter.

Latest Trends

New technologies consider the iodine distribution in the adjacent lung parenchyma at the time of data acquisition. This is not a true perfusion method, as this information is obtained in a single phase by so-called dual energy information. It could be considered as a relevant add-on on dedicated scanner platforms.

Another option is to include the assessment of PE into so-called 'triple rule-out' protocols for assessment of non-traumatic acute chest pain. The exclusion of coronary artery disease is most demanding in this respect, and these protocols should be applied primarily for this purpose. PE can also easily be excluded by these protocols. However, it should be kept in mind that a thorough clinical evaluation is mandatory, given the low prevalence (<1%) of PE and aortic dissection in the studies published so far (Konstantinides *et al.*, 2014).

Cost-effectiveness

In patients with a low/intermediate clinical probability of PE, the most cost-saving strategy involves assessment of plasma D-dimer, a degradation product of cross-linked fibrin. However, the specificity of fibrin for venous thromboembolism is poor. Fibrin is produced in a wide variety of conditions, such as cancer, inflammation,

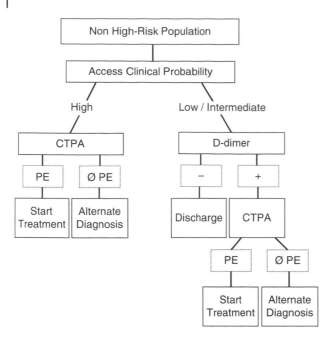

Figure 7.2 Flowchart in patients with suspected PE, classified as non-high-risk patients (modified from Konstantinides *et al.*, 2014). CTPA – computed tomography pulmonary angiography; PE – pulmonary embolism.

infection and necrosis. Additionally, it is not useful in elderly or hospital inpatients, as it is normal in less than 10% of these patient groups.

However, appropriate use of D-dimer testing may reduce the need for unnecessary imaging and irradiation (Konstantinides, 2014), and should therefore be included in the pathway for patients with clinically suspected PE who are not at high-risk (Figure 7.2). Patients clinically classified as low or intermediate risk with a negative D-dimer test may be discharged safely, without further imaging. With a positive D-dimer test, a CTPA is indicated.

Summary

In conclusion, a thorough clinical assessment, in combination with dedicated diagnostic work-up, is required to accurately assess patients presenting with a possible PE. CTPA has become the gold standard for the radiological assessment of a clinically suspected PE in daily practice. Special attention should be given to the clinical impact of incidental and subsegmental emboli.

Key Points

1) CTPA using MSCT is the method of choice, even in critically ill patients.
2) No further examination or treatment is needed for patients with a high-quality negative MSCT PA.
3) Thin sections (≤1 mm) should be used for the detection of PE.
4) Right ventricle : left ventricle ratio greater than 1 represents a well-defined functional parameter for a haemodynamically relevant PE.
5) Dual energy perfusion maps, or integration into triple rule out protocols, are new trends in PE imaging.
6) There is an ongoing debate about the clinical significance of subsegemental emboli.

References

British Thoracic Society Standards of Care Committee Pulmonary Embolism Guideline Development Group (2003). British Thoracic Society guidelines for the management of suspected acute pulmonary embolism. *Thorax* **58**: 470–484.

DeMonaco NA, Dang Q, Kapoor WN, Ragni MV (2008). Pulmonary Embolism incidence is increasing with use of Spiral computed tomography. *The American Journal of Medicine* **121**:611–617.

Goodman LG (2013). In search of venous thromboembolism: The first 2913 years. *American Journal of Roentgenology* **201**:W576–W581

Konstantinides SV (2014). 2014 ESC Guidelines on the diagnosis and management of acute pulmonary embolism. *European Heart Journal* **35**: 3145–3146.

Konstantinides SV, Torbicki A, Agnelli G, Danchin N, Fitzmaurice D, Galiè N, Gibbs JS, Huisman MV, Humbert M, Kucher N, Lang I, Lankeit M, Lekakis J, Maack C, Mayer E, Meneveau N, Perrier A, Pruszczyk P, Rasmussen LH, Schindler TH, Svitil P, Vonk Noordegraaf A, Zamorano JL, Zompatori M; Task Force for the Diagnosis and Management of Acute Pulmonary Embolism of the European Society of Cardiology (ESC) (2014). ESC guidelines on the diagnosis and management of acute pulmonary embolism. *European Heart Journal* **35**: 3033–3080.

Lell MM, Wildberger JE, Alkadhi H, Damilakis J, Kachelriess M (2015). Evolution in computed tomography: The battle for speed and dose. *Investigative Radiology* **50**: 629–644.

Remy-Jardin M, Pistolesi M, Goodman LR, Gefter WB, Gottschalk A, Mayo JR, Sostman HD (2007). Management of suspected acute pulmonary embolism in the era of CT angiography: A statement from the Fleischner Society. *Radiology* **245**: 315–329.

Wiener RS, Schwartz LM, Woloshin S (2013). When a test is too good: how CT pulmonary angiograms find pulmonary emboli that do not need to be found. *BMJ* **347**: f3368.

8

The Antiphospholipid Syndrome

Karen Breen

Dept of Thrombosis, St. Thomas' Hospital, London

The association of antiphospholipid antibodies (aPL) with a variety of clinical features characterised by venous and arterial thrombosis and pregnancy-related morbidity is known as the antiphospholipid syndrome (APS). APS often occurs in patients with other associated autoimmune diseases, particularly systemic lupus erythematosus (previously known as secondary APS), but it can also occur in patients without other associated autoimmune disease (previously known as primary APS).

Specific clinical criteria for diagnosis of APS were originally outlined in the Sapporo criteria (Wilson *et al.*, 1999) and recently updated as the Sydney criteria (see Table 8.1; Miyakis *et al.*, 2006).

Antiphospholipid Antibodies: Epidemiology and Antigenic Specificities

The prevalence of aPL in normal healthy populations have been reported to range between 1.0 and 5.6% (Shi *et al.*, 1990; de Groot *et al.*, 2005) and may increase with age (Richaud-Patin *et al.*, 2000). APL have been reported to be present in up to 14% of patients presenting with either venous or arterial thrombosis (de Groot *et al.*, 2005; Lim *et al.*, 2006; Erkan and Lockshin, 2004) and a prevalence of 20% in patients presenting with recurrent pregnancy losses (Rai *et al.*, 1995; Out *et al.*, 1991). Female-to-male ratios of patients with APS ranging from 2 : 1 to 5 : 1 have also been observed (Jara *et al.*, 2005). The actual prevalence of primary APS in the general population is unknown and, although it is not inherited, familial clustering has been recognised (Hellan *et al.*, 1998), in addition to presence of HLA linkages, namely HLA-DR4, DR7, DR53 and DRB-1 (Wilson and Gharavi, 1996; Sebastiani *et al.*, 1996), suggesting there may be a genetic predisposition.

Transient aPL can occur in association with bacterial, viral, and parasitic infections, such as TB, hepatitis B and C, HIV, syphilis, leptospirosis, malaria and leishmaniasis (Santiago *et al.*, 2001). These antibodies recognise phospholipid directly, do not appear to be associated with the clinical manifestations of APS, and are usually transient. The inclusion of the need for persistent presence of aPL on two occasions greater than 12 weeks apart in the Sydney criteria (Miyakis *et al.*, 2006), therefore, aims to exclude patients with transient aPL. aPL can also occur in association with medications such as antibiotics, hydralazine, quinine and procainamide, and in patients with tissue damage secondary to myocardial infarction or stroke.

Population studies have shown that the presence of the lupus anticoagulant is associated with a high risk of thrombosis (Galli *et al.*, 2003) and recurrent miscarriage (Opatrny *et al.*, 2006). The association of anticardiolipin antibodies with a first thrombotic event is not consistent (Galli *et al.*, 2003), but high titres of anticardiolipin antibodies are associated with a risk of venous and arterial thrombosis (Ginsburg *et al.*, 1992) and

Table 8.1 Criteria for diagnosis of APS (Miyakis *et al.*, 2006).

Clinical criteria	Definition
Vascular thrombosis	One or more episodes of vascular thrombosis (arterial, venous, or small vessel thrombosis) in any tissue or organ. Thrombosis must be confirmed by objective validated criteria (i.e. unequivocal findings of appropriate imaging studies or histopathology). For histopathologic confirmation, thrombosis should be present without significant evidence of inflammation in the vessel wall.

Pregnancy morbidity	One or more unexplained deaths of a morphologically normal foetus at or beyond the 10th week of gestation, with normal foetal morphology documented by ultrasound or by:
	
	a) direct examination of the foetus; or
	b) one or more premature births of a morphologically normal neonate before the 34th week of gestation because of:
	  i) eclampsia or severe preeclampsia defined according to standard definitions, or
	  ii) recognised features of placental insufficiency; or
	c) three or more unexplained consecutive spontaneous abortions before the 10th week of gestation, with maternal anatomic or hormonal abnormalities and paternal and maternal chromosomal causes excluded.

Laboratory criteria	1) Lupus anticoagulant (LA) in plasma, on two or more occasions at least 12 weeks apart, detected according to the guidelines of the International Society on Thrombosis and Haemostasis (Scientific Subcommittee on LAs/phospholipid-dependent antibodies); or 2) Anticardiolipin (aCL) antibody of IgG and/or IgM isotype in serum or plasma, present in medium or high titre (i.e. > 40 GPL or MPL, or > the 99th percentile), on two or more occasions, at least 12 weeks apart, measured by a standardised ELISA (Tincani *et al.*, 2001); or 3) Anti-β2 glycoprotein-I antibody (anti- β2 GPI) of IgG and/or IgM isotype in serum or plasma (in titre > the 99th percentile), present on two or more occasions, at least 12 weeks apart, measured by a standardised ELISA (Reber *et al.*, 2004).

recurrent miscarriage (Opatrny *et al.*, 2006), although a higher risk is associated with presence of lupus anticoagulant (Opatrny *et al.*, 2006).

Reported associated risks for thrombosis with the presence of anti-β2 GPI antibodies vary (de Groot *et al.*, 2005; Petri, 2010; Meroni *et al.*, 2007; Urbanus and de Groot, 2011). Double positivity for lupus anticoagulant and anticardiolipin antibodies (Forastiero *et al.*, 2005) or anti β2-glycoprotein-I (Galli *et al.*, 2007), as opposed to single aPL positivity, has an associated higher risk of thrombosis (Forastiero *et al.*, 2005), and the highest associated risk of aPL associated complications is associated with triple aPL positivity (Pengo *et al.*, 2005). Patients with triple aPL positivity have a high risk of recurrent thromboembolic events (Pengo *et al.*, 2010).

The best predictor of future risk of thrombosis or obstetric outcome is the previous history (Lima *et al.*, 1996) – that is, a history of previous arterial thrombosis was predictive of recurrent arterial events and previous venous thrombosis was predictive of recurrent venous events (Neville *et al.*, 2009).

Antiphospholipid antibodies (aPL) recognise a variety of phospholipid-binding plasma proteins, such as β2-glycoprotein-1 (β2-GPI), prothrombin, annexin A5, and phospholipids expressed on platelets, monocytes and trophoblast cells (Rand, 2002). Other antigenic targets include factor V, protein C, and protein S (de Groot *et al.*, 1996). Some antiphospholipid antibodies directly recognise phospholipids such as cardiolipin and phosphatidylserine. β2-GPI and prothrombin are the main antigenic targets in APS, with β2-GPI, a complement control protein, thought to be the most important antigenic target.

Detection of antiphospholipid antibodies are based on laboratory assays. Lupus anticoagulant testing is based on coagulation assays, and involves an initial detection stage, followed by a confirmation stage (Brandt *et al.*, 1995; Pengo *et al.*, 2009). In the initial detection phase, aPL compete with coagulation factors for the negatively charged phospholipid surface, resulting in prolongation of a phospholipid dependent coagulation test. In the confirmation stage, addition of negatively charged phospholipid removes the antibody and, thus, there is shortening of the coagulation time. The assay is qualitative, and does not give any information on the antigen involved. Treatment with heparin, Vitamin K antagonists and direct oral anti-coagulants interferes with detection of lupus anticoagulants.

Guidelines for detection of lupus anticoagulant have recently been updated (Pengo *et al.*, 2009), and advocate testing only patients who have a significant probability of having APS, or who have an otherwise unexplained prolonged aPTT.

Anticardiolipin antibodies and anti B2GP-1 antibodies are detected by solid phase immunoassay (standardised ELISA). Anticardiolipin antibodies should be of IgG and/or IgM isotype in serum or plasma, present in medium or high titre (i.e. > 40 GPL or MPL, or > the 99th percentile) (Miyakis *et al.*, 2006). Anti-β2 glycoprotein-I antibody should be of IgG and/or IgM isotype in serum or plasma (in titre > the 99th percentile) (Miyakis *et al.*, 2006). While there have been several attempts to standardise these assays, significant inter-laboratory variation in test results from different manufacturers still exists (Kutteh and Franklin, 2004; Audrain *et al.*, 2004).

Thrombosis

Vascular thrombosis is defined in the Sydney classification criteria as one or more clinical episodes of arterial, venous, or small vessel thrombosis, in any tissue or organ (Miyakis *et al.*, 2006). Thrombosis is the most common aPL-associated complication (Cervera *et al.*, 2002), and any vessel can be affected by thrombosis in APS. Sydney criteria suggest females under 65 years or males under 55 years presenting with unprovoked thrombosis should be screened for aPL (Miyakis *et al.*, 2006), and recent guidance from the National Institute for Clinical Excellence (NICE) recommends screening patients with unprovoked VTE for aPL (Chong *et al.*, 2012). Deep vein thrombosis is the most commonly observed thrombotic complication of APS, followed by cerebrovascular disease (Cervera *et al.*, 2002), manifested mainly as typical presentations of stroke or transient ischaemic attacks (TIA). Thrombotic myocardial infarction also occurs in association with aPL, and coronary vessels in these patients are typically unaffected by atherosclerosis (Cervera *et al.*, 2002).

Renal thrombotic complications include renal arterial thrombosis, thrombotic microangiopathy and renal vein thrombosis (Tektonidou *et al.*, 2004). Patients may present with peripheral arterial occlusions, mesenteric ischaemia, thrombosis of retinal artery or vein, and bone necrosis due to thrombosis of the supplying arteries or microvasculature.

Less than 1% of patients with APS may present with catastrophic APS (CAPS), which is the rapid development of thrombosis in the small vessels, resulting in multi-organ failure.

Management of APS

The main goals of treatment are prevention of further thrombosis and pregnancy related complications.

The current recommendations for treatment is for lifelong anticoagulation, with a therapeutic target INR of 2–3 (Keeling *et al.*, 2012). Patients with anticardiolipin antibodies have been shown to have a higher incidence of recurrent events after cessation of anticoagulation six months from an acute event, compared with those who were negative for ACA (Schulman *et al.*, 1998). Similarly, patients with LA had an increased risk of recurrence if they discontinued warfarin at three months (Kearon *et al.*, 1999). For patients who had a transient reversible risk factor, such as surgery or immobilisation, optimal duration of anticoagulation is unknown.

The intensity of anticoagulation has also been debated: should patients with APS and previous thrombosis have a higher target INR, or should this only be applied to patients with a previous arterial event, rather than venous thrombotic event? Some studies have suggested patients with APS have a lower risk of recurrence with a higher target INR, compared with those with a lower target INR (<2), but these have been mainly retrospective (Khamashta *et al.*, 1995).

Two randomised clinical trials directly compared regular (target INR range 2–3) and high-intensity warfarin therapy in patients with APS (Crowther *et al.*, 2003; Finazzi *et al.*, 2005) but, when recurrent venous thromboembolic events on treatment were excluded, patients had a short duration of follow-up and, in some, no information on INR at time of recurrent event was given in this study (Finazzi *et al.*, 2005). So, for now, current recommendations are that patients be anticoagulated with a target INR between 2–3 (Keeling *et al.*, 2012).

Several new direct oral anticoagulants (DOACs) are now licensed and NICE-approved for use in management of acute VTE. These include dabigatran, a direct oral thrombin inhibitor, and rivaroxaban, apixaban and edoxaban – direct oral anti-Xa agents. None of the Phase 3 trials, assessing the efficacy of these agents compared to current standard treatment of LMWH and a vitamin K antagonist, included patients with APS. Results of a study recently comparing use of a direct oral anticoagulant, Rivaroxaban, to vitamin K antagonists in patients with APS and a previous history of venous thrombosis, are awaited (Cohen *et al.*, 2015). For those patients who require an INR target range between 3–4, the use of DOACs cannot currently be recommended.

Options for those who have experienced further thrombotic events despite optimal anticoagulation include addition of aspirin, hydroxychloroquine or a statin and switching to an alternative anticoagulant although there are no studies investigating any of these options.

Management of Pregnancy

Studies of women with aPL-related complications show that women with thrombotic complications of APS have higher rates of pre-term delivery (Lima *et al.*, 1996; Branch *et al.*, 1992; Rosove *et al.*, 1990; Lockshin *et al.*, 1989; Bramham *et al.*, 2009) and pre-eclampsia (Branch *et al.*, 1992), some despite treatment with aspirin and/or heparin.

The American College of Chest Physicians (ACCP), the American College of Obstetricians and Gynecologists (ACOG Practice Bulletin #68, 2005) and the Royal College of Obstetricians and Gynaecologists Guidelines recommend women with previous thrombotic complications, are treated with both heparin and aspirin during pregnancy (Bates *et al.*, 2008). Warfarin is teratogenic in weeks 6–12 of pregnancy, and is therefore discontinued on confirmation of a positive pregnancy test and switched to heparin. There is no current consensus on heparin dosing regimens, and choice of dose is usually according to previous history of either arterial or venous events.

Thromboprophylaxis is advised in the post-partum period for four to six weeks for those women with aPL and no previous thrombotic event (Bates *et al.*, 2008). Both heparin and warfarin are safe for breast-feeding (Ostensen *et al.*, 2006), so women on long-term warfarin can be switched back to warfarin soon after delivery. Since there have been no randomised controlled trials, recommendations for management of acute thrombosis in patients with aPL are based on guidelines for treatment of thrombosis in pregnancy (Bates *et al.*, 2008).

Women with APS need close monitoring throughout pregnancy. Uterine artery Doppler scanning is recommended at 20–24 weeks, to check for evidence of bilateral uterine arterial notching, which has been shown to be predictive of placental dysfunction in women with APS (Le Thi Huong *et al.*, 2006; Papageorghiou and Leslie, 2007). If bilateral notching is detected, serial growth scans are performed to monitor for intrauterine growth restriction.

Management of Catastrophic APS

Catastrophic APS is a rare manifestation of APS, and a high index of suspicion is required to make a diagnosis. Patients present with multi-organ failure due to widespread thrombosis, and there is an associated high mortality rate (up to 50%). Patients require aggressive management, usually in an intensive care setting, with a combination of steroids, anticoagulation and/or plasma exchange. Some case reports suggest that rituximab may be of use in this situation (Rubenstein *et al.*, 2006).

Key Points

- Thrombosis or pregnancy morbidity, in association with persistently elevated antiphospholipid antibodies, are key diagnostic criteria.
- Main treatment goals are prevention of further thrombosis and pregnancy morbidity.
- Consideration should also be given to the presence of co-existent autoimmune disease in patients with a diagnosis of antiphosphospholipid syndrome.
- Catastrophic disease that presents as multi-organ failure occurs in fewer than 1% of patients.
- There should be a high index of suspicion for an underlying diagnosis of antiphospholipid syndrome in a young patient (under 50 years) presenting with arterial thrombosis.

Review Articles

Ruiz-Irastorza G, Crowther M, Branch W, Khamashta MA (2010). Antiphospholipid syndrome. *Lancet* **376**: 1498–509.

Guidelines

Miyakis S, Lockshin MD, Atsumi T, et al. (2006). International consensus statement on an update of the classification criteria for definite antiphospholipid syndrome (APS). *Journal of Thrombosis and Haemostasis* **4**: 295–306.

Keeling D, Mackie I, Moore GW, Greer IA, Greaves M (2012). Guidelines on the investigation and management of antiphospholipid syndrome. *British Journal of Haematology* **157**(1): 47–58.

References

ACOG Practice Bulletin #68 (2005). Antiphospholipid syndrome. *Obstetrics & Gynecology* **106**: 1113–21.

Audrain MA, Colonna F, Morio F, Hamidou MA, Muller JY (2004). Comparison of different kits in the detection of autoantibodies to cardiolipin and beta2glycoprotein 1. *Rheumatology (Oxford)* **43**: 181–5.

Bates SM, Greer IA, Pabinger I, Sofaer S, Hirsh J (2008). Venous thromboembolism, thrombophilia, antithrombotic therapy, and pregnancy: American College of Chest Physicians Evidence-Based Clinical Practice Guidelines (8th Edition). *Chest* **133**: 844S–86S.

Bramham K, Hunt BJ, Germain S *et al.* (2009). Pregnancy outcome in different clinical phenotypes of antiphospholipid syndrome. *Lupus* **19**(1): 58–64.

Branch DW, Dudley DJ, Scott JR, Silver RM (1992). Antiphospholipid antibodies and fetal loss. *New England Journal of Medicine* **326**: 952; author reply 3–4.

Brandt JT, Triplett DA, Alving B, Scharrer I (1995). Criteria for the diagnosis of lupus anticoagulants: an update. On behalf of the Subcommittee on Lupus Anticoagulant/Antiphospholipid Antibody of the Scientific and Standardisation Committee of the ISTH. *Thrombosis and Haemostasis* **74**: 1185–90.

Cervera R, Piette JC, Font J *et al.* (2002). Antiphospholipid syndrome: clinical and immunologic manifestations and patterns of disease expression in a cohort of 1,000 patients. *Arthritis & Rheumatology* **46**: 1019–27.

Chong LY, Fenu E, Stansby G, Hodgkinson S (2012). Management of venous thromboembolic diseases and the role of thrombophilia testing: summary of NICE guidance. *BMJ* **344**: e3979.

Cohen H, Dore CJ, Clawson S *et al.* (2015). Rivaroxaban in antiphospholipid syndrome (RAPS) protocol: a prospective, randomized controlled phase II/III clinical trial of rivaroxaban versus warfarin in patients with thrombotic antiphospholipid syndrome, with or without SLE. *Lupus* **24**: 1087–94.

Crowther MA, Ginsberg JS, Julian J *et al.* (2003). A comparison of two intensities of warfarin for the prevention of recurrent thrombosis in patients with the antiphospholipid antibody syndrome. *New England Journal of Medicine* **349**: 1133–8.

de Groot PG, Horbach DA, Derksen RH (1996). Protein C and other cofactors involved in the binding of antiphospholipid antibodies: relation to the pathogenesis of thrombosis. *Lupus* **5**: 488–93.

de Groot PG, Lutters B, Derksen RH, Lisman T, Meijers JC, Rosendaal FR (2005). Lupus anticoagulants and the risk of a first episode of deep venous thrombosis. *Journal of Thrombosis and Haemostasis* **3**: 1993–7.

Erkan D, Lockshin MD (2004). What is antiphospholipid syndrome? *Current Rheumatology Reports* **6**: 451–7.

Finazzi G, Marchioli R, Brancaccio V *et al.* (2005). A randomized clinical trial of high-intensity warfarin vs. conventional antithrombotic therapy for the prevention of recurrent thrombosis in patients with the antiphospholipid syndrome (WAPS). *Journal of Thrombosis and Haemostasis* **3**: 848–53.

Forastiero R, Martinuzzo M, Pombo G *et al.* (2005). A prospective study of antibodies to beta2-glycoprotein I and prothrombin, and risk of thrombosis. *Journal of Thrombosis and Haemostasis* **3**: 1231–8.

Galli M, Borrelli G, Jacobsen EM *et al.* (2007). Clinical significance of different antiphospholipid antibodies in the WAPS (warfarin in the antiphospholipid syndrome) study. *Blood* **110**: 1178–83.

Galli M, Luciani D, Bertolini G, Barbui T (2003). Lupus anticoagulants are stronger risk factors for thrombosis than anticardiolipin antibodies in the antiphospholipid syndrome: a systematic review of the literature. *Blood* **101**: 1827–32.

Ginsburg KS, Liang MH, Newcomer L *et al.* (1992). Anticardiolipin antibodies and the risk for ischemic stroke and venous thrombosis. *Annals of Internal Medicine* **117**: 997–1002.

Hellan M, Kuhnel E, Speiser W, Lechner K, Eichinger S (1998). Familial lupus anticoagulant: a case report and review of the literature. *Blood Coagulation & Fibrinolysis* **9**: 195–200.

Jara LJ, Medina G, Vera-Lastra O, Barile L (2005). The impact of gender on clinical manifestations of primary antiphospholipid syndrome. *Lupus* **14**: 607–12.

Kearon C, Gent M, Hirsh J *et al.* (1999). A comparison of three months of anticoagulation with extended anticoagulation for a first episode of idiopathic venous thromboembolism. *New England Journal of Medicine* **340**: 901–7.

Keeling D, Mackie I, Moore GW, Greer IA, Greaves M (2012). Guidelines on the investigation and management of antiphospholipid syndrome. *British Journal of Haematology* **157**(1): 47–58.

Khamashta MA, Cuadrado MJ, Mujic F, Taub NA, Hunt BJ, Hughes GR (1995). The management of thrombosis in the antiphospholipid-antibody syndrome. *New England Journal of Medicine* **332**: 993–7.

Kutteh WH, Franklin RD (2004). Assessing the variation in antiphospholipid antibody (APA) assays: comparison of results from 10 centers. *American Journal of Obstetrics & Gynecology* **191**: 440–8.

Le Thi Huong D, Wechsler B, Vauthier-Brouzes D *et al.* (2006). The second trimester Doppler ultrasound examination is the best predictor of late pregnancy outcome in systemic lupus erythematosus and/or the antiphospholipid syndrome. *Rheumatology (Oxford)* **45**: 332–8.

Lim W, Crowther MA, Eikelboom JW (2006). Management of antiphospholipid antibody syndrome: a systematic review. *JAMA* **295**: 1050–7.

Lima F, Khamashta MA, Buchanan NM, Kerslake S, Hunt BJ, Hughes GR (1996). A study of sixty pregnancies in patients with the antiphospholipid syndrome. *Clinical and Experimental Rheumatology* **14**: 131–6.

Lockshin MD, Druzin ML, Qamar T (1989). Prednisone does not prevent recurrent fetal death in women with antiphospholipid antibody. *American Journal of Obstetrics & Gynecology* **160**: 439–43.

Meroni PL, Peyvandi F, Foco L *et al.* (2007). Anti-beta 2 glycoprotein I antibodies and the risk of myocardial infarction in young premenopausal women. *Journal of Thrombosis and Haemostasis* **5**: 2421–8.

Miyakis S, Lockshin MD, Atsumi T *et al.* (2006). International consensus statement on an update of the classification criteria for definite antiphospholipid syndrome (APS). *Journal of Thrombosis and Haemostasis* **4**: 295–306.

Neville C, Rauch J, Kassis J *et al.* (2009). Antiphospholipid antibodies predict imminent vascular events independently from other risk factors in a prospective cohort. *Thrombosis and Haemostasis* **101**: 100–7.

Opatrny L, David M, Kahn SR, Shrier I, Rey E (2006). Association between antiphospholipid antibodies and recurrent fetal loss in women without autoimmune disease: a metaanalysis. *Journal of Rheumatology* **33**: 2214–21.

Ostensen M, Khamashta M, Lockshin M *et al.* (2006). Anti-inflammatory and immunosuppressive drugs and reproduction. *Arthritis Research & Therapy* **8**: 209.

Out HJ, Bruinse HW, Christiaens GC *et al.* (1991). Prevalence of antiphospholipid antibodies in patients with fetal loss. *Annals of the Rheumatic Diseases* **50**: 553–7.

Papageorghiou AT, Leslie K (2007). Uterine artery Doppler in the prediction of adverse pregnancy outcome. *Current Opinion in Obstetrics & Gynecology* **19**: 103–9.

Pengo V, Biasiolo A, Pegoraro C, Cucchini U, Noventa F, Iliceto S (2005). Antibody profiles for the diagnosis of antiphospholipid syndrome. *Thrombosis and Haemostasis* **93**: 1147–52.

Pengo V, Ruffatti A, Legnani C *et al.* (2010). Clinical course of high-risk patients diagnosed with antiphospholipid syndrome. *Journal of Thrombosis and Haemostasis* **8**: 237–42.

Pengo V, Tripodi A, Reber G *et al.* (2009). Update of the guidelines for lupus anticoagulant detection. *Journal of Thrombosis and Haemostasis* **7**: 1737–40.

Petri M (2010). Update on anti-phospholipid antibodies in SLE: the Hopkins' Lupus Cohort. *Lupus* **19**: 419–23.

Rai RS, Regan L, Clifford K *et al.* (1995). Antiphospholipid antibodies and beta 2-glycoprotein-I in 500 women with recurrent miscarriage: results of a comprehensive screening approach. *Human Reproduction* **10**: 2001–5.

Rand JH (2002). Molecular Pathogenesis of the Antiphospholipid Syndrome. *Circulation Research* **90**: 29–37.

Reber G, Tincani A, Sanmarco M, de Moerloose P, Boffa MC (2004). Proposals for the measurement of anti-beta2-glycoprotein I antibodies. Standardization group of the European Forum on Antiphospholipid Antibodies. *Journal of Thrombosis and Haemostasis* **2**: 1860–2.

Richaud-Patin Y, Cabiedes J, Jakez-Ocampo J, Vidaller A, Llorente L (2000). High prevalence of protein-dependent and protein-independent antiphospholipid and other autoantibodies in healthy elders. *Thrombosis Research* **99**: 129–33.

Rosove MH, Tabsh K, Wasserstrum N, Howard P, Hahn BH, Kalunian KC (1990). Heparin therapy for pregnant women with lupus anticoagulant or anticardiolipin antibodies. *Obstetrics & Gynecology* **75**: 630–4.

Rubenstein E, Arkfeld DG, Metyas S, Shinada S, Ehresmann S, Liebman HA (2006). Rituximab treatment for resistant antiphospholipid syndrome. *Journal of Rheumatology* **33**: 355–7.

Santiago M, Martinelli R, Ko A *et al.* (2001). Anti-beta2 glycoprotein I and anticardiolipin antibodies in leptospirosis, syphilis and Kala-azar. *Clinical and Experimental Rheumatology* **19**: 425–30.

Schulman S, Svenungsson E, Granqvist S (1998). Anticardiolipin antibodies predict early recurrence of thromboembolism and death among patients with venous thromboembolism following anticoagulant therapy. Duration of Anticoagulation Study Group. *American Journal of Medicine* **104**: 332–8.

Sebastiani GD, Galeazzi M, Morozzi G, Marcolongo R (1996). The immunogenetics of the antiphospholipid syndrome, anticardiolipin antibodies, and lupus anticoagulant. *Seminars in Arthritis and Rheumatology* **25**: 414–20.

Shi W, Krilis SA, Chong BH, Gordon S, Chesterman CN (1990). Prevalence of lupus anticoagulant and anticardiolipin antibodies in a healthy population. *Australian and New Zealand Journal of Medicine* **20**: 231–6.

Tektonidou MG, Sotsiou F, Nakopoulou L, Vlachoyiannopoulos PG, Moutsopoulos HM (2004). Antiphospholipid syndrome nephropathy in patients with systemic lupus erythematosus and antiphospholipid antibodies: prevalence, clinical associations, and long-term outcome. *Arthritis & Rheumatology* **50**: 2569–79.

Tincani A, Allegri F, Sanmarco M *et al.* (2001). Anticardiolipin antibody assay: a methodological analysis for a better consensus in routine determinations – a cooperative project of the European Antiphospholipid Forum. *Thrombosis and Haemostasis* **86**: 575–83.

Urbanus RT, de Groot PG (2011). Antiphospholipid antibodies – we are not quite there yet. *Blood Reviews* **25**: 97–106.

Wilson WA, Gharavi AE (1996). Genetic risk factors for aPL syndrome. *Lupus* **5**: 398–403.

Wilson WA, Gharavi AE, Koike T *et al.* (1999). International consensus statement on preliminary classification criteria for definite antiphospholipid syndrome: report of an international workshop. *Arthritis & Rheumatology* **42**: 1309–11.

Section III

Treatment

9

Inpatient or Outpatient Anticoagulation

Lauren Floyd[1] and Jecko Thachil[2]

[1] *Core Trainee, Manchester Royal Infirmary, Manchester, UK*
[2] *Department of Haematology, Manchester Royal Infirmary, Manchester, UK*

Introduction

Many patients with venous thromboembolism (VTE) present to the hospital with symptoms which may be chronic, and not significant enough to require hospitalisation. In addition, individuals can present with a deep vein thrombosis or pulmonary embolism at a younger age, when they may prefer treatment as an outpatient if possible, and it is not likely to have an impact on their long-term health. The advent of direct oral anticoagulants has also simplified outpatient anticoagulation management, in that patients may not require injections. However, it is necessary that patients for outpatient management are carefully selected, to ensure that appropriate treatment and plans are put in place for good follow-up.

Deep Vein Thrombosis

Patients with suspected DVT tend to attend their family physicians and, in some cases, the hospital, to confirm or exclude the diagnosis. Due to the fact that missing the diagnosis of a DVT can be both dangerous and have huge medico-legal implications, physicians tend to have a very low threshold for investigating suspected DVT. Many recent studies have shown that only about 20% of cases suspected to have a DVT have radiological confirmation of the thrombosis.

In the majority of these cases, the presenting symptoms may be attributable to musculoskeletal causes. In the minority of cases, where DVT may be confirmed then, if the patient can mobilise without support, it may be reasonable to manage the patient as an outpatient. Two follow-up arrangements may be made in such cases – the first one to assess the patient to ensure the symptoms are improving (if possible in a week), and the second after an interval of three months, to decide on the duration of anticoagulation. If the symptoms have not improved, assessment by a physician experienced in the management of VTE is ideal.

In the cases of suspected DVT, it is important to bear in mind that prescribing DOACs prior to the confirmation of the thrombus is unlicensed and, if done, should be explained to the patient. Otherwise, low molecular weight heparin injections should be prescribed at treatment dose, until the radiological investigations have been performed. If the scans are negative, the injections may be stopped if the degree of suspicion for DVT is not high. If the scans confirm a DVT, low molecular weight heparin is continued and switched to warfarin, or a DOAC such as dabigatran or edoxaban. If the patient was prescribed rivaroxaban or apixaban at the onset, the dose needs to be reduced after an interval (apixaban 10 mg BD to 5 mg BD after seven days, and rivaroxaban 15 mg BD to 20 mg OD after three weeks). Detailed explanations for DOAC use are given in chapter 12.

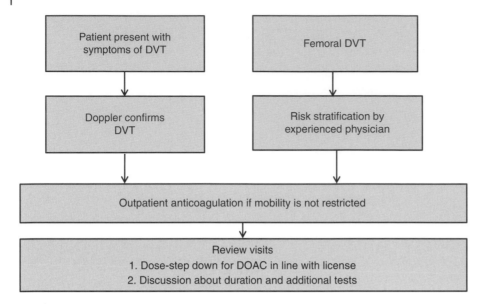

Figure 9.1 Algorithm for managing DVT as an outpatient.

Patients who come to hospital may have more extensive DVT or more severe symptoms. These patients may require hospitalisation. Also, those individuals who have poor mobility would require hospitalisation for the investigations and treatment for DVT. An algorithm for managing DVT as an outpatient is given in Figure 9.1.

Pulmonary Embolism

The latest European Society of Cardiology guidelines categorise PE into high-risk, intermediate-risk and low-risk types, with the low-risk patients being appropriate for outpatient care in the presence of adequate follow-up services. Two criteria are helpful in this risk stratification. The first of these is the PESI score (Pulmonary Embolism Severity Index) and its simplified version, and the second one is the HESTIA criteria.

Aujesky *et al.* (2011) undertook a multinational, open-label, randomised trial where patients with symptomatic PE with PESI score of I or II were randomised to outpatient (discharged from hospital within 24 hours) or inpatient treatment with low molecular weight heparin, followed by oral anticoagulation. Out of the 344 patients, one out of the 171 outpatients developed recurrence of the PE, compared with none of the 168 inpatients. One each in both groups died within 90 days, and two outpatients and no inpatients had major bleeding within the first two weeks. The authors concluded that, in selected low-risk patients with PE, outpatient management is possible safely and effectively.

The HESTIA study was a prospective cohort study of patients from 12 hospitals in the Netherlands, which included 297 patients. Six patients had recurrent VTE, including five PEs, three patients died within 90 days but none from a PE, and two patients had major bleeding. This, again, suggests that selected patients with PE can be treated with anticoagulants on an outpatient basis.

A meta-analysis has confirmed the same findings. The analysis included 13 studies with over 1600 patients where discharge was within 24 hours (outpatient), three studies with about 250 patients discharged within 72 hours (early discharge), and five studies with nearly 400 inpatients. The incidence of recurrent VTE was 1.7%, 1.1% and 1.2%, respectively, while that of major bleeding was 0.97%, 0.78% and 1.0%, respectively. Mortality was 1.9% in the outpatients, 2.3% in early discharge, and 0.74% in the inpatients. Although the safety and efficacy has been proven for outpatient PE care with low-risk patients, the use of DOACs in this setting is yet to be confirmed. The MERCURY PE (Multicenter trial of Rivaroxaban for early discharge of pulmonary embolism from the Emergency Department) study is designed to test this hypothesis, and the results are awaited.

Sub-segmental Pulmonary Embolism

Computerised tomography (CT) scans have become increasingly sensitive in recent years. The thinner slices mean that increasing numbers of smaller PE are being detected. These are usually found in the smaller branches of pulmonary vasculature, especially the segmental and subsegmental vessels. There is currently a lot of debate about whether these should be treated or not and trials are undergoing in this area (discussed in detail in Chapter 29). Until the results of these are available, the current recommendation is that such patients, in the presence of symptoms and co-morbidities, should be treated. The majority of such individuals may be candidates for outpatient treatment and, after detailed discussion, can be considered for DOAC treatment. It should be remembered, however, that DOACs are not licensed in the presence of a VTE related to an underlying malignancy.

The Importance of a VTE Clinic

VTE is often considered as an acute disease, but many patients with a DVT or PE or thrombosis which develops in a different venous circulation can have both short-term and long-term requirements. In the short term, the patients who have been prescribed DOACs will need a dose change in the case of Apixaban or Rivaroxaban while, in the case of patients on low molecular weight heparin, it will be a transition clinic to ensure appropriate switch to Dabigatran or Edoxaban or warfarin. In addition, the clinic could be used as the follow-up site for patients with VTE, who often have to be managed by family physicians who have limited resources and time. One of the crucial decisions which needs to be made, and is probably best done through the VTE clinic, is the decision about the duration of anticoagulation, based on whether the first clot was provoked or unprovoked. An algorithm to guide this decision is given in Figure 9.2.

Chronic complications also can be a problem in VTE patients. For example, post-thrombotic syndrome is not an uncommon complication of a DVT which was extensive at presentation or was diagnosed late. Similarly, pulmonary hypertension can develop in up to 5% of patients who developed a PE in the previous months. Another complication of PE is 'post-PE syndrome', which has been observed in a few patients who develop exertional breathlessness a few weeks to months after a PE. It is useful for such patients to be monitored in a VTE clinic for the development of such symptoms, and arrangements made for the appropriate investigations and referral to specialist centres (e.g. for pulmonary hypertension). Of course, bleeding risks need to be assessed regularly in patients on anticoagulation, which may also come under the remit of such a specialised clinic.

Thus, the VTE clinic will have the expertise for understanding the caveats which may be associated with the VTE diagnosis, the ability to monitor patients who have already commenced treatment, the facilities to arrange appropriate investigations for chronic complications, and making the decision about the duration of the anticoagulation.

Cost-effectiveness

Managing patients in the outpatient setting not only avoids unnecessary hospital admissions and the bed costs associated with this, it also prevents costs relating to hospital-acquired infection or unnecessary investigations. A recent study carried out at a district general hospital over two months showed that, if all low-risk PE patients were managed as an outpatient, there would have been a total saving of 17 bed nights.

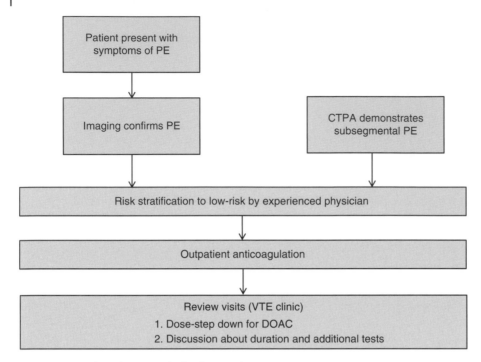

Figure 9.2 An algorithm to guide the decision for managing PE as an outpatient.

Investigation of low-risk patients in an ambulatory, outpatient setting is also extremely cost-effective. Many patients are now able to receive a dose of LMWH and can then be discharged with an outpatient appointment for further imaging and investigation. A study of 35 patients showed that those managed as outpatients created a total saving of £9,800, based on time to imaging.

Summary

Outpatient management of VTE is certainly possible but a good risk assessment is crucial in this regard. The arrival of DOACs have made this process much easier, but input from a VTE clinic may have the advantage of expertise and appropriate follow-up.

Further Reading

Zondag W, Mos IC, Creemers-Schild D *et al.* (2011). Outpatient treatment in patients with acute pulmonary embolism: the Hestia Study. *Journal of Thrombosis and Haemostasis* **9**: 1500–1507.

den Exter PL, van Es J, Klok FA *et al.* (2013). Risk profile and clinical outcome of symptomatic subsegmental acute pulmonary embolism. *Blood* **122**: 1144–1149.

Aujesky D, Roy PM, Verschuren F *et al.* (2011). Outpatient versus inpatient treatment for patients with acute pulmonary embolism: an international, open-label, randomised, non-inferiority trial. *Lancet* **378**: 41–48.

Zondag W, Kooiman J, Klok FA *et al.* (2013). Outpatient versus inpatient treatment in patients with pulmonary embolism: a meta-analysis. *European Respiratory Journal* **42**: 134–144.

Lakhanpal A, Watters C, Hughes C, Iyer S, Babores M (2013). Outpatient Management of Pulmonary Embolism-Patient characteristics and Outcomes. *Thorax* **68**: A145.

Benjamin JA, Griffiths A, Power S, Kidner E (2012). Outpatient management of suspected pulmonary embolism at a district general hospital: a two month review. *Thorax* **67**: A122–A123.

10

An Anticoagulant Service in Practice

Kathy Macintosh, Dawn Kyle and Linda Smith

Team Leaders, Glasgow and Clyde Anticoagulation Service, Glasgow, UK

Greater Glasgow & Clyde Health Board (NHSGGC) is the largest health board in NHS Scotland. Glasgow and Clyde Anticoagulant Service (GCAS) currently monitors 12 500 patients who are prescribed a Vitamin K Antagonist, primarily warfarin. This is predominantly a nurse-led service with haematology medical support. This chapter will explore the GCAS service model and discuss the challenges and successes it has experienced in recent years.

History

The Glasgow Anticoagulation Service (GAS) was successfully introduced in the Greater Glasgow area in 2002, after the introduction of new atrial fibrillation (AF) guidelines, and local general practitioners (GPs) opted to commit funding to a dedicated, centralised anticoagulant service. The overall aim of the service was to reduce the incidence of stroke, and to reduce hospital admissions of patients with high INRs.

The service uses a capillary sampling system, termed Point Of Care (POC) testing, which improves productivity and provides a quicker and more direct level of patient care.

In 2009, the Greater Glasgow Health Board merged with Clyde Health Board to form NHSGGC, serving a population of 1.2 million, and the anticoagulation service became Glasgow & Clyde Anticoagulant Service (GCAS). This increased patient numbers substantially which, in turn, required increased resources, mainly in the form of staffing and equipment.

To incorporate the large extended geographical area, the service was reshaped as follows:

- increased recruitment of staff;
- increased numbers of outreach clinics;
- increased numbers of domiciliary visits, to reduce patient transport numbers;
- standardisation of referral procedures and equipment used by GCAS staff.

The service was divided into three teams, with each team covering a particular geographical area (North/South/City). These teams were each headed by a team leader with their own designated staff, with one lead nurse having overall responsibility for all staff throughout the service, ensuring compliance with GCAS policy and procedure.

Handbook of Venous Thromboembolism, First Edition. Edited by Jecko Thachil and Catherine Bagot.
© 2018 John Wiley & Sons Ltd. Published 2018 by John Wiley & Sons Ltd.

At its peak in 2013/14, GCAS was monitoring 15 000 patients, which put the service under great pressure. At the same time, the service moved from the NHSGGC Diagnostic Directorate to the Regional Directorate, with a management structure change and a service redesign, in order to combat the many challenges facing GCAS and to streamline the service for patients and reduce pressure on staff. The service also took part in a 'Kaizen' event.

As a result, certain changes were made to the running of the service:

- streamlining and organising the delivery of stock to local areas to prevent staff travelling to a central pick up point, thereby reducing travelling and ensuring more effective time management;
- setting up a definitive 'did not attend' (DNA) policy for clinics;
- producing a domiciliary referral procedure;
- extension to clinics' times and adjustment of appointment slots to accommodate patients more effectively.

These, along with other minor changes, allowed the service to evolve to what it is today. Furthermore, with the introduction of the direct oral anticoagulants (DOACS), the patient numbers are now more manageable.

Current Organisation

Currently GCAS has three team leaders, with 29 full-time equivalent specialist nurses and a clerical team of five, with one office manager. The service operates Monday to Friday, running 87 clinical sessions and 47 domiciliary sessions per week. GCAS team leaders are responsible for the weekly planning of clinical/domiciliary sessions and allocation of staff.

All GCAS nurses have a three-month intensive training period under the direct supervision of an allocated mentor, learning all aspects of anticoagulation, including the education, induction, monitoring and maintenance dosing of vitamin K antagonists, along with the care and safety of all patients on oral anticoagulants, while having to pass various competencies throughout. At the end of the training period, the new nurse will undergo a competency test and a practical clinical session with their team leader, before being signed off as suitable to practice.

All GCAS staff are required to sit and pass a competency test every two years. They also attend quarterly internal staff study/training sessions, as well as any relevant external courses/training days. All staff actively participate in annual audits, and the service subscribes to a National External Quality Assurance programme (NEQAS), which is carried out six times per year and is overseen by the NHSGGC haemostasis laboratory. Staff are also encouraged to participate in their ongoing learning, and that of others, by preparing and delivering presentations, and to keep up to date with their Professional Development Plan (PDP) by carrying out e-learning modules and undertaking annual Education and Knowledge Skills Framework (EKSF) reviews with their line manager.

GCAS is primarily a nurse-led service. However, there is input from haematology consultants, and the GCAS team leaders attend quarterly operational group meetings to discuss any issues involving the service. The team leaders also attend the quarterly venous thrombosis (VTE) safety group meeting, where all anticoagulant incidents throughout the Health Board are discussed. There is also a representative from GCAS on the NHSGGC thrombosis committee.

Referral Process

When the service was established in 2002, the main referral process from both primary and secondary care was via completion of a GCAS paper form, which would be faxed to the central office and the information entered by clerical staff onto the DAWN AC software programme (Anticoagulation Server). The patients would either be sent an appointment, or the discharging ward would be phoned and the clinic appointment details given. This process created a number of issues, including incomplete or incorrect referral forms, resulting in GCAS clerical staff chasing medical staff for the correct information, which had a significant impact on the efficiency of the service and, to a certain extent, the safety of patients on Vitamin K antagonists.

In 2014/2015, GCAS investigated ways to improve the referral service to make it safer and more efficient. After various meetings and discussions, it was decided that all secondary referrals would be via the hospital electronic patient record system, Trakcare, and that completion of certain areas on this form (i.e. demographics, ward, contact number, indication, warfarin dose and INR results) would be obligatory for successful electronic submission to the anticoagulant office and the subsequent allocation of an anticoagulation appointment. This process commenced in March 2016, and has greatly improved the referral service within secondary care.

Within primary care, referrals are processed via the electronic Scottish Care Information (SCI) gateway to the central anticoagulation office. Once received, the team leaders vet the referrals and the clerical staff send out appointments and enter the patients' demographics, indication for anticoagulation, appointment date, etc. onto the Dawn AC computerised dosing system, ready for the nurse carrying out the clinic. It is the anticoagulant nurses' responsibility to check that this information is correct during the patient's first clinic visit.

Patients are given their first clinic appointment in the nearest hospital-based GCAS clinic, depending on their address. Thereafter, patients are transferred to an outreach clinic of their choice, if deemed suitable.

Induction Appointments

When a patient is referred to the service for induction onto warfarin, they are sent an appointment to attend a hospital induction session within two weeks of receiving the referral. The patient is encouraged to bring a relative or carer with them. This first appointment can take up to 45 minutes.

During the patient's first visit to the anticoagulant clinic, the specialist nurse will complete a patient education/counselling form (Figure 10.1), which is fully completed and scanned onto the patient's file for future reference.

The patient is educated in all aspects of warfarin therapy, including diet, lifestyle and interaction with other medicines, and is also given a patient information booklet specific to GCAS, along with the generic National Patient Safety Agency (NPSA) yellow oral anticoagulant information pack. The patient is commenced on warfarin by the anticoagulation specialist nurse, using the appropriate induction regimen (e.g. Oates, or Tait & Sefcick) depending on the underlying diagnosis, INR, and if awaiting any cardiac procedures (e.g. DC cardioversion or cardiac radiofrequency ablation). The INR and dosing instructions are documented in the patient's yellow record book, and they are advised to carry this with them at all times and bring it to every clinic appointment. There is a contact number for the GCAS central office, and also an out-of-hours number for NHS 24.

The GCAS specialist nurses are not prescribers; hence, the GP will already have been sent a letter requesting a prescription for 1 mg and 3 mgs of warfarin, to be issued to the patient, who is advised to bring this medication to their anticoagulant appointment. Future prescriptions for warfarin are also organised via the patient's GP.

The timing of the next appointment is dependant on the induction regimen used (i.e. Oates, 7 days; Tait & Sefcick, 5 days). A letter is sent from GCAS central office to the patient's GP after this clinic visit. This will then be followed up with six-monthly reports.

GLASGOW ANTICOAGULATION SERVICE

NEW PATIENT COUNSELLING FORM

		TICK
PATIENT DETAILS	CHI NUMBER	
	SURNAME	
	FORENAME	
	DOB	
	TEL NUMBER	
GP DETAILS	NAME	
	ADDRESS	
	TEL NUMBER	
ACTION OF WARFARIN	Explain how warfarin affects blood clotting	
REASON FOR AC THERAPY	Ensure patient understands reason for AC	
MONITORING OF THERAPY	Explain how & why warfarin needs monitoring	
LENGTH OF THERAPY	Confirm with patient length of time they will be on warfarin	
HOW TO TAKE MEDICATION	Best time to take medication (6pm)	
HOW DOSE IS WRITTEN	Explain weekly dosing	
HOW TO MAKE UP DOSES	Discuss different strengths of tablets	
SIDE EFFECTS	Explain symptoms to look for	
	What to do/who to contact in event of a problem	
CLINIC	Discuss clinic options, including outreach clinic availability	
INFORMATION NEEDED AT EACH CLINIC VISIT	Bleeding/bruising problems	
	Hospital admission/treatment	
	Changes to medication	
	Missed doses	
	Check dosage patient has been taking	
YELLOW BOOK	Stress importance of carrying yellow book at all times	
DRUG INTERACTIONS	Discuss problems with drug interactions	
DIETARY EFFECTS	Explain the effect diet can have on warfarin therapy	
ALCOHOL EFFECTS	Explain the effects of alcohol with warfare therapy	
	How many units of alcohol weekly	
CONTRACEPTION/PREGNANCY	Discuss issues concerning pregnancy and contraception	

Figure 10.1 Counselling form used by GCAS when commencing patient on Vitamin K antagonist.

GLASGOW ANTICOAGULATION SERVICE

RISK FACTORS

AGE	NO	YES
DIABETES Diet/Tablet/Insulin		What medication
HYPERTENSION On medication		What medication
ACTIVE CANCER Chemo/Radiotherapy		Treatment duration
PEPTIC ULCER On medication/last bleeding incident		What medication
CARDIAC CONDITIONS Angina/IHD/MI		What medication
PREVIOUS TIA/CVA How many/When?		
PREVIOUS VTE Where treated		
ANAEMIA Previous transfusions/iron tablets		What medication
REGULAR STEROIDS How often/Treating what condition?		What medication
REGULAR ANTIBIOTICS How often/Treating what condition?		What medication
COMPLIANCE ISSUES Dosette boxes/Family support		
HISTORY OF FALLS How many in last 6 months		
ALCOHOL EXCESS How many units weekly?		
OTHER MEDICATIONS Please list on DAWN		
VITAMINS/HERBAL MEDICATIONS Discuss the effects these can have on warfarin.		

DATE: COUNSELLORS SIGNATURE:

Figure 10.1 (Continued)

Hospital Discharge Patients

A hospital discharge patient who has recently been commenced onto warfarin (generally using the Fennerty regimen) will be seen at a hospital-based GCAS clinic within seven days of discharge, and all education carried out as with an induction patient, with the timing of the subsequent appointment dependent on the patient's INR. The GP will receive a letter regarding the patient's anticoagulation management once the patient has been seen by GCAS.

If the patient is already managed by GCAS prior to the hospital admission, the patient is re-referred via the Trakcare referral system, and is given an appointment to attend their regular hospital or outreach clinic again within seven days of discharge. The anticoagulation nurse specialist will update the patient's DAWN AC file with relevant information and any changes of medication, and INR results from admission as per the hospital discharge letter, which can be accessed via the electronic NHSGGC clinical portal system.

Anticoagulant Clinic Structure

GCAS carry out 87 anticoagulant clinics per week throughout NHSGGC, either hospital-based or at an outreach clinic in the community. Each clinic runs on an appointment basis for patients, either in the morning or afternoon, and GCAS staff are allocated a weekly rota for clinics on specific days and areas each week.

Before the specialist nurse commences their clinic, they collect thromboplastin reagent from a local hospital laboratory. On arrival in the clinic, the nurse will set up the clinic room with all the equipment required, which they carry with them. Each nurse uses a whole blood coagulometer, which undergoes internal quality control prior to each clinical session. A capillary whole blood sample is taken from each patient, added to the thromboplastin reagent in a cuvette in the coagulometer, and the patient's prothrombin time measured. The patient's INR result is displayed on the screen of the coagulometer and, from this result, the nurse can subsequently dose the patient.

GCAS uses computerised dosing management software (DAWN AC), and each patient has an individual file which contains information on that patient's diagnosis, commencement date of warfarin, duration of therapy, INR target and therapeutic range, along with other relevant demographic and clinical details.

Once the INR result has been obtained, the nurse enters this into the DAWN AC software, which will provide a warfarin dosing regimen for the patient. This dosing advice can be overridden by the specialised nurse if required – for example, if the patient has had a change to their medication which may result in an out-of-range INR.

Alongside taking the patient's capillary sample, the nurse will also ask six key questions:

- Have there been any medicine changes?
- What dose of warfarin is the patient taking?
- Does the patient have any bruising or bleeding?
- Has the patient been in hospital since the last clinic visit?
- Has the patient missed any doses of warfarin?
- Does the patient have any pending procedures?

The DAWN AC file also calculates each patient's time in therapeutic range (TTR), and GCAS will specifically target reviews of patients with a TTR < 60% and the reasons for this (e.g. non-compliance). The nurse may consider discussing with the patient's GP if a DOAC may be more suitable.

Depending on the INR, the nurse will then dose the patient, taking into account the answers to the above questions, and will then allocate the next clinic appointment. If the patient has their warfarin medication added to a dossette/blister pack administered by a pharmacy, then the nurse will call the pharmacy (telephone number on patient file) and instruct pharmacy staff what dose the patient is to receive, along with the date of the next appointment.

At the end of each clinical session, the DAWN AC system will display the name and patient identification number of every patient who has not attended for their anticoagulant appointment, and the GCAS DNA (did not arrive) procedure is followed. Alternatively, the nurse may phone the patient, depending on the previous INR result or other relevant information within the DAWN AC file.

GCAS also carry out home visits (47 sessions per week) for patients who are housebound, for which there are criteria that a patient needs to fulfil. A risk and domiciliary assessment is also carried out on the first visit (Figure 10.2). GCAS use a Coaguchek XS Plus (Roche Diagnostics 2017) coagulometer to monitor housebound patients' INR results. This machine undergoes quality control on a weekly (internal) and quarterly (external (Neqas, POC)) basis and uses Coaguchek strips (i.e. no 'wet' reagent is required).

NHS
Greater Glasgow and Clyde

GCAS First Home Visit Risk Assessment

(This form should be used in conjunction with the guidance given on risk assessment as outlined within the risk management manual)

GCAS	HOME VISITS:

Patient:	Individual(s) exposed to the risk:
CHI Number:	Anticoagulant Nurse
Tel. Number:	
GP:	
NOK/ carer Tel:	

Risk assessment carried out by:	Date completed:	Review date:

		Comment where appropriate	Assess the degree of risk after considering your existing control measures (✓)			
1. Before Visit	Previous Experience/Knowledge (e.g. violence/ aggression/ drink/ drugs)					
	Do you know the location?					
	Does the patient know you are coming?					
	Is the visit during unsocial hours or during hours of darkness?					
	Do you require a key or code? (key holder/ key safe)					
	Do you have contact telephone numbers the patient or carer?					
2. On Arrival	Parking					
	Lighting					
	Access to property					
	House Type (Detached ~ Semi ~ Tenement ~ Multi Storey ~ Other)					
	Lift (operational?) Stairs (Number of flights?)					
3. On Entry	Groups Gathering/ Loitering					
	Front Door Security					
	Concierge Service					
	Mobile phone signal					
	Condition of House					
	Hazards (e.g. electricity/ passive smoking)					
	Client Behaviour					
	Behaviour of others					
	Pets Type Are they secured (Y/N)					
	Ease of escape					
4. Post Visit	Felt safe					
	Felt threatened/ intimidated					
	Would not revisit alone?					
	Would not revisit					
5. Other Factors (Include any other information not covered above)						

Figure 10.2 GCAS risk assessment form for patients requiring domiciliary visits for INR testing.

Home or Community Risk Assessment ~ First Visit (Cont.)

Comment on any actions that could eliminate or reduce the risk to a safe level?
Before Visit:
On Arrival:
On Entry:
Post Visit:
Other Factors:

What will the overall level of risk be when additional control measures have been implemented
Low ⬛   Medium ☐   High ⬛   Very High ⬛
Remember risk levels that are high or very high indicate that lone working should not take place ~ action must be taken to reduce the level of risk

Figure 10.2 (Continued)

Self-testing Patients

Prior to the current service setup, there were approximately 30–40 patients who owned a Coaguchek coagulometer and self-tested via support from their GPs. However, there was no formal policy or procedure in place. GCAS has now developed a self-testing policy, in conjunction with a consultant haematologist, which addresses self-testing criteria and patient and staff training. The team leaders of GCAS have all completed an accredited self-testing training programme, and now train appropriate patients in self-testing, enabling more patients to join this programme, while working in partnership with GPs. At present, GCAS monitors 131 self-testing patients.

The criteria for this programme include patients who work away from home, find it difficult to attend clinics, and young adults with congenital heart conditions who have self-tested since childhood. Once the patient expresses an interest in self-testing, the team leaders assess the patients' suitability using established GCAS criteria. The patient is responsible for purchasing their own Coaguchek machine, unless provided by a charity (e.g. Congenital Cardiac Society). The INR monitoring strips are either purchased by the patient, or prescribed by their GP.

Once the patient has been deemed suitable, they are trained in all aspects of self-testing, which includes a practical demonstration and educational session with patient participation. The patient/relative/carer will then sign a GCAS agreement (Figure 10.3). The patient will be given a date to self-test, and advised to either phone/email GCAS with the INR result and provide answers to the six key questions, as outlined in the section 'Anticoagulation Clinic Structure'. A GCAS team leader will, in turn, reply with dosing advice and the next test date.

Patients are advised to contact GCAS within specified times if there are any changes in their medications or clinical condition, such as bleeding. One of the requirements of the self-testing agreement is that the patients must attend a clinic for a comparison test between the patient's Coaguchek and a GCAS Coaguchek for quality assurance every six months, where the nurse will review the patients' technique/ previous INRs and yellow book to ensure all records are up to date.

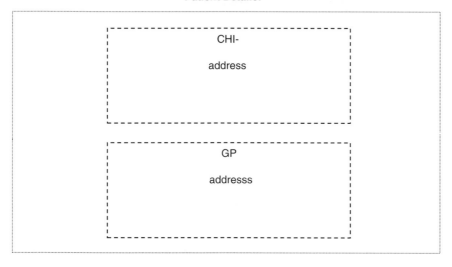

GLASGOW & CLYDE ANTICOAGULANT SERVICE

Anticoagulation Clinic & Patient Agreement

Agreement for the Use of a CoaguChek XS Machine for Self Testing INR

This is an agreement for self-testing between Glasgow & Clyde Anticoagulant Service and:
Patient Details:

CHI-

address

GP

addresss

Patient Anticoagulation History:

Indication of Anticoagulation:	
Target INR range:	
Type of Anticoagulant/strength:	
Start date of Anticoagulation:	
Start date of self testing:	

POCT ANALYSER NUMBER :

Patient email address:

If self testing; the patient is responsible for testing his/her INR. The patient is not responsible for dosing. The dosing remains the responsibility of the Anticoagulation Clinic.

Figure 10.3 GCAS protocol outlining patient and GCAS responsibilities, and signed agreement form for INR self-testing.

CoaguChek XS Agreement

Patient Training Record

Patient Name: _____

Trainer Name: _____

The training session is being carried out to ensure the correct use of the CoaguChek XS monitoring device. Please check off boxes to confirm the following information has been given, and sign to confirm this:

Criteria	✓
Meter Set Up	
Batteries	
Display check	
Date Format	
Date Setting	
Time Format	
Time Setting	
Set Test Measurement	
Beep Tone	
Therapeutic Range	
CoaguChek XS Test Strips	
Storage conditions	
Handling test strip	
Calibration Code Chip	
Changing Code Chip	
Onboard Quality Control	
Sample dosing area	

Criteria	✓
Performing a Test	
Switch meter on	
Checking screen	
Insertion of test strip	
Confirm code lot number	
Strip warming	
Operation of Softclix Device	
Device components	
Removal of protective	
Insertion of lancet	
Priming device	
Depth setting	
Firing lancet	
Ejecting lancet	

Criteria	✓
Obtaining a Finger Prick Sample	
Hand washing	
Sites for taking a sample	
Time limits	
Sampling problems	
Recording Results	
Anticoagulation Record	
Memory	
Retrieving saved results	
Maintenance & Troubleshooting	
Cleaning meter	
Common error codes	

I confirm that I have received the information on the above criteria from the above named trainer. I confirm that I should still read the user manual accompanying my CoaguChek XS device in conjunction with this training.

Date: _____

Patient Sign: _____

Trainer Sign: _____

Figure 10.3 (Continued)

CoaguChek XS Agreement
Patient Responsibilities

- I have a CoaguChek XS monitor. To ensure my own safety I agree to work in partnership with Glasgow & Clyde Anticoagulation Service.

- I have been trained in the use of the CoaguChek XS machine.

- I will perform INR tests at mutually agreed intervals and will inform the Anticoagulation Clinic of the results via the email or phone.

- I will be contactable on the day of my blood test by phone .

- I will repeat any test if my INR is less than 1.5 or greater than 5.

- If my INR is less than 1.8 and I have a mechanical heart valve I will contact an anticoagulation nurse via the GCAS office number xxx.

- If my INR is greater than 8 or un-recordable I will inform an anticoagulation nurse immediately via the GCAS office number xxx.

- I will act on the advice given by the anticoagulation nurses with regard to dosages and test interval. I understand that the maximum permitted interval for testing is 12 weeks.

- I understand that it is my responsibility to order supplies of test strips and finger prick lancets from the manufacturer or obtain them under prescription, as appropriate. Maintenance of the machine is also my responsibility.

- I will dispose of used lancets, other sharps and contaminated waste carefully.

- I will inform the anticoagulation nurses if starting new medications (conventional and unconventional), before and after dental and surgical procedures, changes in medications/diet/alcohol/herbal remedies, missed doses, recent hospital admissions, if unwell/diarrhoea and vomiting.

- If I do experience any unexplained or excessive bleeding or bruising I will contact the Anticoagulation Clinic for advice.

- I will attend the Anticoagulation Clinic for follow up appointments every 6 months or sooner if the Anticoagulation Clinic requires. At all appointment I will bring my CoaguChek XS machine and test strips currently in use, for a comparative venous / capillary blood sample.

- I will inform the Anticoagulation Clinic if I intend to travel abroad and self test.

- I will inform the Anticoagulation Clinic if I decide to stop self-testing or move house to a different area so that arrangements can be made for alternative management of my treatment.

Any bleeding or bruise which occurs out of hours the patient should attend A & E or phone NHS 24 on 111

Figure 10.3 (Continued)

CoaguChek XS Agreement

Anticoagulation Clinic Responsibilities

- The Anticoagulation Clinic agrees to support the above named patient with his / her self-testing provided that the conditions listed above are met.

- The Anticoagulation Nurses will be available during normal office hours for help and advise.

- After the patient has contacted the Anticoagulation Clinic with a result, advice on dosing will be given the same day via email or phone.

- The Anticoagulation Clinic will provide an external quality control by comparative testing of patient's capillary blood INR by the patients own CoaguChek XS and the Anticoagulation Clinic method (Merlin or KC1 analyser). Patients will be sent an appointment for review every 6 months by email.

- In the event that conditions are not met; the Anticoagulation Clinic will offer the patient a normal clinic service without any regard to self testing.

- The Anticoagulation Clinic will inform the patient General practitioner of his/her intentions to start self testing, stop self testing or of any failure to comply with this agreement.

- The patient has been supplied with a customs letter.

Figure 10.3 (Continued)

In summary, then, self-testing patients are responsible for testing their INR at home using capillary sampling and the POC Coaguchek testing device, internal quality control, external quality assessment, and general maintenance of the POC device and test strips. Dosing of warfarin and frequency of testing remains the responsibility of the healthcare professional, who is clinically responsible for their management.

GCAS is currently developing a patient self-management programme (where a patient has responsibility for both INR testing and warfarin dosing), following guidance from Health Improvement Scotland (HIS) and a published systematic review, that INR self-management is safer and more efficient than self-testing or standard clinic care.

Direct Oral Anticoagulants (DOACs)

In recent years, with the introduction of the DOACs, the number of referrals to GCAS of patients with venous thromboembolism has reduced significantly with these patients being treated with a DOAC rather than warfarin.

DOACs are also used for the prevention of stroke in non-valvular atrial fibrillation but, with warfarin continuing to be one of the first line treatments alongside the DOACs, GCAS has not seen such a substantial drop in these referrals. However, the 2016 European Society of Cardiology (ESC) guidelines are now recommending DOACs in preference to warfarin, and this, in turn, may affect future UK guidelines.

Furthermore, GCAS nurses can refer patients whose INR TTR is less than 60% to their GP, for consideration of switching to a DOAC if they meet certain criteria, including non-valvular AF, recurrent VTE, INR target range 2–3, or anticoagulation required for greater than six months. Before contacting the GP, the nurse first undertakes a number of actions to try and improve patient TTR (e.g. family/carer involvement, dossette/blister pack, medication prompting, setting an alarm, visual reminders). Switching to a DOAC is also dependent on adequate renal function.

DOACs can also be considered in patients who require frequent administration of vitamin K, or regular DNA GCAS clinic appointments, as long as they are compliant with taking their anticoagulation. Patients with cognitive impairment, with no family or carer support, may also benefit switching to a DOAC, which can be added to a dossette/blister pack by the pharmacy. The final decision rests with the GP regarding whether their patient is suitable for a DOAC. However, if this decision is made, GCAS will facilitate the transfer of warfarin to a DOAC.

Interestingly, although there has been a small overall fall in the number of patients attending GCAS over the last year, the service has also seen some patients re-referred GCAS to switch back from a DOAC to warfarin, either due to re-thrombosis or DOAC side-effects.

The Future of GCAS

Despite the initial thinking that, with the introduction of the DOACs, this would decrease the need for an anticoagulant service, to date this has been shown not to be the case. Although GCAS referral numbers have dropped, the service still receives approximately 30–40 new referrals per month. This is likely due to a combination of reasons, such as clinicians' familiarity with warfarin, patient preference and anticoagulant indication. For example, DOACs are not licensed for patients with mechanical heart valves, and these patients will remain on warfarin for the foreseeable future.

As familiarity with DOACs increases, and with the recent change in the ECS guidelines, recommending the use of a DOAC over warfarin in patients with non-valvular AF, it is likely that, over time, new referrals to GCAS will decline further. Therefore, in the future, there is the potential for GCAS to become more involved in patient education with the use of DOACs.

Overall, the service will continue to adapt to the ever-changing anticoagulant needs of the patients.

Key Points

1) A region-wide, centralised anticoagulant monitoring service can be highly effective at providing safe, efficient and effective anticoagulation to a large patient population. It enables standardisation of patient management, staff training and INR monitoring.
2) Patient INR self-management is one of the current challenges to try to optimise INR control for those patients who may not be able to adapt to clinic attendance. GCAS hope to develop a framework for self-monitoring that could subsequently receive national approval.
3) Other challenges for GCAS currently include trying to achieve maximum efficiency in the service, by reducing domiciliary visits through transfer of appropriate patients onto a DOAC and closely auditing reagent stock.
4) The potential for greater numbers of patients in the future to receive a DOAC, rather than a vitamin K antagonist, means that centralised anticoagulant services such as GCAS will likely need to adapt and evolve in the future, and to become involved in the education of patients in the safe use of DOACs and remain as facilitators in the safe conversion from one oral anticoagulant to another.

Further Reading

ESC (2016). ESC Guidelines for the management of atrial fibrillation developed in collaboration with EACTS. *European Heart Journal* **37**: 2893–2962.

Fitzmaurice DA, Gardiner C, Kitchen S, Mackie I, Murray ET, Machin SJ (2005) An evidence- based review and guidelines for patient self-testing and management of oral anticoagulation anticoagulation. *British Journal of Haematology* **131**: 156–165.

National Institute for Clinical Excellence (2014). *Atrial Fibrillation Management, Clinical Guideline 180*. Updated August 2014. https://www.nice.org.uk/guidance/CG180.

Scottish Intercollegiate Guidelines Network (SIGN) (2014). Guidelines – Prevention of stroke in patients with atrial fibrillation. Updated January 2014. http://www.sign.ac.uk/pdf/AF_publication.pdf.

Sharma P, Scotland G, Cruickshank M *et al.* (2015). Is self-monitoring an effective option for people receiving long term vitamin K antagonist therapy? A systematic review and economic evaluation. *BMJ Open* **5**: e007758. doi:10.1136/bmjopen-2015-007758.

11

Point of Care Testing

Dianne Patricia Kitchen

Point of Care, UK NEQAS for Blood Coagulation, Sheffield, UK

International Normalised Ratio (INR)

Patients undergoing vitamin K antagonist therapy are monitored using the INR. This was introduced in the late 1980s in order to standardise the many reagents used to perform this test. Prior to its introduction, patients were monitored using the prothrombin time ratio (patients PT : control PT), but this meant that a test performed using one reagent might give quite different results compared with another reagent. The introduction of the INR, using the international sensitivity index (ISI), allows measurement of different PT reagents to give comparable results. The INR is calculated using the equation:

$$INR = (\text{patient prothrombin time} / \text{mean normal prothrombin time})^{\wedge} ISI$$

The International Sensitivity Index (ISI) is calculated by measuring the prothrombin time of a series of 60 or more stable patients (on vitamin K anticoagulant therapy) in the range 1.5–4.5, together with 20 or more control subjects not on oral vitamin K antagonists, using the reagent and a reference thromboplastin. These results are plotted, and the log of the slope of the plot is the ISI value. The very first reference thromboplastin was given an ISI of 1.0, and all other thromboplastins were measured and assigned ISIs by calibrating against this reference thromboplastin. When the reference thromboplastin stocks were running low, a new reference thromboplastin was developed and given an ISI by calibrating against the original.

The manufacturer of the reagent performs this ISI calculation and set the ISI value for their reagents. Although some larger laboratories may have the capacity to perform an ISI calibration, very few do so. For POC devices, the manufacturer sets the ISI and the device makes the calculations, so there is no possibility of the user being able to adjust this calculation.

Figure 11.1 shows calibration of a new reagent using reference thromboplastin. The values are plotted on log paper, and the slope of the trend line multiplied by the ISI of the reference preparation is the new reagent's ISI value.

The introduction of the INR system meant that a patient's INR could be measured anywhere in the world, and a consistent INR result would be achieved. However, the equation that the INR is based upon only works in the range of 1.5–4.5, due to the fact that only patients in this range are used for the ISI calculation. Patients outside of this criteria range may not get similar results between methods. The measurement of the INR was traditionally performed in a laboratory setting by laboratory staff, using anticoagulated venous samples. In the last decade or so, some countries, including the United Kingdom, have seen a movement towards performing INR tests using Point Of Care (POC) devices, and with the majority of tests being performed by non-laboratory staff.

Figure 11.1 Calibration of a new reagent using reference thromboplastin.

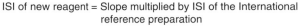
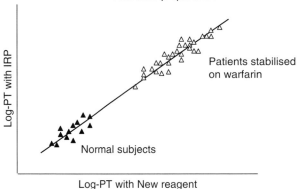

ISI of new reagent = Slope multiplied by ISI of the International reference preparation

These POC devices are designed to be small, portable and easy to use. Although the POC INRs are not tested in a laboratory setting using laboratory staff, we still need to ensure that the quality of the result is maintained. Although the POC devices have the INR equation within their software, it is important that users understand the principle of the INR, and that different methods should give similar results. Agreement between methods is accepted as up to 0.5 INR units, and it should be realised that, although the INR system works well, exact agreement between methods should not be expected in all patients.

POC INR devices currently available for INR testing are as follows:

- CoaguChek XS
- CoaguChek XS Plus
- CoaguChek XS Pro
- Hemochron citrated cuvettes and non-citrated cuvettes
- INRhythm
- I-STAT
- MicroINR
- Xprecia Stride
- INRatio

Most share common features in that the majority use non-anticoagulated capillary whole blood, taken directly from a finger stick, and this is applied to a single-use test strip. The exception to this would be the Hemochron device, which can use both non-citrated or citrated venous whole blood. As these POC devices have developed, the amount of blood required has been reduced, and the newer technology now requires only a very small amount of blood. (approximately <10 μl). There has also been an increase in memory storage capacity, and additional features, such as quality control lockouts and operator ID access restrictions (this means that there is a list of approved operators who are allowed to use the device but, without the appropriate passwords, the device will not perform a test). The QC lockouts can allow a device to be locked, so that further tests cannot be carried out until a QC sample has been completed. Table 11.1 shows a comparison of the features of INR POC testing devices.

In order to obtain a quality result (i.e. an INR value in which the user has full confidence), we require a quality sample and a method upon which we can rely. The quality of the sample is achieved by training the staff how to acquire the sample, and this applies in both venepuncture samples and finger stick samples. There are more pre-analytical issues with venepuncture samples than finger stick samples, as patients that have been on Vitamin K antagonists for many years have poor venous access and can be difficult to bleed, leading to poorly filled samples or haemolysed samples. Both of these issues can affect the INR results.

Table 11.1 Point of care devices available and their characteristics.

	Test strip storage	Sample volume	Sample type	IQC available	Keypad patient ID entry?	End point detection	Operator lockouts?	Memory storage
CoaguChek XS	Room temp	8 μl	Native capillary or venous whole blood	Onboard QC	No	Electro-chemical cleavage	No	300
CoaguChek XS Plus	Room temp	8 μl	Native capillary or venous Whole Blood	Onboard QC and liquid IQC	Yes	Electro-chemical cleavage	Yes	2000 patient tests 500 liquid controls
CoaguChek XS Pro	Room temp	8 μl	Native capillary or venous whole blood	Onboard QC and liquid IQC	Bar code reader and manual entry	Electro-chemical cleavage	Yes	2000 patient tests, 500 liquid controls
Hemochron Signature Series	Room temp storage up to three months, 2–8 °C up to 12 months	15 μl	Native or citrated Whole Blood	Electronic simulator and liquid IQC at two levels	Bar code reader and manual entry	Optical detection of mechanical clot technology	Yes	600 patient results, 600 QC results
i-STAT	2–8 °C two weeks upon removal from refrigerator	17 μl	Native capillary whole blood	Electronic simulator and liquid IQC at two levels	Bar code reader and manual entry	Electro-chemical cleavage	Yes	5000
INRatio2	Room temp	15 μl	Native whole blood	Onboard and electronic QC	No	Impedance	No	120
INRhythm	Room temp storage	13 μl	Native whole blood	Onboard QC and liquid IQC at two levels	Bar code reader and manual entry	Mechanical clot-based technology	No	1200 results
Xprecia Stride	Room temp	6 μl	Native capillary whole blood	Onboard QC and Liquid IQC at two levels	Bar code reader and manual entry	Electro-chemical detection of thrombin generation	Yes	640 patient results, 300 liquid controls

A finger stick sample needs to be acquired quickly as, once the skin has been pierced, the clotting process will commence. This means that if a sample takes several minutes to obtain, it may not properly represent the level of anticoagulation happening within that patient. It is important that the amount of blood required is obtained, as too small a sample will give an error. If this occurs, a new finger stick sample should be obtained, using a different finger, as coagulation will have already started at the original site. It is, therefore, better to be thorough and to obtain enough blood on the first attempt, rather than to waste a test strip and have to perform a second finger stick.

Some devices have been assessed for use with non-anticoagulated venous whole blood, and this can be useful for patients for whom it is difficult to obtain a finger stick sample, such as patients with very poor circulation or very calloused fingertips. 0.5 ml of venous blood is acquired using a needle and syringe, the needle is then discarded, and the syringe is gently depressed in order to apply a drop of blood onto the test strip. However, it is essential to check with the manufacturers of the devices to ensure that venous blood can be used. Training of staff is essential, so that they are able to obtain good quality samples, and this applied equally to venepuncture or finger stick samples. Staff should undergo training and be signed off as competent to perform this task.

The device needs to be CE marked for sale in the UK, and FDA approved for sale in the USA. However, when considering which device to purchase, it is well worth checking scientific reviews and peer-reviewed journals, to get a true feel of how well the devices perform. It is also advisable to assess the ease of use of the device before committing to a purchase. There have been many published studies, usually comparing a POC device and a lab method. In these studies, it is usually assumed that the laboratory method is correct and the POC system either agrees or is incorrect. However, this does not really tell us how well the POC system is performing, as the assumption that the laboratory system gives the true INR may not be the case.

A more appropriate study would also include a reference thromboplastin that gives the true INR results, and to which both the POC system and the laboratory method can be compared. Nevertheless, published studies have shown that POC devices are accurate and reliable, and can be reliably used to monitor vitamin K antagonist therapy patients by both healthcare professionals and patient self-testers. POC devices have also been used extensively in studies looking at patient self-testing versus standard care. These studies have shown that POC devices for patient self-testing are a reliable alternative to standard care. Some have shown better Time in Therapeutic Range (TTR) than standard care, but some of this effect may be due to more frequent testing in the self-testing arm of the study, compared to the standard care. Comparing TTR as a measure of how well the system is working is useful but, as these studies have been performed in many different countries, it must be remembered that some countries have better TTRs than others. It is, therefore, important to look at the data, and not simply the conclusions.

Quality Control

To ensure a reliable result in either a laboratory test or POC test requires quality control. A quality control system needs both internal quality control (IQC) and external quality assurance (EQA). The two forms of quality control work together to ensure that the method is accurate and precise. The IQC is a constant monitoring of the system, and this ensures that the method is consistent. The EQA is provided by an external organisation, and checks that the method is accurate (i.e. is giving the correct result). The EQA is provided at regular intervals, so is providing a spot check of the method.

For example, the UK National External Quality Assessment Scheme (NEQAS) for blood coagulation provides an EQA programme for POC INR testing, whereby four sets of two samples are provided annually. If a series of three INR tests are performed on the same patient on the same day, a precise and accurate method would get the same correct result all three times. This is illustrated in figure 11.2a, where the bull's-eye is the true INR result. If the precision is good but accuracy is poor, then we get three similar results, but all would be incorrect, as shown in figure 11.2b. If both precision and accuracy are poor, then the results would be scattered around the bull's-eye, with the three results all different and no result correct as, shown in figure 11.2c.

(a) (b) (c)

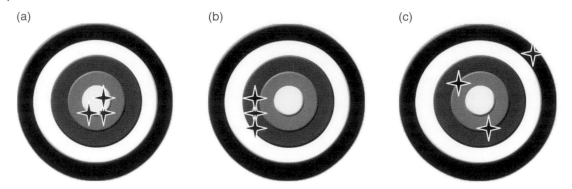

Figure 11.2 Comparison of three INR tests performed on the same patient on the same day: (a) shows results which are accurate and precise; (b) shows results that are inaccurate but precise; (c) shows inaccurate and imprecise results.

It is recommended in the UK guidelines for patient self-testers, and in a recent review of POC tests for haemostasis by Perry *et al.*, that both IQC and EQA are undertaken. A robust QC package (regular IQC and EQA, with thorough documentation) is essential in order to protect the patient by ensuring accurate and reliable results. The evidence (documentation) of a robust QC system also protects the user of the device, should any untoward events occur, in that they can show that all the correct measures were in place. It is essential that all users follow QC SOPs, and that all are aware of where these QC records are stored.

Internal Quality Control (IQC)

IQC (sometimes called liquid QC) is purchased from the manufacturer of the device, and should be tested at the start of a new batch of test strips and once per clinic, if the clinic is relatively small (i.e. 20–30). If the POC device is used in a setting whereby many more patients attend clinic then as a general rule, one IQC should be tested per 20 patient tests. If only a very small number of tests are performed per week (e.g. a device used for home visits with five visits per week), then one IQC test can be performed per week.

These QC tests need to be documented, and all users should know where these results are stored and should check that the required IQC test has been completed before using the device. If a IQC results falls outside the acceptable range, a second vial should be tested. If this second vial is outside of the accepted range, all patient testing using the system should be suspended until the problem has been investigated.

External Quality Assessment (EQA)

EQA is provided by an external organisation and is a spot check on the test system. A test sample will be distributed at regular intervals (UK NEQAS BC provide two samples every three months), and the user should test and return the results. The EQA provider will analyse the data, and issue a report stating whether the test system is within the acceptable range or not. The principle of this EQA is that if the same sample is tested by very many users of the same type of device, then the results should be similar, and an acceptable range is created, to which each centre's test result are compared. The samples distributed should be as close as possible to that for which the test is designed.

In the case of INR POC testing, the sample that the systems are designed for is fresh native whole blood; however, EQA samples are usually freeze-dried, citrated plasma samples. Although there are differences in the EQA sample and the patients' samples, the most appropriate EQA material should be sourced from patients that are undergoing vitamin K antagonist therapy. Not all EQA providers use material sourced in this way, and users should check with their EQA providers that appropriate samples are distributed.

Within Europe, there is a variation between many aspects of EQA provision, such as frequency of test, source of EQA material and performance assessment of these samples. However, many of the EQA providers use 15% deviation from a median or mean result to calculate the acceptable limits to apply to their samples. If a centre's EQA is out of the acceptable range, a repeat sample should be tested. If this second sample is out of range, the system should be investigated.

It is vital, when a centre is assessing whether to provide POC INR monitoring, that the costing should include the cost of both the IQC and EQA for the device.

Comparison with Laboratory Results

The most common question that occurs in POC INR monitoring is that of comparison with a laboratory test. Frequently, any difference seen in patients samples between POC and laboratory methods is assumed to be due to an inaccurate POC method. This is not necessarily the case, but the laboratory is generally considered to be the expert, and this can lead to loss of confidence in the POC system. If performing comparison studies between a POC and a laboratory method, it must be remembered that the INR system does not give agreement between methods outside the therapeutic range. Therefore, any patients that are over-anticoagulated are not suitable to use to check the method. In fact, any results over 4.5 on the POC device should be re-checked using the POC device, and then treated appropriately. Only results over >8.0 should have a venous check sent to the laboratory.

When comparing any two INR methods, we need to look at several patients' samples and look at the relationship overall (at least 20–30 patients in the therapeutic range are needed). It must also be remembered that venous samples are more prone to pre-analytical changes, due to delay in analysing the sample or, perhaps, if the sample was haemolysed. Therefore, if an occasion comparison check sample is quite different from the laboratory results (and differences of up to 0.5 are acceptable), it is worth checking a second sample on that particular patient.

Any changes that the patient is undergoing in their therapy that may make their INR unstable (such as introduction of a new antibiotic) may show a difference between test methods. If, however, there is a genuine difference between the POC and laboratory methods that is present in the majority of patients, this only tells us that there is a difference, and not which is the true INR. The use of comparison checks with a laboratory are not considered to be an acceptable form of QC, as we would simply be checking one system with another without knowing whether either is performing adequately.

Limitations of POC Devices

There are limitations to the POC INR testing devices which users should be aware of. The manufacturers provide literature enclosed with the test strips that will detail the level of haematocrit (a very low haematocrit is present in anaemia, and a very high haematocrit is present in polycythemia), the bilirubin levels and triglyceride levels at which the devices will give accurate results, and the levels of each at which the results may become inaccurate. These levels are only found in extreme cases, and the vast majority of patients will be suitable to be tested using POC devices. The presence of antiphospholipid antibodies can make the INR very difficult to monitor, as these antibodies can interact with the reagents in both POC and in laboratory testing. It is generally recognised that these patients are best monitored in secondary care by laboratory methods and, in some very difficult cases, factor assays may be performed to assess the level of anticoagulation.

POC INR devices are not useful for assessing whether a patient is adequately anticoagulated on the direct oral anticoagulants (DOACs). Indeed, patients that are on these DOACS may well have a low INR result, but this does not mean they are not anticoagulated.

POC D-dimer Tests

In the last decade, the use of the D-dimer test has been used to aid in the diagnosis of VTE. The D-dimer test has already been covered in a previous chapter. However, it is included here as, recently, there has been a movement to perform the D-dimer in a POC setting, such as general practitioners' offices or emergency departments.

There are several POC D-dimer methods currently, with more in development. The Roche cobas h232 and the Alere Triage are both hand-held devices with disposable test cuvettes that give a quantitative result in around 15 mins. There is also the Alere Clearview and Ciga Suresign, which are single-use qualitative test kits that show a control line and a patient test giving a positive result; if no line is present, the test is negative (providing that a control line present). These four methods all use capillary blood samples, and any of these could be suitable for use in a GP setting. There are also some tabletop devices, such as the AQT90, which uses a venous whole blood sample taken into EDTA, citrate or heparin lithium, and takes around 15 minutes to produce results. These may be better suited to an emergency department setting.

However, D-dimer testing is complicated by the fact that there is no standardisation, and there is a range of different units in use, both within and between methods. This can lead to problems when running two different methods in the same hospital, and comparing the laboratory method with a POC method, as might happen in emergency departments. The laboratory will have a D-dimer method and have a normal range and a cut-off for VTE prediction, as the D-dimer test is also used in other clinical situations as well as VTE prediction.

However, POC D-dimer tests are generally only used for VTE prediction and, therefore, only require a cut-off value. Staff using these devices need to be trained in the use of the device, and also in interpretation of the test when coupled with a suitable clinical prediction score, such as the Wells score or similar. The use of these POC D-dimer tests can reduce the number of patients who require further tests which, in turn, reduces the anxiety of the patients and also reduces the cost. Of course, we want to achieve this, but do not want to miss any patients that might have a VTE.

D-dimer manufacturers state the specificity and sensitivity of their method so that users can decide how well they can perform, and can compare different methods. A reagent with 100% specificity means that no patient with a VTE will be missed (so no false negatives). A method with 100% sensitivity means that no patient will be referred for further tests unnecessarily (so no false positives). Therefore, a perfect method would have 100% specificity and 100% sensitivity. Unfortunately, however, this method does not exist at present, and a reasonable method now would have 100% specificity and around 98% sensitivity. This means that no patient with a VTE will be missed, and only a small number of false positives will occur.

Key Learning for POC INR Testing

- POC devices are small, portable, easy-to-use devices that can give accurate precise results.
- They give an INR result in around three minutes, so that the patients' dosage can be reviewed and adjusted there and then.
- Training is required to ensure that the finger stick procedure is as required to produce a small drop of whole blood to apply to the device. It is important that the whole blood is acquired quickly as, once the skin is pierced, this will trigger the coagulation process.
- A quality control system is required in the form of both IQC and EQA. The IQC is required to ensure the precision (consistency) of the system, whereas the EQA ensures the accuracy of the system. Any QC tests should be fully documented, and these records should be kept for at least eight years (guidance from The Royal College of Pathologists: *The retention and storage of pathological records and specimens, 5th edition*).

- Comparison checks between the POC and laboratory system are not suitable as a form of QC and any differences that are shown may lead to loss of confidence in the POC system, due to a general assumption that the laboratory is always correct – which is not always the case.
- POC D-dimer testing is now occurring in the UK, and can be used effectively to exclude VTEs if used with a clinical prediction score. Again, staff need to be trained in the use of the devices, in the QC required for the tests (IQC and EQA), and in the interpretation of these results in conjunction with a clinical prediction score (for example, the Wells score).

Further Reading

Jennings I, Kitchen D, Keeling D, Fitzmaurice D *et al.* (2014). Patient self-testing and self-management of oral anticoagulant with vitamin k antagonists: guidance from the British Committee for Standards in Haematology. *British Journal of Haematology* **167**(5): 600–7.

Keeling D, Baglin T, Tait C, Watson H *et al.* (2011). Guidelines on oral anticoagulation with warfarin – fourth edition. *British Journal of Haematology* **154**: 311–324.

Kitchen DP, Kitchen S, Jennings I *et al.* (2012). Point of Care INR testing devices: performance of the Roche CoaguChek XS and XS Plus in the UK NEQAS BC external quality assessment programme for healthcare professionals: four years' experience. *Journal of Clinical Pathology* **65**: 1119–112.

Purchasing and supply agency centre for evidence-based purchasing (2010). *Market review: D-dimer test for the exclusion of deep vein thrombosis.* nhscep.useconnect.co.uk.

Medical Devices Agency (2010). *Management and Use of IVD Point of Care Test Devices.* Medical Devices Agency Bulletin 2010: wwwmhra.gov.uk

Perry DJ, Fitzmaurice DA, Kitchen S, Mackie I, Mallett S (2010). Point-of care testing in haemostasis. *British Journal of Haematology* **150**: 501–514.

12

Direct Oral Anticoagulants in the Prevention and Management of Venous Thromboembolism

Yen-Lin Chee[1] and Henry G. Watson[2]

[1] *Consultant Haematologist, Department of Hematology-Oncology, National University Cancer Institute, Singapore*
[2] *Consultant Haematologist and Honorary Professor of Medicine, Aberdeen Royal Infirmary, Foresterhill Health Campus, Aberdeen, Scotland, UK*

DOACs in Treatment and Prevention of Venous Thromboembolism: Introduction

The last ten years has seen the development of a number of direct-acting oral anticoagulants (DOACs). These drugs directly inhibit the active site of either thrombin or FXa, unlike the vitamin K antagonists (VKA), which work indirectly by inhibiting the production of functional vitamin K dependent clotting factors. DOACs are not only as effective and safe as VKAs, but have many favourable characteristics. These include the lack of food interactions, few drug interactions and predictable dose-anticoagulant response, allowing fixed doses to be administered without monitoring of anticoagulant effect. DOACs have rapid onset of action ($\approx$2–4 hours), which is similar to that of low molecular weight heparin (LMWH), and a short half-life ranging from 5–17 hours. All are partially cleared renally, with the risk of accumulation in renal impairment.

The European Medicines Agency (EMA) and US Food and Drug Administration (FDA) currently approve four DOACs: the direct thrombin inhibitor (DTI), dabigatran (Pradaxa®); and three direct FXa inhibitors – rivaroxaban (Xarelto®), apixaban (Eliquis®) and edoxaban (Lixiana®), for use in venous thromboembolism (VTE). Large multi-centre Phase 3 clinical trials to evaluate their efficacy and safety are summarised below. These trials primarily aimed to demonstrate non-inferiority of DOACs compared with standard treatment.

In the orthopaedic trials, the primary efficacy outcome was a composite of any DVT, nonfatal PE and all-cause mortality, and the primary safety outcome was major bleeding. Two enoxaparin dosing regimens were used: the North American 30 mg twice daily (for total knee replacements only); and the European 40 mg once daily dose (UK licensed dose for orthopaedic surgery). In the treatment of VTE and prevention of recurrent VTE studies, the primary outcome was a composite of symptomatic VTE or VTE-related death while the primary safety outcome was major bleeding.

In the VTE treatment trials, initial parenteral heparin was given in the dabigatran and edoxaban studies, while apixaban and rivaroxaban were used from the start of treatment, without any bridging strategy. The DOACs were given at fixed doses, while VKAs were dose-adjusted to achieve an INR target of 2.5.

Current approved indications for DOACS are summarised in Table 12.1.

Table 12.1 Current approved indications for DOACs from FDA, EMA and Health Canada.

	US Food and Drug Administration (FDA)	European Medicines Agency (EMA)	Health Canada
Dabigatran	NVAF Prophylaxis for VTE after hip replacement surgery only Treatment and secondary prevention of VTE	NVAF Prophylaxis for VTE after elective total hip or knee replacement surgery Treatment and secondary prevention of VTE	NVAF Prophylaxis for VTE after elective total hip or knee replacement surgery Treatment and secondary prevention of VTE
Rivaroxaban	NVAF Prophylaxis for VTE after elective total hip or knee replacement surgery Treatment and secondary prevention of VTE	NVAF Prophylaxis for VTE after elective total hip or knee replacement surgery Treatment and secondary prevention of VTE	NVAF Prophylaxis for VTE after elective total hip or knee replacement surgery Treatment and secondary prevention of VTE
Apixaban	NVAF Prophylaxis for VTE after elective total hip or knee replacement surgery Treatment and secondary prevention of VTE	NVAF Prophylaxis for VTE after elective total hip or knee replacement surgery Treatment and secondary prevention of VTE	NVAF Prophylaxis for VTE after elective total hip or knee replacement surgery Treatment and secondary prevention of VTE
Edoxaban	NVAF Treatment and secondary prevention of VTE	NVAF Treatment and secondary prevention of VTE	Not available

NVAF – non-valvular atrial fibrillation; VTE – venous thromboembolism.

Oral Direct Thrombin Inhibitors

Prophylaxis

Dabigatran was assessed in four large Phase 3 orthopaedic surgery trials (RE-NOVATE and RE-NOVATE II in hip arthroplasty, and RE-MODEL and RE-MOBILIZE in knee arthroplasty). These studies compared two doses of dabigatran (220 mg and 150 mg once daily) against enoxaparin 40 mg once daily (RE-NOVATE, RE-NOVATE II and RE-MODEL), or 30 mg twice daily (RE-MOBILIZE). Both doses were non-inferior to enoxaparin for the primary efficacy outcome, with similar major bleeding, except in RE-MOBILIZE, where non-inferiority was not met. Dabigatran is approved at 220 mg once daily by the English National Institute for Health and Care Excellence (NICE) and the Scottish Medicines Consortium (SMC) for prevention of VTE after hip or knee arthroplasty, with a recommended dose of 150 mg once daily in patients over 75 years and in those with CrCl 30-50 ml/min.

Treatment

Two replicate trials (RE-COVER and RE-COVER II) randomised patients with acute symptomatic VTE to dabigatran 150 mg twice daily, or dose-adjusted VKA for six months. All patients received initial parenteral anticoagulation for a median of nine days. A pooled analysis by Schulman *et al.* (2014) showed dabigatran was non-inferior to VKA for the primary efficacy outcome with similar rates of major bleeding. There was significantly more dyspepsia in dabigatran recipients.

Dabigatran was evaluated in extended treatment for prevention of recurrent VTE in two studies. RE-MEDY compared dabigatran 150 mg twice daily with VKA for a further 6–36 months, after an initial 3–12 months of anticoagulation. Dabigatran was non-inferior to VKA for the primary efficacy outcome, with similar rates of major bleeding. RE-SONATE compared dabigatran 150 mg twice daily with placebo for a further 6–12 months, after an initial 6–18 months of anticoagulation. Dabigatran had superior efficacy to placebo but, as expected, with higher rates of bleeding. Dabigatran is approved by NICE and SMC at 150 mg twice daily after initial parenteral anticoagulation for at least five days for treatment of VTE, and at 150 mg twice daily for prevention of recurrent VTE. A dose of 110 mg twice daily is recommended by the summary product characteristic (SPC) for patients aged over 80 years.

Oral Xa Inhibitors

Rivaroxaban

Prophylaxis
Rivaroxaban 10 mg once daily was studied in four Phase 3 trials for prevention of VTE after total hip (RECORD 1 and 2) or knee arthroplasty (RECORD 3 and 4), compared with enoxaparin 40 mg once daily (RECORD 1–3) or 30 mg twice daily (RECORD 4). A pooled analysis by Turpie *et al.* (2011) showed superior efficacy for rivaroxaban with similar major bleeding, but significantly more major plus clinically relevant non-major bleeding, compared with enoxaparin. Rivaroxaban is approved by SMC and NICE at 10 mg once daily for prevention of VTE in patients undergoing total hip or knee arthroplasty.

MAGELLAN compared an extended course of rivaroxaban 10 mg once daily for 35 days to enoxaparin 30 mg twice daily for 10–14 days in acutely ill medical patients. The primary efficacy outcome was a composite of asymptomatic proximal DVT, symptomatic VTE and VTE-related death. Rivaroxaban was non-inferior to enoxaparin for the first ten days, and superior to placebo at day 30–35, but major bleeding was increased. Rivaroxaban is not approved for thromboprophylaxis in medical in-patients.

Treatment
In EINSTEIN-DVT and EINSTEIN-PE, patients with acute symptomatic DVT or PE were randomised to rivaroxaban (15 mg twice daily for three weeks, then 20 mg once daily) or dose-adjusted VKA for 3, 6 or 12 months. In a pre-specified pooled analysis by Prins *et al.* (2013), rivaroxaban was non-inferior to VKA for the primary efficacy outcome, with reduced major bleeding.

Rivaroxaban has also been evaluated in extended treatment for prevention of recurrent VTE. EINSTEIN-EXT compared rivaroxaban 20 mg once daily with placebo for a further 6–12 months, after an initial 6–12 months of anticoagulation for a first VTE. Rivaroxaban was superior to placebo, with no difference in major bleeding, but was associated with significantly higher rates of major plus clinically relevant non-major bleeding. SMC and NICE have approved rivaroxaban at 15 mg twice daily for three weeks, then 20 mg once daily for treatment of acute VTE without initial parenteral anticoagulation, and at 20 mg once daily for extended treatment for prevention of recurrent VTE.

Apixaban

Prophylaxis
Apixaban has been evaluated in three Phase 3 trials for prevention of VTE after total knee arthroplasty (ADVANCE 1 and 2) or hip arthroplasty (ADVANCE 3) at a dose of 2.5 mg twice daily, compared with enoxaparin 40 mg once daily (ADVANCE 2 and 3) or enoxaparin 30 mg twice daily (ADVANCE 1). ADVANCE-1 failed to meet non-inferiority, while ADVANCE 2 and 3 showed superior efficacy in favour of apixaban, with no difference in major bleeding. In a pooled analysis of ADVANCE 2 and 3 by Raskob *et al.* (2012), apixaban

was superior to enoxaparin for the primary efficacy outcome of major VTE (composite of adjudicated total proximal DVT, non-fatal PE and VTE-related death), with similar major bleeding. Apixaban is approved by SMC and NICE for prevention of VTE after total hip or knee arthroplasty, at a dose of 2.5 mg twice daily.

ADOPT compared an extended course of apixaban at a dose of 2.5 mg twice daily for 30 days to enoxaparin 40 mg once daily for 6–14 days in acutely ill medical patients. Apixaban failed to show superiority for the primary efficacy outcome, and was associated with more major bleeding. Apixaban is not approved for thromboprophylaxis in the medical in-patient setting.

Treatment

AMPLIFY randomised patients with acute VTE to apixaban 10 mg twice daily for seven days, then 5 mg twice daily or dose-adjusted VKA for six months. Apixaban was non-inferior to VKA for the primary efficacy outcome, with significantly less major bleeding. AMPLIFY–EXT randomised patients with a first VTE after 6–12 months of anticoagulation to receive two different doses of apixaban (2.5 mg or 5 mg twice daily) or placebo for a further 12 months. Both doses of apixaban were superior to placebo, with no difference in major bleeding. Apixaban is approved by SMC and NICE for acute VTE treatment without initial parenteral anticoagulation at 10 mg twice daily for seven days, then 5 mg twice daily for at least three months. The dose for extended treatment for the prevention of recurrent VTE is 2.5 mg twice daily.

Edoxaban

Prophylaxis

Edoxaban has been assessed in two relatively small Japanese Phase 3 trials for prevention of VTE in total hip and total knee arthroplasty, at a dose of 30 mg once daily, compared with enoxaparin 20 mg twice daily. Edoxaban significantly reduced the primary efficacy outcome, with similar bleeding compared with enoxaparin.

Treatment

Hokusai-VTE randomised patients with acute VTE to receive edoxaban 60 mg once daily (or 30 mg once daily in patients with CrCl 15–50 ml/min or weight < 60 kg), or dose-adjusted VKA for 3–12 months. All patients had initial parenteral anticoagulation, for a median of seven days. Edoxaban was non-inferior to VKA for the primary efficacy outcome, with no difference in major bleeding. Edoxaban is approved by NICE and SMC for treatment of acute VTE at a dose of 60 mg once daily after initial use of parenteral anticoagulation for at least five days, and in extended treatment for the prevention of recurrent VTE at a dose of 60 mg once daily. A dose reduction to 30 mg is recommended in patients with CrCl 15–50 ml/min, weight < 60 kg and concomitant use of some P-gp inhibitors.

Systematic Reviews and Meta-analyses of DOACs

In the absence of clinical trials directly comparing the relative efficacy and safety of DOACs, simple indirect treatment comparisons (ITC) and, increasingly, adjusted indirect comparisons in the form of network meta-analyses (NMA), are performed. However, treatment effects should be interpreted with caution, due to the inherent assumptions underlying indirect comparisons, including that of homogeneity and similarity of trials.

Prevention of VTE in Total Hip or Knee Arthroplasty

Gomez-Outes *et al.* (2012) compared the clinical outcomes of dabigatran, rivaroxaban and apixaban with enoxaparin in their study of 16 phase 2 and 3 trials with 38 747 patients. Compared with enoxaparin, symptomatic VTE was significantly lower with rivaroxaban, but similar for dabigatran and apixaban. However, rivaroxaban was associated with a trend for more major bleeding, which was not seen with dabigatran or apixaban. Indirect treatment comparisons found that rivaroxaban was associated with the lowest risk for symptomatic VTE, while apixaban had the lowest risk for clinically relevant bleeding.

Treatment of Acute VTE and Extended Treatment for Prevention of Recurrent VTE

Van der Hulle *et al.* included five Phase 3 acute VTE trials with 24 455 patients in their meta-analysis comparing dabigatran (RE-COVER), rivaroxaban (EINSTEIN-PE AND -DVT), apixaban (AMPLIFY) and edoxaban (HOKUSAI-VTE) with dose-adjusted VKA. All combined relative risks (RRs) for recurrent VTE, and fatal PE and overall mortality were similar between the DOACs and VKA. The combined RRs for major bleeding, clinically relevant non-major bleeding, non-fatal intracranial bleeding and fatal bleeding were significantly reduced in favour of the DOACs. However, the number of patients needed to be treated to prevent one major bleed was relatively high (56 to prevent one clinically relevant non-major bleed, and 1111 to prevent one fatal bleed).

Gomez-Outes *et al.* included six Phase 3 acute VTE trials (RE-COVER and RE-COVER II, EINSTEIN DVT and PE, AMPLIFY and HOKUSAI-VTE) in their meta-analysis of 27 127 patients. The primary efficacy outcome was recurrent symptomatic VTE, defined as a recurrent or new episode of symptomatic DVT or PE, and the primary safety outcome was major bleeding. DOACs were as effective as VKA in preventing recurrent VTE, with reduced major bleeding compared with VKA. A significant reduction in relative risk of intracranial haemorrhage and fatal bleeding was observed for DOACs, compared with VKA.

Practical Issues for DOAC Usage

While the introduction of the DOACs as an alternative for the management and prevention of VTE has simplified patient care in some key respects, it has complicated it in other ways. The key areas where there is lack of clarity and/or controversy in the management of VTE using DOACs include:

- monitoring, or lack of it;
- interpretation of routine coagulation tests performed on patients using DOACs;
- accurate measurement of drug concentrations;
- management of surgery and bleeding episodes.

Monitoring

One of the major issues for practitioners, and also for patients who have previously been anticoagulated with warfarin, is the step away from the need to routinely monitor the anticoagulant effect of the drug. In our experience, this lack of routine blood test monitoring is one of the key reasons given by our patients for choosing DOAC treatment over warfarin. It is worth noting that, although routine testing of anticoagulant effect is no longer required, this does not mean that there is no need or benefit in continuing to monitor these patients in other ways. A recent study of patients' anticoagulated with dabigatran, for example, showed that pharmacist-led adherence monitoring and reporting of adverse events improved compliance with therapy.

The outcome data from Phase 3 trials indicate that the DOACs at fixed dose are at least as efficacious and as safe as warfarin therapy. However, there is a wide range in the peak and trough levels of the DOACs between individuals, and several patient characteristics that predict high plasma drug levels have been identified. The key patient features that are associated with high drug concentrations include old age, low body weight, and impaired renal function. This has prompted suggestions that it may be possible, by making a small number of measurements of drug levels, to tailor dosing to individuals in order to optimise treatment. At present, however, fixed dose treatment should be combined with routine patient follow-up, to include review of any bleeding or thrombotic events, review of drug therapies for potential interactions, and routine assessment of renal function.

Interpretation of Routine Coagulation Tests

This is a major issue surrounding the safe use of the DOACs. The key problem is that, whereas warfarin produces a predictable effect on the prothrombin time that can be standardised by the use of the INR, the same is not the case for the DOACs. As a result, the interpretation of routine coagulation tests, such as the prothrombin time (PT) and the activated partial thromboplastin time (aPTT), is not straightforward in patients on DOACs, which is a potential safety issue.

Several studies have now shown the variable sensitivity of different PT and aPTT reagents to dabigatran, apixaban and rivaroxaban. In general, it appears that, for most reagents, dabigatran causes a prolongation of the aPTT with less effect on the PT, while the reverse is true for rivaroxaban. Both tests appear fairly insensitive to apixaban, which causes minimal or no prolongation of either test even at peak levels. To further complicate things for users, different reagents have different sensitivities, so that experience is not always transferable between centres, and this is particularly an issue for junior doctors on training rotations.

UK NEQAS coagulation have published their data on the sensitivities of different aPTT and PT assays to plasma samples spiked with different concentrations of dabigatran and rivaroxaban. Local laboratories may be able to use these to give guidance on approximate drug levels to users.

Accurate Measurement of Anticoagulant Drug Levels

There are several situations where it might be valuable to accurately measure the levels of a DOAC in plasma. These include:

- life-threatening haemorrhage;
- emergency surgery;
- acute renal failure;
- thrombotic event sustained during anticoagulation.

The specific laboratory assays that can be used to more accurately measure drug levels are given in Table 12.2.

At present, the quality assurance data for these assays are not completely reassuring, and further work needs to be done in this field.

Management of the Peri-surgical Period and Bleeding

Idarucizumab (Praxbind®), a humanized anti-dabigatran monoclonal antibody, is EMA and FDA-licensed as a specific reversal agent for dabigatran. A site-inactivated Xa molecule, andexanet alfa has been submitted to the FDA for approval as a universal antidote for factor Xa inhibitors. Published data for both of these agents are promising, with both molecules producing immediate, and almost complete, reversal of the anticoagulant effect of their respective targets.

The approach to peri-surgical management of patients on DOACs where a specific reversal agent is not available is based on adequate discontinuation of the drug prior to the planned procedure. The duration of

Table 12.2 Specific laboratory assays that can be used to more accurately measure drug levels.

Drug	Assay
Dabigatran	Ecarin clotting time, dilute thrombin time
Rivaroxaban	Calibrated anti-Xa
Apixaban	Calibrated anti-Xa
Edoxaban	Calibrated anti-Xa assay

discontinuation is determined by the bleeding risk of the surgery and by the calculated half-life of the drug, which is based primarily on renal function (see manufacturers' SPC).

In the absence of specific antidotes for the DOACs, the approach to bleeding has been to encourage local methods to stop bleeding, such as endoscopic intervention or simple surgical procedures. This is combined with the use of pro-haemostatic agents, such as tranexamic acid and prothrombin complex concentrates (PCCs). The use of activated charcoal, taken up to 3–6 hours post-ingestion of a DOAC, appears to reduce drug absorption. The evidence for these approaches is very much based on *ex vivo* and animal model work, and the general consensus is that the use of PCC should be confined to life- and limb-threatening bleeding.

DOAC Use in Specific Patient Subgroups

The extrapolation of results from DOAC trials to the general population should always take into account the stringent inclusion/exclusion criteria and underrepresented subgroups in the trial population. These include patients at extremes of weight, extremes of age, liver impairment, and those at high risk of bleeding. Other specific subgroups are discussed below.

Renal Impairment

All the DOACs are partially renally cleared, with a risk of accumulation in renal impairment. Patients with a CrCl ≤ 30 ml/min were excluded from the trials of orthopaedic prophylaxis after arthroplasty. In acute VTE trials with dabigatran, rivaroxaban and edoxaban, patients with CrCl ≤30 ml/min were excluded, while the apixaban trial excluded patients with CrCl ≤25 ml/min. However, the SPC for rivaroxaban, apixaban and edoxaban only contraindicates DOACs at a CrCl <15 ml/min. This is based on pharmacokinetic, and not clinical, data.

Cancer

NICE did not make specific recommendations for DOAC use in patients with active cancer, as this patient group was underrepresented in the Phase 3 acute VTE trials. Furthermore, there is no comparison with the standard of care, LMWH. The British Committee for Standards in Haematology (BCSH) recommends VKA or DOAC only for patients who cannot have or tolerate LMWH.

Complicated VTE

Patients with massive PE who were candidates for thrombolysis or thrombectomy were excluded from acute VTE treatment trials. Furthermore, DOACs have not been adequately studied in patients with antiphospholipid antibody syndrome, heparin-induced thrombocytopenia, or other complicated thrombophilia.

Key Points

1) NICE and SMC currently approve dabigatran, rivaroxaban, apixaban and edoxaban for the treatment of acute VTE and prevention of recurrent VTE. Dabigatran, rivaroxaban and apixaban are also licensed for the prevention of VTE in elective hip and knee arthroplasty.
2) Meta-analyses of acute VTE trials show that, as a class, DOACs have significantly less major bleeding, intracranial haemorrhage and fatal bleeding, compared with VKA. However, recommendations cannot be made for one DOAC over another, due to the lack of direct comparison.
3) Rivaroxaban and apixaban are approved for use in acute VTE as monotherapy, while dabigatran and edoxaban require at least five days of parenteral anticoagulation prior to starting the DOAC.

4) Health care practitioners should be aware that all DOACs can affect both routine and specialised coagulation tests.
5) Idarucizumab (Praxbind®) is EMA/FDA licensed as a specific dabigatran reversal agent, and andexanet alfa, a site-inactivated Xa molecule, is pending EMA/FDA approval for specific reversal of factor Xa inhibitors.
6) DOACs should be used with caution in specific patient subgroups, including those with renal impairment, cancer and complicated VTE.

Further Reading

EMA (2015). European Medicines Agency 1995–2015 [accessed 07 Jul 2015]. Available from: http://www.ema. europa.eu/ema/.

Gómez-Outes A, Terleira-Fernández AI, Lecumberri R, Suárez-Gea ML, Vargas-Castrillón E (2014). Direct oral anticoagulants in the treatment of acute venous thromboembolism: a systematic review and meta-analysis. *Thrombosis Research* **134**(4): 774–82.

Gómez-Outes A, Terleira-Fernández AI, Suárez-Gea ML, Vargas-Castrillón E (2012). Dabigatran, rivaroxaban, or apixaban versus enoxaparin for thromboprophylaxis after total hip or knee replacement: systematic review, meta-analysis, and indirect treatment comparisons. *BMJ* **344**: e3675.

Kitchen S, Gray E, Mackie I, Baglin T, Makris M (2014). Measurement of non-coumarin anticoagulants and their effects on tests of Haemostasis: Guidance from the British Committee for Standards in Haematology. *British Journal of Haematology* **166**(6): 830–41.

NNIoHaCE (2014). NICE: National Institute of Health and Care Excellence 2004 [accessed 07 Jul 2014]. Available from: https://www.nice.org.uk.

Prins MH, Lensing AW, Bauersachs R, van Bellen B, Bounameaux H, Brighton TA, Cohen AT, Davidson BL, Decousus H, Raskob GE, Berkowitz SD, Wells PS; EINSTEIN Investigators (2013). Oral rivaroxaban versus standard therapy for the treatment of symptomatic venous thromboembolism: a pooled analysis of the EINSTEIN-DVT and PE randomized studies. *Thrombosis Journal* **11**(1): 21.

Raskob GE, Gallus AS, Pineo GF, Chen D, Ramirez LM, Wright RT, Lassen MR (2012). Apixaban versus enoxaparin for thromboprophylaxis after hip or knee replacement: pooled analysis of major venous thromboembolism and bleeding in 8464 patients from the ADVANCE-2 and ADVANCE-3 trials. *Journal of Bone and Joint Surgery (British Volume)* **94**(2): 257–64.

Sardar P, Chatterjee S, Mukherjee D (2013). Efficacy and safety of new oral anticoagulants for extended treatment of venous thromboembolism: systematic review and meta-analyses of randomized controlled trials. *Drugs* **73**(11):1171–82.

Schulman S, Kakkar AK, Goldhaber SZ, Schellong S, Eriksson H, Mismetti P, Christiansen AV, Friedman J, Le Maulf F, Peter N, Kearon C and for the RE-COVER II trial investigators (2014). Treatment of Acute Venous Thromboembolism with Dabigatran or Warfarin and Pooled Analysis. *Circulation* **129**(7): 764–72.

SMC (2015). Scottish Medicines Consortium [accessed 7 Jul 2015]. Available from: https://www. scottishmedicines.org.uk/.

Turpie AGG, Lassen MR, Eriksson BI, Gent M, Berkowitz SD, Misselwitz F, Bandel TJ, Homering M, Westermeier T, Kakkar AK (2011). Rivaroxaban for the prevention of venous thromboembolism after hip or knee arthroplasty. *Thrombosis and Haemostasis* **105**(3): 444–453.

UFaDA (2015). US Food and Drug Administration [accessed 07 Jul 2015]. Available from: http://www.accessdata. fda.gov/scripts/cder/drugsatfda/index.cfm.

van der Hulle T, Kooiman J, den Exter PL, Dekkers OM, Klok FA, Huisman MV (2014). Effectiveness and safety of novel oral anticoagulants as compared with vitamin K antagonists in the treatment of acute symptomatic venous thromboembolism: a systematic review and meta-analysis. *Journal of Thrombosis and Haemostasis* **12**(3): 320–8.

Watson HG, Keeling DM, Laffan M, Tait RC, Makris M (2015). Guideline on aspects of cancer-related venous thrombosis. *British Journal of Haematology* **170**(5): 640–8.

13

The Role of Thrombolysis in the Management of Venous Thromboembolism

Carlos J. Guevara and Suresh Vedantham

Interventional Radiology Section, Mallinckrodt Institute of Radiology, Washington University in St. Louis, USA

Introduction

The use of thrombolysis in the treatment of venous thromboembolism (VTE) began with the use of systemic thrombolytic therapy, but has evolved substantially to include both pharmacological and mechanical methods, of which some are delivered via a small catheter. The first description of catheter-directed thrombolysis (CDT) for the treatment of venous thrombosis came about in 1991 (Okrent *et al.*, 1991). Clinical experience was initially directed at the most dire manifestations of VTE, but has gradually evolved to encompass less severely affected patients as well. Rigorous clinical studies, including the NIH-sponsored ATTRACT Trial (Acute Venous Thrombosis: Thrombosis Removal with Adjunctive Catheter-Directed Thrombolysis), are currently under way to better characterize the risks and benefits of CDT in patients with VTE (Vedantham *et al.*, 2013).

Rationale Behind CDT for Acute DVT

The development of thrombus in the deep venous system of the lower extremities impedes the natural pathways of blood flow, with increased drainage by collateral veins. In the acute setting, thrombus formation leads to vein inflammation, which can lead, in turn, to venous valve injury and incompetence. This process is more dramatic as the thrombus extends into the central veins (common femoral vein, external and common iliac veins and inferior vena cava). When these central veins are involved, blood flow from the lower extremities has a very complex route in order to complete its return to the IVC and, eventually, the heart.

As the thrombus matures from the acute event it can:

1) become fibrotic and scar down the vein;
2) become partially re-canalised with partial and abnormal flow through the vein, which might injure the valves; or
3) resolve completely by the body's own fibrinolytic system.

If the thrombus does not resolve, or there is valve damage, venous hypertension develops. Ultimately, this can lead to a constellation of symptoms known as post thrombotic syndrome (PTS). PTS most commonly presents as lower extremity pain, swelling, heaviness and fatigue, which can progress to venous stasis skin changes, dermatitis and ulcers (Table 13.1).

Handbook of Venous Thromboembolism, First Edition. Edited by Jecko Thachil and Catherine Bagot.
© 2018 John Wiley & Sons Ltd. Published 2018 by John Wiley & Sons Ltd.

Table 13.1 Extremity signs and symptoms of post-thrombotic syndrome.

Pain
Swelling
Fatigue
Heaviness
Paresthesias
Varicosities
Stasis dermatitis
Hyperpigmentation
Subcutaneous fibrosis
Skin ulceration

It is estimated that 25–50% of patients with DVT will develop PTS (Kahn *et al.*, 2008a), while severe PTS will occur in 5–10% of patients. Patients with PTS have a poor quality of life, comparable with chronic lung disease, diabetes, while patients with severe PTS have a quality of life similar to cancer and congestive heart failure patients (Kahn *et al.*, 2008b), so the importance of preventing PTS cannot be overemphasized.

Both the inflammatory changes and the venous lumen occlusion contribute to the pathophysiology of PTS. Larger and more central thrombi are less likely to re-canalise than peripheral and smaller thrombus (Markel *et al.*, 2003). Venous valve damage from the thrombus leads to reflux, and it is theorized that rapid resolution of the thrombus may preserve valvular function (O'Shaughnessy and FitzGerald, 2001; Meissner *et al.*, 1993).

The goal of CDT in most patients with extensive lower extremity DVT is to remove the thrombus and restore physiological and anatomical venous flow, to decrease the inflammatory changes, increase the likelihood of vessel patency, preserve venous valvular function and, ultimately, limit PTS development. At approximately two weeks, the thrombus begins to organise, and the likelihood of obtaining complete thrombus resolution decreases.

The standard of care, systemic anticoagulation, relies on the body's own fibrinolytic system to degrade and resolve the thrombus. Anticoagulation medications do not play an active role in thrombolysis but, rather, prevent thrombus propagation. Studies have demonstrated the addition of CDT to anticoagulation allows for earlier and more complete lysis (Elsharawy and Elzayat, 2002) when compared to anticoagulation alone, as well as decreased venous reflux (Laiho *et al.*, 2004), decrease in venous obstruction and an overall decreased incidence of PTS (Enden *et al.*, 2009).

Pre-procedural Evaluation and Indications

The use of thrombolytic agents carries a small, but real, risk of haemorrhage. Bleeding is most often localised to the venous puncture site but can involve the retroperitoneum, GI tract, brain, or spinal cord. Therefore, the patient's clinical status, medical history, symptomatology, thrombus load and risk of haemorrhage must be carefully assessed, and a personalised risk/benefit analysis should be made prior to embarking in the use of thrombolytics. Overall, the risk of major bleeding is probably between 3–7%, with intracranial bleeding around 0.5% (Mewissen *et al.*, 1999; Bjarnason *et al.*, 1997). Fatal pulmonary embolism and death are also rare complications (<0.5%).

On one end of the spectrum, there are patients with symptoms of venous congestion (pain, swelling) with central DVT that has not improved after anticoagulation, and with low risk of haemorrhage. On the opposite end of the spectrum, there are patients with massive lower extremity DVT that has progressed to include acute skin changes, blisters and signs of acute limb threat (arterial compromise, severe oedema, cyanosis, blistering, neurologic dysfunction and pain), known as Phlegmasia Cerulea Dolens (Table 13.2), for which

Table 13.2 Signs and symptoms of Phlegmasia Cerulea Dolens.

Acute skin changes (blisters, cyanosis)
Severe oedema
Extreme pain
Arterial compromise
Neurological dysfunction

rapid intervention might be needed to prevent limb loss or progression to systemic inflammatory response syndrome (SIRS) or sepsis. These two extreme examples illustrate how each patient is different, and how clinical judgment has to be employed in each case.

Many patients will present with symptomatic lower extremity DVT that has not improved (or worsened) on anticoagulation. The best candidates for CDT have involvement of the common femoral vein, iliac vein, and/ or IVC, and a low projected risk of bleeding. In contrast, the possible benefits of CDT are not likely to out-weigh the risks in patients with isolated calf DVT (Yamaki and Nozaki, 2005). It is important to remember that, while DVT symptoms and PTS are important to patients, they are not life-threatening conditions and, therefore, a low threshold should be employed to exclude patients who are at higher risk of bleeding.

A small minority of patients will present with Phlegmasia Cerulea Dolens, which should be considered a medical emergency. Limb salvage is the indication in this situation, and a more 'aggressive' approach to the risk profile might be accepted. However, the risk should remain low. If haemorrhage is a concern, then surgical thrombectomy might be the best option.

Contraindications

Major contraindications to CDT are any state that would predispose to haemorrhage, particularly in the central nervous system. Major criteria include active internal haemorrhage or DIC, recent stroke, TIA, neurosurgery or intracranial trauma within three months. Other states that place the patient at an increased risk for haemorrhage include recent CPR, abdominal surgery, solid organ biopsy, trauma or eye surgery, any CNS tumour (including the spinal cord), seizure disorder, uncontrolled hypertension (>180/110), recent major GI haemorrhage, allergic reaction to contrast agents, thrombocytopenia, right to left shunt, massive PE with tenuous hemodynamics, or concern for infected thrombus. (Table 13.3) Elderly patients (e.g. > 65 years of age) and those with liver dysfunction, renal failure, pregnancy, bacterial endocarditis, infectious thrombophlebitis and diabetic hemorrhagic retinopathy, may also be more likely to experience CDT-related complications.

Table 13.3 Contraindications to catheter-directed thrombolysis.

Major contraindications to CDT	Relative contraindications to CDT
Recent stroke, neurosurgery, CNS tumor	Age > 70
Recent major abdominal surgery (<3 months)	Liver dysfunction
Active hemorrhage, thrombocytopenia	Pregnancy
Uncontrolled hypertension	Solid organ biopsy
Sepsis, DIC	Diabetic retinopathy
Right to left shunt	
Septic thrombus	

Technical Aspects of CDT

CDT is routinely performed while the patient is under conscious sedation and, in most circumstances, in prone position. Therefore, patients should be able to breathe while prone and cooperate while sedated. Under ultrasound guidance, puncture of the popliteal vein or small saphenous vein is performed with a micropuncture needle. It is important to know the anatomy of the popliteal region, to avoid arterial puncture or nerve injury. A diagnostic venogram is performed to evaluate the extent of thrombus and obtain the appropriate catheter length needed for thrombolytic infusion (Figures 13.1 to 13.6). Non-ionic contrast agents are needed to thoroughly evaluate the veins and the response to therapy. Adequate renal function is required, so that contrast agents can be used.

The traditional CDT techniques involves starting with overnight pharmacological thrombolysis, followed by mechanical thrombolysis (if needed) the following day. There are physicians that employ mechanical thrombectomy or perform pharmacomechanical thrombolysis prior to overnight chemical thrombectomy, and therefore this should be left up to the physician's experience and comfort level.

Through the popliteal infusion catheter, recombinant tissue plasminogen activator (rt-PA) is initially infused for approximately 6–18 hours at 0.01 mg/kg/hr, not to exceed 1 mg/hr. At the same time, systemic anticoagulation is given. Generally speaking, an agent that can be reversed readily is preferred – either intravenous unfractionated heparin (often deliberately targeting a sub-therapeutic level – aiming at 1.2–1.7 times the control PTT, or empirically using 6–12 units/kg/hr), or twice-daily injections of a low molecular weight heparin.

Baseline CBC, PT, PTT and fibrinogen is obtained prior to rt-PA infusion. It is the author's practice to monitor the fibrinogen level and decrease the rt-PA dose if the fibrinogen falls rapidly or to a level below 100 mg/dl. Although there is no clear data to support this or any other threshold value, many physicians do believe that hypofibrinogenaemia may predict bleeding.

Patients undergoing thrombolytic infusion should be monitored in an ICU or step-down unit, so that any sign of haemorrhage can be immediately identified and appropriate steps taken to prevent catastrophic complications. In addition, frequent blood draws are needed to monitor red blood cell counts, coagulation

Figure 13.1 Initial venogram via a popliteal vein catheter, demonstrating acute thrombus in the femoral vein with increased flow through deep perforator branches, and the greater saphenous vein (GSV).

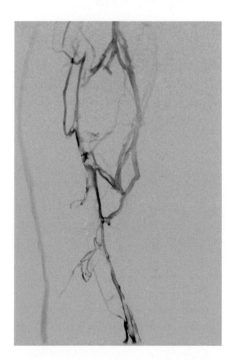

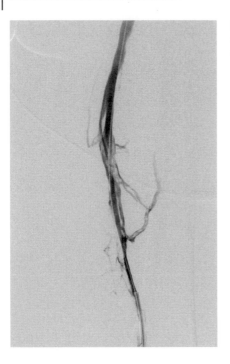

Figure 13.2 Follow-up venogram after 12-hour CDT rt-PA infusion demonstrates minimal residual thrombus with preferential flow through the femoral vein and decreased flow through perforators. The GSV is no longer visualised.

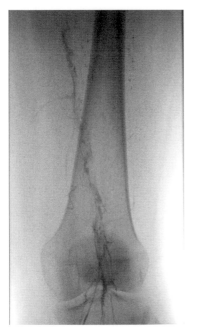

Figure 13.3 Venogram through popliteal catheter demonstrates acute thrombus in the popliteal and femoral vein.

parameters and fibrinogen during therapy. If there are any signs of bleeding, coagulation parameters should be obtained immediately, and the thrombolytic infusion should be stopped.

After initial thrombolysis, mechanical thrombectomy can then be used to remove any residual acute thrombus. Mechanical thrombectomy involves the use of devices that macerate or aspirate the thrombus. In certain circumstances, stents might be placed, particularly in chronically narrowed or thrombosed veins in the pelvis

Figure 13.4 Venogram after overnight CDT rt-PA infusion demonstrates complete thrombus resolution.

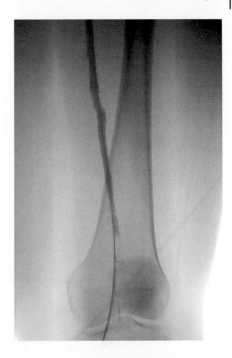

Figure 13.5 Pelvic venogram through right femoral catheter demonstrates acute on chronic thrombus extending to the IVC filter. Contrast surrounds the acute thrombus in the IVC and right iliac veins.

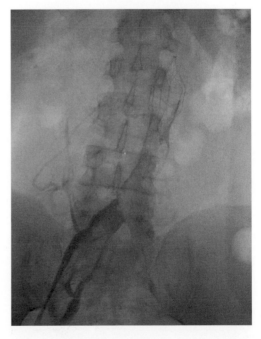

(Figure 13.7). It is the author's experience that most cases of unilateral CDT can be performed with one session of overnight rt-PA infusion, followed by definitive treatment with mechanical thrombectomy and, if needed, stent placement.

Prophylactic placement of an IVC filter has been considered optional. It is left to the physician's assessment of the patient to decide if the risk of pulmonary embolus is high, or the patient's clinical status is tenuous enough to require filter placement. Routine placement of an IVC filter is not recommended, as studies have

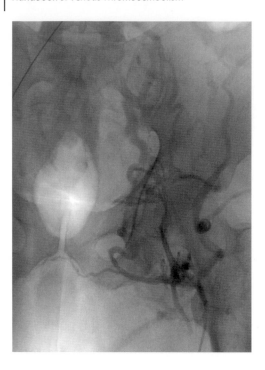

Figure 13.6 Left pelvic venogram through left common femoral vein catheter, collateral veins due to acute on chronic thrombus of the left iliac system.

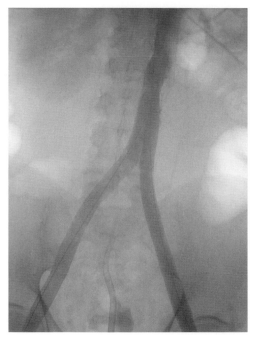

Figure 13.7 Overnight, CDT dissolved acute thrombus. However, there was residual high grade thrombus so, therefore, stenting of the iliac veins and IVC was performed. The final angiogram demonstrates anatomic flow without stenosis.

demonstrated that the risk of PE in patients undergoing CDT is similar to that of patients receiving anticoagulation alone. If a filter is placed, it is crucial to provide regular clinical follow-up and remove the filter as soon as appropriate.

Following completion of the intervention, the patient should be closely monitored for at least 6–12 hours, to ensure there is no bleeding. The patient will remain on therapeutic anticoagulation for at least three months, with the specific duration dependent upon the underlying risk factors for re-thrombosis. Outpatient follow-up will usually involve visits at one month, six months, one year, and yearly thereafter. Patients should be educated on the common signs of re-thrombosis, and encouraged to contact the physician quickly if symptoms recur.

CDT Pros and Cons

Potential benefits of CDT include providing earlier relief of presenting symptoms, decreasing the incidence of PTS, improving long-term quality of life, and (in rare patients who present with DVT causing acute limb-threatening circulatory compromise) limb salvage. Drawbacks to CDT are mainly related to the thrombolytic infusion which can lead to haemorrhage, which is most commonly minor and limited to the venous access site. However, the risk of major haemorrhage varies between 3–7% (Vedantham *et al.*, 2009). The risk of bleeding can be lessened by appropriate patient selection, meticulous procedural technique to minimise puncture site bleeding, and close monitoring during thrombolytic infusions.

Moderate sedation and its associated risks (over-sedation, aspiration, paradoxical reaction), and the inconveniences of undergoing an endovascular procedure, are other drawbacks of CDT. Patients who receive stents should be aware of the possible risks of late stenosis, re-thrombosis, migration, and malposition, as well as their nature as permanent implants, and the paucity of long-term information on their fate.

The cost of the endovascular procedure and the need for overnight ICU or step-down admission, make the expense a potential drawback of CDT. However, when this is compared to the decrease in productivity and need for medical attention in patients with PTS, it is possible that prevention of PTS by CDT may be cost-effective. This point remains to be proven.

Outcomes for CDT in DVT

To date, there have been several retrospective studies that have demonstrated improved outcomes in patients treated with CDT (without mechanical thrombectomy), when compared with systemic fibrinolysis, and CDT compared with anticoagulation alone. Elsharawy and Elzayat (2002) compared patients that had CDT versus anticoagulation alone, and demonstrated improved thrombus lysis in the CDT out to six months, as well as decreased obstruction and reflux in the CDT group (28% vs 88% in the anticoagulation group). A retrospective study by Laiho *et al.* (2004) demonstrated improved valvular competence in the CDT but similar disability scores. However, these studies had important methodological deficiencies.

The CaVent study (Enden *et al.*, 2012) was a multi-centre, randomised clinical trial from Norway that compared CDT plus anticoagulation to anticoagulation alone, and found a statistically significant reduction in PTS at two years in CDT recipients (26% relative risk reduction), with 3% major bleeding (and no intracranial bleeding or procedure-related death). As mentioned previously, the ATTRACT trial has completed patient recruitment, and results are expected in 2017.

Thrombolysis in Pulmonary Embolism

150 000–200 000 deaths are attributed to pulmonary embolus (PE) in the USA (Wood, 2002), and massive PE is associated with a 52% three-month mortality rate (Kucher *et al.*, 2006). Patients with massive and sub-massive embolus are managed with anticoagulation, and are sometimes considered for CDT. Clinically, the primary difference between massive and sub-massive PE is the presence of hemodynamic instability (i.e. persistent hypotension or bradycardia) in massive PE, in addition to the signs of right heart strain that are commonly seen in both groups of patients.

Therapy can be escalated in patients with massive PE, with the goal of preventing immediate death and reversing hemodynamic deterioration. In current practice, this usually consists of systemic intravenous administration of rt-PA, at the FDA-approved dosing of 100 mg. In some centres, either surgical thrombectomy or endovascular therapy may also be used in selected cases; when endovascular therapy is performed, the methods tend to vary considerably among different operators in different centres. For sub-massive PE, treatment can be escalated after careful individualised patient assessment, with the dual goals of preventing short-term clinical decompensation and improving long-term quality of life.

In 2014, three systematic meta-analyses were published, summarising the results of 16 randomised clinical trials evaluating the use of systemic thrombolysis for treatment of massive or sub-massive PE. These analyses demonstrated that the risk : benefit ratio of systemic thrombolysis is, indeed, very finely balanced, with a very small mortality benefit being counterbalanced by significant increases in major and intracranial bleeding in systemic thrombolysis recipients. The impact of these studies upon clinical practice remains to be seen. For patients with massive PE, the preponderance of evidence suggests that the use of systemic thrombolysis to prevent further clinical decompensation and (perhaps to a lesser extent) death may be more reasonable than previously appreciated. On the other hand, the increased bleeding risk may reduce enthusiasm for the use of systemic thrombolysis for stable patients with sub-massive PE, especially patients over 65 years of age, in whom bleeding is more frequent.

These findings have increased interest in carefully evaluating catheter-based PE treatment options, and in considering also the long-term patient consequences of the initial choice of PE therapy. Similar to lower extremity DVT, CDT of PE has the potential benefit of allowing greater efficacy (i.e. faster restoration of pulmonary artery flow and reduction of right heart strain) with use of reduced rt-PA dosage. While no randomised controlled studies have evaluated outcomes of CDT in PE, a pooled analysis of patients with massive PE who received some form of CDT observed clinical improvement (defined by improvement in hemodynamics, hypoxia and survival) in 87% of patients, with major complications in 2.4% (Kuo *et al.*, 2009). It must be noted, however, that this analysis included mostly case series, with few prospective studies, and that publication bias may have excluded patients with poor outcomes from the literature.

In recent years, the use of ultrasound-accelerated CDT for patients with massive or sub-massive PE has been studied with somewhat more rigour. With this method, a specialised catheter (EkoWave, EKOS Corporation, Bothell, WA) that emits low-power ultrasound is used to achieve the intra-thrombus drug delivery and to enhance thrombolysis via ostensibly improved drug dispersion. Available studies, which include one small RCT, have found ultrasound-accelerated CDT to successfully lyse pulmonary thrombi, and achieve faster resolution of right heart hemodynamics, than anticoagulation alone (Bagla *et al.*, 2015; Kucher *et al.*, 2014; Lin *et al.*, 2010). To date, there are no published PE studies comparing use of the ultrasound catheter with a standard multi-sidehole catheter.

CDT may have an important role in the treatment of massive and sub-massive PE, although precise estimates of safety and efficacy are not yet available. The available studies are quite heterogeneous in terms of the patients and specific treatments studied, precluding easy comparison. It is the author's belief that it is reasonable to consider use of CDT and related methods for patients with massive PE, if there is an experienced interventionalist available, the procedure area can be activated quickly, and staff availability and expertise permit close monitoring of critically ill patients. For sub-massive PE, randomised trials are badly needed to enable better assessment of risk and benefit. In the meantime, careful risk stratification, and a balanced discussion of options and expectations with the patient, is recommended.

Upper Extremity DVT

Patients with a history of central line placement or venous thoracic outlet syndrome (TOS) are at risk of developing thoracic central vein stenosis/occlusion with development of DVT, causing upper extremity pain and swelling.

Historically, these patients have been treated with anticoagulation and removal of the central venous catheter, if present. In carefully selected patients who are felt to be at low risk for bleeding, CDT has been employed to eliminate any acute thrombus, using techniques very similar to that of CDT for lower extremity DVT. Because the volume of thrombus is smaller, it is often possible to complete acute clot lysis in a single procedure session. Depending on the aetiology of the underlying venous stenosis, further therapy usually consists of immediate balloon angioplasty (for catheter-related stenoses) or surgical thoracic outlet decompression (generally performed 6–12 weeks later). Stents are generally contraindicated for sub-clavian vein placement, due to the likelihood of stent fracture. Aggressive angioplasty is not recommended for patients with thoracic outlet syndrome, since it may just aggravate the venous trauma from the surrounding compressive structures.

There have been no trials comparing anticoagulation alone against anticoagulation with CDT. Most experienced groups approach these patients in a multidisciplinary manner, involving haematology (anticoagulation), interventional radiology (prompt CDT) and vascular surgery (surgical decompression in the case of TOS). This type of approach was utilised by Melby *et al.* (2008) while treating competitive athletes with TOS, with 100% of the patients resuming their athletic activity after the comprehensive evaluation and treatment.

Key Points

- CDT permits intra-thrombus fibrinolytic drug delivery, enabling improved clot removal efficacy, a decreased drug dose and, probably, a decreased risk of major bleeding, compared with systemic delivery of fibrinolytic drugs.
- All patients being considered for CDT should undergo a careful individualised assessment of the potential for clinical benefit versus potential risks of bleeding and other complications. Because thrombolytic therapy increases the risks of major and catastrophic bleeding, careful patient selection and close monitoring in an advanced care unit are essential. Immediate physician evaluation is required if there are any signs of haemorrhage.
- Phlegmasia Cerula Dolens and massive PE are medical emergencies, for which either CDT or surgical thrombectomy (depending upon presence of contraindications to CDT and the type of local expertise) should be considered immediately.
- CDT of acute DVT involving the IVC, iliac vein, and/or common femoral vein may be considered for purposes of limb salvage (for patients with acute limb threat), prevention of PE (for patients with rapid caval progression despite initial anticoagulation) and/or relief of severe DVT symptoms that have progressed, or are not improving on anticoagulation.
- In patients with extensive acute proximal DVT, CDT has the potential to improve long-term venous patency, reduce venous valvular reflux and reduce the development of PTS.
- CDT may be used to treat sub-massive PE, but risks and benefits are finely balanced, so careful risk stratification and individualised patient assessment should be performed.
- CDT should not be used for chronic femoropopliteal DVT or isolated calf vein thrombosis.
- CDT can rapidly restore central venous patency in axillosubclavian venous thrombosis, and may be effective as part of an interventional-surgical strategy for venous TOS.

Further Reading

Baldwin MJ1, Moore HM, Rudarakanchana N, Gohel M, Davies AH (2013). Post-thrombotic syndrome: a clinical review. *Journal of Thrombosis and Haemostasis* **11**(5): 795–805.

Birn J, Vedantham S (2015). May-Thurner syndrome and other obstructive iliac vein lesions: Meaning, myth, and mystery. *Vascular Medicine* **20**(1): 74–83.

Lee L, Kavinsky CJ, Spies C (2010). Massive pulmonary embolism: review of management strategies with a focus on catheter-based techniques. *Expert Review of Cardiovascular Therapy* **8**(6): 863–73.

Thompson JF, Winterborn RJ, Bays S, White H, Kinsella DC, Watkinson AF (2011). Venous thoracic outlet compression and the Paget-Schroetter syndrome: a review and recommendations for management. *CardioVascular and Interventional Radiology* **34**(5): 903–10.

References

Bagla S, Smirniotopoulos JB, van Breda A, Sheridan MJ, Sterling KM (2015). Ultrasound-Accelerated Catheter-Directed Thrombolysis for Acute Submassive Pulmonary Embolism. *Journal of Vascular and Interventional Radiology* **18**: S1051–0443.

Bjarnason H, Kruse JR, Asinger DA, *et al.* (1997). Iliofemoral deep venous thrombosis: safety and efficacy outcome during 5 years of catheter-directed thrombolytic therapy. *Journal of Vascular and Interventional Radiology* **8**: 405–418.

Elsharawy M, Elzayat E (2002). Early results of thrombolysis vs anticoagulation in iliofemoral venous thrombosis: a randomised clinical trial. *European Journal of Vascular and Endovascular Surgery* **24**: 209–214.

Enden T, Haig Y, Kløw NE, Slagsvold CE, Sandvik L, Ghanima W, Hafsahl G, Holme PA, Holmen LO, Njaastad AM, Sandbæk G, Sandset PM; CaVenT Study Group (2012). Long-term outcome after additional catheter-directed thrombolysis versus standard treatment for acute iliofemoral deep vein thrombosis (the CaVenT study): a randomized controlled trial. *Lancet* **379**(9810): 31–8.

Enden T, Kløw NE, Sandvik L, Slagsvold CE, Ghanima W, Hafsahl G, Holme PA, Holmen LO, Njaastad AM, Sandbaek G, Sandset PM (2009). Catheter-directed thrombolysis vs. anticoagulant therapy alone in deep vein thrombosis: results of an open randomized, controlled trial reporting on short-term patency. *Journal of Thrombosis and Haemostasis* **7**: 1268–75.

Kahn SR, Shbaklo H, Lamping DL *et al.* (2008b). Determinants of health-related quality of life during the 2 years following deep vein thrombosis. *Journal of Thrombosis and Haemostasis* **6**: 1105–1112.

Kahn SR, Shrier I, Julian JA, *et al.* (2008a). Determinants and time course of the postthrombotic syndrome after acute deep venous thrombosis. *Annals of Internal Medicine* **149**: 698–707.

Kucher N, Boekstegers P, Müller OJ, Kupatt C, Beyer-Westendorf J, Heitzer T, Tebbe U, Horstkotte J, Müller R, Blessing E, Greif M, Lange P, Hoffmann RT, Werth S, Barmeyer A, Härtel D, Grünwald H, Empen K, Baumgartner I (2014). Randomized, controlled trial of ultrasound-assisted catheter-directed thrombolysis for acute intermediate-risk pulmonary embolism. *Circulation* **129**(4): 479–86.

Kucher N, Rossi E, De Rosa M, Goldhaber SZ (2006). Massive pulmonary embolism. *Circulation* **113**(4): 577–582.

Kuo WT, Gould MK, Louie JD, Rosenberg JK, Sze DY, Hofmann LV (2009). Catheter-directed therapy for the treatment of massive pulmonary embolism: systematic review and meta-analysis of modern techniques. *Journal of Vascular and Interventional Radiology* **20**(11): 1431–1440.

Laiho MK, Oinonen A, Sugano N *et al.* (2004). Preservation of venous valve function after catheter-directed and systemic thrombolysis for deep venous thrombosis. *European Journal of Vascular and Endovascular Surgery* **28**: 391–396.

Lin PH, Annambhotla S, Bechara CF, Athamneh H, Weakley SM, Kobayashi K, Kougias P (2010). Comparison of percutaneous ultrasound-accelerated thrombolysis versus catheter-directed thrombolysis in patients with acute massive pulmonary embolism. *Vascular* **17**(Suppl 3): S137–47. Erratum in: *Vascular* **18**(1): 62.

Markel A, Meissner M, Manzo RA, Bergelin RO, Strandness DE Jr. (2003). Deep venous thrombosis: rate of spontaneous lysis and thrombus extension. *International Angiology* **22**: 376–82.

Meissner M, Manzo RA, Bergelin RO, Markel A, Strandness DE Jr. (1993). Deep venous insufficiency: the relationship between lysis and subsequent reflux. *Journal of Vascular Surgery* **18**: 596–608.

Melby SJ, Vedantham S, Narra VR, Paletta GA Jr, Khoo-Summers L, Driskill M, Thompson RW (2008). Comprehensive surgical management of the competitive athlete with effort thrombosis of the subclavian vein (Paget-Schroetter syndrome). *Journal of Vascular Surgery* **47**(4): 809–820; discussion 821.

Mewissen MW, Seabrook GR, Meissner MH, *et al.* (1999). Catheter-directed thrombolysis for lower extremity deep venous thrombosis: report of a national multicenter registry. *Radiology* **211**: 39–49.

O'Shaughnessy AM, FitzGerald DE (2001). The patterns and distributions of residual abnormalities between the individual proximal venous segments after an acute deep vein thrombosis. *Journal of Vascular Surgery* **33**: 379–84.

Okrent D, Messersmith R, Buckman J (1991). Transcatheter fibrinolytic therapy and angioplasty for left iliofemoral venous thrombosis. *Journal of Vascular and Interventional Radiology* **2**: 195–200.

Vedantham S, Goldhaber SZ, Kahn SR, Julian J, Magnuson E, Jaff MR, Murphy TP, Cohen DJ, Comerota AJ, Gornik HL, Razavi MK, Lewis L, Kearon C (2013). Rationale and design of the ATTRACT Study: A multicenter randomized trial to evaluate pharmacomechanical catheter-directed thrombolysis for the prevention of postthrombotic syndrome in patients with proximal deep vein thrombosis. *American Heart Journal* **165**(4): 523–553.

Vedantham S, Thorpe PE, Cardella JF, Grassi CJ, Patel NH, Ferral H, Hofmann LV, Janne d'Othée BM, Antonaci VP, Brountzos EN, Brown DB, Martin LG, Matsumoto AH, Meranze SG, Miller DL, Millward SF, Min RJ, Neithamer CD Jr, Rajan DK, Rholl KS, Schwartzberg MS, Swan TL, Towbin RB, Wiechmann BN, Sacks D; CIRSE and SIR Standards of Practice Committees (2009). Quality improvement guidelines for the treatment of lower extremity deep vein thrombosis with use of endovascular thrombus removal. *Journal of Vascular and Interventional Radiology* **20**(7 Suppl): S227–39.

Wood KE (2002). Major pulmonary embolism: review of a pathophysiologic approach to the golden hour of hemodynamically significant pulmonary embolism. *Chest* **121**(3): 877–905.

Yamaki T, Nozaki M (2005). Patterns of venous insufficiency after an acute deep vein thrombosis. *Journal of the American College of Surgeons* **201**: 231–8.

14

Inferior Vena Cava Filters in the Management of Venous Thromboembolism

Anita Rajasekhar and Molly W. Mandernach

University of Florida College of Medicine, Gainesville, Florida, USA

Introduction

Venous thromboembolism (VTE), including deep vein thrombosis (DVT) and pulmonary embolism (PE), is a major cause of morbidity, mortality, and increased health care costs. Anticoagulants are the standard of care for both prevention and treatment of VTE (Geerts *et al.*, 2008); however, alternative mechanical prophylaxis is employed in those with active or perceived high risk of bleeding. In these scenarios, clinicians are faced with the decision of whether or not to utilise an inferior vena cava filter (IVCF) to prevent a potentially fatal PE. Since FDA approval of the first retrievable IVCF (rIVCF), utilisation has increased dramatically in the United States (Stein *et al.*, 2011). The largest proportional increase has been in patients at risk for PE, but who have neither PE nor DVT (i.e. prophylactic IVCFs).

The purpose of this chapter is to provide a comprehensive overview of the role of inferior vena cava filters (IVCFs) in the prevention or treatment of VTE. Where possible, evidence-based practice recommendations will be provided to address common clinical questions surrounding IVCF use. However, there is a lack of strong evidence in many areas related to IVCFs, in which case expert opinion will be highlighted.

Evidence for IVCFs

An IVCF is designed to capture a DVT in order to prevent it from travelling to the pulmonary circulation, thereby preventing a PE. However, unlike anticoagulant therapy, whose efficacy and safety have been demonstrated in prospective randomised controlled trials (RCTs), the benefit derived from IVCFs remains unproven. To date, the only RCTs evaluating the efficacy of IVCFs in the management of VTE are the PREPIC and PREPIC2 studies (Decousus *et al.*, 1998; PREPIC Study Group, 2005; Mismetti *et al.*, 2015).

In both studies, patients with acute proximal DVT were randomised to therapeutic anticoagulation alone versus anticoagulation and the placement of an IVC filter. These trials reported mixed results, with regards to prevention of PE and DVT in the filter groups. However, overall survival was no different, in either trial, between the filter group and non-filter group.

The results of PREPIC and PREPIC2 do not provide justification for routine placement of IVCFs in patients with proximal DVT. Unfortunately, because all patients received therapeutic anticoagulation, these data offer no insight into the outcome of the typical patient who has had an IVCF placed – namely, those who have contraindications to anticoagulant therapy. Nevertheless, in the absence of a randomised

Handbook of Venous Thromboembolism, First Edition. Edited by Jecko Thachil and Catherine Bagot.
© 2018 John Wiley & Sons Ltd. Published 2018 by John Wiley & Sons Ltd.

comparison between IVCFs and anticoagulation for treatment of VTE, these data are the principal available means by which filter efficacy and safety can be assessed.

A plethora of observational studies evaluating the benefit of IVCFs in various patient populations have been published, most with methodological limitations, and many with conflicting results. Unfortunately, these studies form the basis of variable practice patterns revolving around the use of IVCFs.

Complications of IVCFs

IVCF placement is usually performed through common femoral or jugular vein access. Most of the data on IVCF complications comes from case reports and case series. The Manufacturer and User Facility Device Experience (MAUDE) database is a web-accessible database established by the United States Food and Drug Administration (FDA) to compile voluntary reporting of adverse events associated with medical devices. From 2000–2010, over 842 IVCF- related complications were reported to the MAUDE database. Immediate procedure-related complications are uncommon (<1.0% of insertions), and include IVCF misplacement, pneumothorax, local haematoma, air embolism, carotid artery puncture, and arterio-venous (AV) fistula formation.

The reported frequency of long-term complications vary widely in the literature. These include inferior vena cava (IVC) thrombosis (2–30%), filter fracture (2–10%), filter migration (0–18%) and IVC perforation or penetration (0–86%) (Caplin *et al.*, 2011; Durack *et al.*, 2012; Oh *et al.*, 2011). The most reliable data for the frequency of DVT following filter placement come from the PREPIC study, which noted an 8.5% cumulative incidence of DVT at one year, 20.8% at two years and 35.7% at eight years, despite 35% of patients in the PREPIC study being on anticoagulation for the duration of follow-up (Decousus *et al.*, 1998; PREPIC Study Group, 2005).

In addition, a systematic review revealed that patients who received an IVCF for secondary VTE prevention (i.e. those with known VTE) had a higher risk of post-thrombotic syndrome than those who received an IVCF for primary prevention (Fox and Kahn, 2008). A recently recognised long-term complication of IVCFs is the entrapment of guide wires used to place vascular access catheters (Streib and Wagner, 2000). In several instances, forceful attempts to remove guide wires have led to filter displacement (Browne and Estrada, 1998; Loesberg *et al.*, 1993).

IVCF Retrieval

The rationale for using retrievable rIVCFs is to offer mechanical protection against PE during the limited high-risk period, when anticoagulation may be contraindicated. More than half of IVCFs are placed for temporary prophylaxis and, therefore, are candidates for retrieval (Kaufman *et al.*, 2009; Helling *et al.*, 2009; Tschoe *et al.*, 2009; Athanasoulis *et al.*, 2000). However, a systematic review showed an average retrieval rate of only 34% (Angel *et al.*, 2011). If attempted, approximately 85–90% of IVCF retrievals are successful (Thoung Van Ha, 2011; Uberoi *et al.*, 2011).

The optimal time frame for successful retrieval of IVCFs remains undefined, although retrieval is typically most successful within 9–12 weeks of insertion before filter adherence to the caval wall occurs (Thoung Van Ha, 2011; Uberoi *et al.*, 2011). Clinical factors that influence whether or not IVCF retrieval is attempted include comorbidities, concurrent anticoagulation, primary indication for placement, and documented plans for removal at the time of insertion or when the patient is discharged (Sarosiek *et al.*, 2013; Mission *et al.*, 2010; Irwin *et al.*, 2010). On August 8, 2010, the FDA issued a safety alert encouraging timely removal of IVCFs in order to avoid long-term complications (http://www.fda.gov.). Thus, strategies to increase retrieval rates are needed.

IVCFs and Anticoagulation

While IVCFs may protect against PE in the short term, prolonged indwelling IVCFs are associated with thrombotic complications, most commonly DVT and IVC thrombosis. Whether or not those with long-term indwelling IVCFs (either those with permanent IVCFs or with rIVCFs that were never removed) should remain on indefinite anticoagulation is a common clinical question. In the PREPIC study, 35% of patients in both the IVCF group and non-filter group remained on anticoagulation during the entire eight-year follow-up. While 15% of patients in the IVCF group experienced major bleeding events, there was no difference in mortality between the IVCF and non-filter group (PREPIC Study Group, 2005). Clinical outcomes based on presence or absence of continued anticoagulant therapy were not reported.

Retrospective studies addressing this clinical question have reported conflicting results (Billett *et al.*, 2004; Narayan *et al.*, 2009). A meta-analysis addressed the need for anticoagulation following IVCF placement (Ray and Prochazka, 2008). Data from nine studies indicated that anticoagulation after filter placement resulted in a trend towards decreased VTE, although this did not achieve statistical significance (OR 0.639; 95%CI 0.351–1.159, $p = 0.14$). However, due to methodological limitations of the individual studies, the authors concluded that routine long-term anticoagulation following IVCF placement can neither be supported nor refuted. Therefore, the benefit of continued anticoagulation with a long-term indwelling IVCF is unknown.

In considering long-term anticoagulation in patients with an IVCF, clinicians must weigh the risks (bleeding) and benefits (prevention of thrombotic events) of anticoagulation. As the risk of recurrent VTE declines over time, while the risk of bleeding with anticoagulant therapy remains constant (major bleeding risk on vitamin K antagonist is 2% per year), the risk : benefit ratio of long-term anticoagulation likely worsens as time passes (Carrier *et al.*, 2010; Palareti *et al.*, 1996). This conclusion may change with the emergence of target specific oral anticoagulants that appear at least as effective as warfarin in the treatment of VTE, with less bleeding (Schulman *et al.*, 2009; Bauersachs *et al.*, 2010; Buller *et al.*, 2012; Agnelli *et al.*, 2013; Hokusia-VTE Investigators, 2013). Until additional data are available, the duration of anticoagulation for patients with IVCFs should be determined on the basis of individualised assessment of the risk of bleeding and thrombosis, and not solely on the presence of a filter (Kearon *et al.*, 2012).

Specific Indications for IVCF Placement

Several professional medical societies have published practice-based guidelines or scientific statements addressing the indications for IVCF placement (Kearon *et al.*, 2012; Rogers *et al.*, 2002; Kaufman *et al.*, 2006; Baglin *et al.*, 2006; Jaff *et al.*, 2011; Lyman *et al.*, 2013; Konstantinides *et al.*, 2014; Falck-Ytter *et al.*, 2012; Gould *et al.*, 2012). Controversy exists over the absolute and relative indications for IVCF placement (Table 14.1). This variability likely explains the inconsistency in practice patterns of IVCF placement and retrieval.

Contraindication to or Complication from Anticoagulation

Although the vast majority of patients with an acute VTE can be managed with anticoagulation, anticoagulant therapy is contraindicated in a small subset of patients, usually due to active or high risk of bleeding, or the need for urgent major surgery. Because patients with an acute episode of VTE are at high risk for recurrence in the absence of anticoagulation (40% in the first month; Kearon and Hirsh, 1997; Kearon, 2003) and contraindications to anticoagulation are usually temporary, IVCFs should be considered for this population. In patients with an acute DVT, for example, within last 30 days, who require major surgery where therapeutic anticoagulation is contraindicated postoperatively, a perioperative retrievable IVCF is reasonable. If more than 30 days have passed since the thrombotic event, patients can usually be managed with bridging anticoagulation postoperatively, initially at prophylactic, then therapeutic doses, instead of an IVCF.

Table 14.1 Professional medical society practice-based guidelines for IVCF indications.

Indications	EAST^ 2002	SIR 2006	BSH^ 2006	AHA¥ 2011	ACCP* 2012	ASCO 2013	ESC€ 2014
Acute VTE and contraindication to AC	NR	Yes	Yes (grade B, level III)	Yes (class 1, level B)	Yes (grade 1B)	Yes	Yes (class IIa, level C)
Failure of AC	NR	Yes	Consider (grade C, level IV)	Yes (class IIa, level C)	NR	Consider	Yes (class IIa, level C)
Preoperatively if recent acute VTE (<30 days) and must have AC interrupted for surgery	NR	NR	Yes (grade C, level IV)	NR	NR	NR	NR
As an adjunct to therapeutic AC in acute VTE	NR	NR	No (grade A, level 1b)	No (class III, level C)	No (grade 1B)	NR	NR
Free-floating proximal DVT	NR	Consider	No (grade B, level III)	NR	NR	NR	No
Massive PE or proximal DVT undergoing thrombolysis	NR	Consider	No (grade C, level IV)	Consider (class IIb, level C)	NR	NR	NR
Primary prophylaxis in high-risk surgical patients (e.g. trauma, orthopaedic, or spinal)	Yes, if PP CI (level III)	Consider if PP CI	NR	NR	No (grade 2C)	NR	NR

Adapted with permission from Girard *et al.* (2014)

EAST – Eastern Association for the Surgery of Trauma (Rogers *et al.*, 2002); SIR – Society of Interventional Radiology (Kaufman *et al.*, 2006); BSH – British Committee for Standards in Haematology (Baglin *et al.*, 2006); AHA – American Heart Association (Jaff *et al.*, 2011); ACCP – American College of Chest Physicians (Kearon *et al.*, 2012; Falck-Ytter *et al.*, 2012; Gould *et al.*, 2012); ASCO – American Society of Clinical Oncology (Lyman *et al.*, 2013); ESC– European Society of Cardiology (Konstantinides *et al.*, 2014).

AC – anticoagulation; NR – not reported; PP – pharmacological prophylaxis; CI – contraindicated

Classification of evidence and grading of recommendations based on: * Grading of Recommendations Assessment, Development and Evaluation (GRADE) system, US Agency for Health Care Policy and Research (AHCPR) system. ¥ – American Heart Association Levels of Evidence, € – predefined ESC grading system.

Failure of Anticoagulation

True anticoagulant failure is an uncommon cause of recurrent VTE. RCTs of anticoagulation for VTE demonstrate 95% reduction in recurrent VTE. Furthermore, the PREPIC and PREPIC2 studies showed that IVCFs do not add incremental benefit to standard anticoagulation in the treatment of DVT. Therefore, any patient with recurrent VTE despite anticoagulation should be carefully evaluated for other causes of recurrent VTE prior to considering IVCF placement, such as non-adherence to anticoagulation therapy, inadequate dosing of anticoagulant therapy, or misdiagnosis as acute recurrent VTE when, in fact, it is chronic.

Instead of labelling these as failures of anticoagulation, efforts should be redoubled to maintain the patient in the therapeutic range, or to use an alternative anticoagulant, rather than place an IVCF that may predispose to further thrombosis and promote morbidity if sub-therapeutic anticoagulant therapy continues. If the patient has been clearly therapeutic, investigation for hypercoagulable syndromes, such as antiphospholipid syndrome, Trousseau's syndrome, or heparin-induced thrombocytopenia, should be undertaken (Khamashta *et al.*, 1995; Ruiz-Irastorza *et al.*, 2011; Sack *et al.*, 1977; Ishibashi *et al.*, 2005; Warkentin *et al.*, 2008). Because these syndromes are due to a systemic hypercoagulable state, regional approaches to prevent thromboembolism, such as IVCFs, are never adequate, and may exacerbate thrombotic morbidity and mortality. Instead, these conditions may require more intensive or alternative forms of anticoagulation. Recurrent events in the same location, despite therapeutic anticoagulation, should prompt consideration of anatomic abnormalities such as iliac vein compression (May-Thurner syndrome) or thoracic outlet Paget-Schröetter syndrome.

Massive Pulmonary Embolism

Patients with massive or sub-massive PE with hemodynamic compromise are often considered candidates for IVCF placement. The concern is that, despite therapeutic anticoagulation, even a recurrent small PE could lead to fatal outcomes, due to limited cardiopulmonary reserve. A retrospective analysis from an international registry found that in patients with massive PE (defined as hemodynamic instability on presentation) treated with therapeutic anticoagulation, IVCF insertion reduced 90-day mortality, compared with those that did not receive an IVCF (Kucher *et al.*, 2006). However, only 10% of patients with massive PE received an IVCF, and two-thirds did not receive thrombolysis. Therefore, conclusive evidence in support of IVCFs in this vulnerable population does not exist. The ACCP 2012 guidelines acknowledge that their firm recommendations *against* IVCFs in patients with acute VTE that can be treated with anticoagulation may not apply to this subpopulation with massive PE and hemodynamic compromise (Kearon *et al.*, 2012).

Thrombolysis of Acute Ilio-caval Venous Thrombosis

The principal complications of DVT are PE and post-thrombotic syndrome (PTS). While catheter-directed thrombolysis for DVT does not reduce the risk of PE, studies have shown that thrombolysis decreases the incidence of PTS (Pacouret *et al.*, 1997; Voet and Afschrift, 1991; Elliot *et al.*, 1979; Arnesen *et al.*, 1982; Grossman and McPherson, 1999). Implantation of an IVCF before systemic or catheter-directed thrombolysis to prevent embolisation of thrombotic fragments to the pulmonary circulation has been suggested (Mewissen *et al.*, 1999; Enden *et al.*, 2009). The evidence to support this practice is conflicting, and is based on mostly retrospective data.

In a multicenter registry of catheter directed thrombolysis, only one fatal pulmonary embolus (0.3%) occurred without routine filter use (Mewissen *et al.*, 1999). Therefore, the value of pre-emptive deployment of an IVCF during thrombolysis of DVT remains unproven. Clinicians should consider filters on a case-by-case basis after reviewing the patient's risk for embolisation (e.g., poorly adherent IVC, iliac thrombi) and mortality from PE (e.g., patients with concomitant PE, those with limited cardiopulmonary reserve).

IVCF for Primary PE Prophylaxis

Major Trauma Patients

Without pharmacologic prophylaxis, VTE is a common complication of major trauma, and can occur in up to 58% of patients, with 18% being proximal vein DVTs (Geerts *et al.*, 1994). While pharmacologic prophylaxis remains the mainstay of VTE prevention in this population, it is sometimes contraindicated due to active or high risk of bleeding from traumatic injury (Geerts *et al.*, 1996; Knudson *et al.*, 2004). Furthermore, the use of mechanical prophylaxis, with graduated compression stockings or intermittent pneumatic compression devices, may be precluded due to injury pattern. The rationale for using retrievable IVCFs is to offer mechanical protection against PE during the limited high-risk period when anticoagulation may be contraindicated.

A recent meta-analysis evaluated the evidence for prophylactic IVCFs in trauma patients without known VTE (Rajasekhar *et al.*, 2011). The authors found no RCTs addressing the role of prophylactic IVCFs in *any* patient population. Among observational studies in trauma patients, there was a statistically significant decrease in PE with prophylactic IVCF placement compared to matched controls (OR 0.21, 95% CI 0.09–0.49). However, these studies had significant limitations, most notably the lack of contemporary pharmacological prophylaxis. Thus, no firm recommendations, either for or against the routine use of prophylactic IVCFs in this population, could be made. Another recent meta-analysis confirmed these findings; the authors rated the strength of evidence as low to support the reduction of non-fatal and fatal-PE, insufficient to support a reduction in mortality, and insufficient to determine an increase or decrease in DVT in trauma patients receiving IVCFs versus no IVCFs (Haut *et al.*, 2014). Unfortunately, practice guidelines provide either conflicting or no recommendations on this practice (Table 14.1).

Cancer Patients

Cancer is a well-documented independent risk factor for the development of VTE. Thrombosis is the second cause of death in cancer patients and is predictive of worse short-term and long-term survival (Sorensen HT *et al.*, 2000; Khorana *et al.*, 2007; Khorana, 2010). Pharmacologic prophylaxis and treatment of VTE, specifically with low molecular weight heparin, is the preferred method based on Level 1 evidence (Lee *et al.*, 2003; Deitcher *et al.*, 2006; Iorio *et al.*, 2003). However, cancer patients with VTE being treated with anticoagulant therapy are at particularly high risk for recurrent VTE (hazard ratio of 3.2; 95% CI, 1.9–5.4) and major bleeding, compared with patients without cancer (hazard ratio of 2.2; 95% CI, 1.2–4.1) (Prandoni *et al.*, 2002). IVCFs have been suggested as an alternative or complimentary strategy to anticoagulation.

While case series have reported efficacy and safety of IVCFs in cancer patients with VTE, pooled analysis of comparative studies of filters versus anticoagulation have found an increased risk of symptomatic PE, DVT and IVC thrombosis in filter recipients, and no difference in overall survival between groups. However, the pooled rate of major bleeding was increased (Streiff, 2003) in the anticoagulant treated patients. In patients with cancer, IVCFs are more likely to be placed outside of guideline-supported indications, for example, for primary VTE prophylaxis (Abtahian *et al.*, 2014). In addition, cancer patients were more likely to experience negative clinical outcomes, such as shorter time to DVT, PE, IVC thrombosis and death. Furthermore, retrieval of IVCFs was less likely in cancer patients, compared with non-cancer patients, presumably due to shorter life expectancy (Abtahian *et al.*, 2014).

The effectiveness of IVCFs as an adjunct to therapeutic anticoagulation was studied in a single-centre randomised controlled trial (Barginear *et al.*, 2012). Sixty-four cancer patients with acute DVT were randomised to therapeutic doses of fondaparinux, with or without an IVCF. At three-year follow-up, there was no difference between the two groups in terms of recurrent DVT, PE, or IVCF thrombosis. Although a trend towards decreased survival was seen in the IVCF group, this may have been due to differences in patient characteristics at baseline (e.g. more patients with poor prognosis cancers in the IVCF group).

The hypercoagulable state associated with cancer affects all vascular beds. It would, therefore, ensue that regional approaches to preventing recurrent VTE, such as IVCFs, would not provide adequate protection in these patients, and may actually be harmful. Therefore, pharmacological approaches will continue to be the preferred therapy for most patients with cancer who have VTE. To reflect this approach, recent evidence-based guidelines on the prevention and management of VTE in cancer patients have recommended against the routine use of IVCFs for prevention and treatment of VTE (Table 14.2) (Lyman *et al.*, 2013; Farge *et al.*, 2013).

High-risk Orthopaedic Patients

Patients undergoing orthopaedic surgery, such as total knee arthroplasty (TKA) or total hip arthroplasty (THA), are considered to be at very high risk for the development of VTE, because of a number of factors that contribute to venous stasis, such as older age, position on the operating table, use of thigh tourniquets during knee arthroplasty, long periods of preoperative and postoperative immobility, as well as vascular injury. The prevalence of DVT without pharmacologic prophylaxis in this group of patients is as high as 40–60% (Geerts *et al.*, 2008). With contemporary pharmacological VTE prophylaxis, the rate of symptomatic DVT is estimated at 0.8% and PE at 0.35% (Falck-Ytter *et al.*, 2012). However, in certain orthopaedic populations, such as spinal surgery cases, the incidence of PE has remained high with appropriate pharmacological prophylaxis, and the

Table 14.2 Summary of randomised controlled trials of IVCFs.

Study	Population	Intervention	Comparator	Follow-up	Outcomes	Authors' conclusions
PREPIC (Angel et al. (2011), Thoung Van Ha (2011))	400 adult patients with proximal DVT +/– PE	Therapeutic AC	Therapeutic AC and permanent IVCF	8 years	12 days: PE 1.1%(F) vs. 4.8% (NF). $p = 0.03$ 2 years: DVT 21% (F) vs. 12% (NF), $p = 0.02$ 8 years: 50% in each group still on AC. Sx PE 6.2% (F) vs. 15.1% (NF), $p = 0.008$	In addition to therapeutic AC for acute DVT, IVCFs reduce the risk of short-term symptomatic PE, increase long-term DVT, and provide no mortality benefit.
Usoh et al. (2010)	156 adult patients with DVT or high-risk for DVT	Greenfield filter	TrapEase filter	12 months	IVCT/IVT 0% (G) vs. 6.9% (TF), $p = 0.019$	TrapEase filters increase risk of filter related complications compared with Greenfield filters.
Xiao et al. (2012)	108 adult patients with DVT undergoing catheter-directed thrombolysis	Straight introducer retrievable filter	Curved introducer retrievable filter	Until IVCF retrieval	Severe filter tilt 24.1% (straight) vs. 9.3% (curved), $p = 0.039$	The introducer curving technique minimises filter tilt which may improve filter retrieval
Rajasekhar et al. (2011b)	34 adult trauma patients without VTE	Pharmacologic prophylaxis	Pharmacologic prophylaxis and retrievable IVCF	6 months	Primary feasibility outcomes no different between groups Secondary efficacy outcomes @ 6 months: DVT 0.06% (F) vs. 0% (NF) PE 0% (F) vs. 0.06% (NF)	A large multicenter RCT evaluating IVCFs for primary prophylaxis in trauma patients is feasible
Barginear et al. (2012)	64 adult cancer patients with DVT +/– PE	Fondaparinux	Fondaparinux and IVCF	3 years	No difference in recurrent DVT, PE, or IVCF thrombosis. Trend towards increased survival in filter group	IVCF does not provide additional benefit to anticoagulation in cancer patients with DVT
FILTER-PEVI (Sharifi et al. (2012))	141 adults patients with symptomatic proximal DVT undergoing PEVI and therapeutic AC	IVCF	No IVCF	15 months	Symptomatic PE 1.4% (F) vs. 11.3% (NF) No difference in mortality	IVCF placement prior to PEVI reduced iatrogenic symptomatic PE without mortality benefit.
PREPIC II (Mismetti et al. (2015))	399 adult patients with acute PE + lower limb thrombosis (DVT or SVT) + additional risk factor	Therapeutic AC	Therapeutic AC and retrievable IVCF	6 months	3mos: PE 3%(F) vs. 1.5% (NF), $p = 0.5$ No difference in DVT, bleeding, death at 3 months or 6 months	Retrievable IVCFs are not indicated for routine use in symptomatic acute PE

Adapted with permission from Girard et al. (2014).
DVT – deep vein thrombosis; PE – pulmonary embolism; SVT – superficial vein thrombosis; AC – anticoagulation; IVCF – inferior vena cava filter; F – filter group; NF – non-filter group; IVCF – inferior vena cava filter thrombosis; IVT – iliac vein thrombosis; PEVI – percutaneous endovascular intervention

fear of bleeding (e.g. epidural hematoma) in the operative field due to anticoagulation has led to the consideration of IVCFs for primary prophylaxis. Unfortunately, RCTs in this patient population are likely not feasible and, therefore, clinical practice is based on observational studies with methodological limitations.

In a recent observational study involving more than 9000 orthopaedic patients, 90 patients (0.96%) received an IVCF, 55 (0.6%) for primary prophylaxis of PE. Only 51% of retrievable filters were removed at six months, and two patients (2.2%) encountered complications with the filter (Bass *et al.*, 2010). Glotzbecker and colleagues performed a systematic review of observational studies evaluating the rates of postoperative DVT and PE, with different forms of pharmacological and mechanical prophylaxis in spinal surgery patients. They reported the highest rate of DVT (22%) with use of prophylactic IVCFs, compared with other forms of VTE prophylaxis or no prophylaxis. The authors concluded that there is insufficient evidence to support the routine use of IVCFs in this population outside of consensus indications, namely acute VTE and contraindication to anticoagulation (Glotzbecker *et al.*, 2009).

In the era of targeted oral anticoagulants recently shown to be at least as effective as traditional pharmacological prophylaxis in prevention of VTE after high-risk orthopaedic surgery, the minimal benefit of prophylactic IVCFs is diminishing. Given the low quality of evidence available, potential for adverse events with IVCF placement and non-retrieval, and the efficacy and safety of contemporary pharmacologic prophylaxis, the routine use of IVCFs for primary prevention of PE in major orthopaedic surgery is not recommended (GRADE 2C) (Falck-Ytter *et al.*, 2012).

Bariatric Surgery

Several factors contribute to the increased risk of VTE in bariatric surgery patients: underlying obesity, added risk of surgery, comorbidities such as obesity hypoventilation syndrome and obstructive sleep apnoea, and possible under-dosing with standard fixed-doses of thromboprophylaxis. PE is considered the leading cause of perioperative death in bariatric surgical patients (Byrne, 2001; Eriksson *et al.*, 1997; Melinek *et al.*, 2002; Sapala *et al.*, 2003). The reported incidence of DVT is 1–3% and PE is 0.3–2%; however, mortality in patients with PE may be as high as 30% (Sapala *et al.*, 2003). The optimal drug, timing, dose, frequency, and duration of thromboprophylaxis in bariatric surgery are not established.

A recent survey of the members of the American Society of Metabolic and Bariatric Surgery found that 55% of respondents consider placement of an IVCF for thromboprophylaxis, compared with only 7% in a survey published by the same authors in 2000 (Barba *et al.*, 2009; Wu and Barba, 2000). Data from a prospective national registry reported that approximately 8.5% of 6376 patients who underwent bariatric surgery had an IVCF placed pre-operatively, 65% of which were for primary VTE prophylaxis (Birkmeyer *et al.*, 2010).

Despite this aggressive strategy for VTE prevention, IVC filter patients did not have reduced rates of postoperative VTE (odds ratio 1.28; 95% CI 0.51–3.21), serious complications (adjusted OR, = 1.40; 95% CI, 0.91–2.16), or death/permanent disability (adjusted OR, = 2.49; 95% CI, 0.99–6.26). In fact, 57% of patients with major perioperative complications could be attributed directly to the IVCF. A meta-analysis of IVCFs in bariatric surgery found that IVCFs were associated with a three-fold increased risk of postoperative DVT (RR2.81; 95%CI 1.33–5.97, $p = 0.007$) and death (RR 3.27; 95%CI0.78–13.64, $p = 0.1$), without reducing the risk of PE (RR 1.02; 95%CI 0.31–3.77, $p = 0.09$) (Kaw *et al.*, 2014). Given the poor retrieval rates of IVCFs and the lack of strong evidence for efficacy, IVCFs in this population should not be used routinely for primary VTE prophylaxis.

Conclusion

VTE is a significant public health problem, as PE is the leading cause of preventable hospital death. The standard of care for treatment of VTE is therapeutic anticoagulation. However, a subset of patients is unable to receive anticoagulation due to an increased risk of bleeding. In this patient population, as well as for broader indications, IVCF utilisation has increased exponentially, despite the lack of high-level data to support this practice (Stein *et al.*, 2011; Smouse and Johar, 2010; Girard *et al.*, 2014).

Research in the field of IVCFs is challenging, given the lack of standardised indications for placement and retrieval of these devices, geographical practice pattern variations, differences in the devices themselves, and the heterogeneous population in which these devices are deployed. Multidisciplinary experts have identified several unanswered questions surrounding IVCFs that require dedicated research studies (Kaufman *et al.*, 2009). These questions include:

- Do IVCFs improve mortality in patients with acute VTE and contraindication to anticoagulation?
- Do IVCFs add any benefit in addition to contemporary pharmacologic prophylaxis?
- Are there any populations that would benefit from primary VTE prophylaxis with IVCFs?
- What strategies can maximise removal of retrievable IVCFs?
- What is the ideal removal window for retrievable IVCFs?

Until such studies are carried out, a more restrictive approach to IVCF utilisation should be adopted, to prevent undue harm from these devices.

Key Points

1) The primary method of venous thromboembolism prevention and treatment is pharmacologic anticoagulation.
2) In patients with an acute DVT, where bleeding risk is perceived to be too high for anticoagulation, mechanical prophylaxis with an inferior vena cava filter is often considered.
3) Contraindication to anticoagulation in the setting of acute DVT is a generally agreed-upon indication for inferior vena cava filter placement, while other, more liberal indications are controversial.
4) There is a paucity of high-level evidence showing that inferior vena cava filters improve clinically relevant outcomes.
5) Practice patterns for inferior vena cava filter placement and retrieval vary considerably.
6) Unsubstantiated indications for inferior vena cava filter placement include primary prophylaxis in trauma, orthopaedic surgery, cancer, and bariatric surgery patients.
7) Retrievable inferior vena cava filters are rarely removed, which can lead to long-term sequelae.
8) Further research is needed to guide best practices of inferior vena cava filter placement and retrieval.

Further Reading

British Committee for Standards in Haematology Writing Group, Baglin TP, Brush J, Streiff M (2006).Guidelines on use of vena cava filters. *British Journal of Haematology* **134**(6): 590–595.

Farge D, Debourdeau P, Beckers M, *et al.* (2013). International clinical practice guidelines for the treatment and prophylaxis of venous thromboembolism in patients with cancer. *Journal of Thrombosis and Haemostasis* **11**(1): 56–70.

Kaufman JA, Kinney TB, Streiff MB, Sing RF, Proctor MC, Becker D, Cipolle M, Comerota AJ, Millward SF, Rogers FB, Sacks D, Venbrux AC (2006). Guidelines for the Use of Retrievable and Convertible Vena Cava Filters: Report from the Society of Interventional Radiology Multidisciplinary Consensus Conference. *Journal of Vascular and Interventional Radiology* **17**: 449–459.

Kaw R, *et al.* (2014). Inferior vena cava filters and postoperative outcomes in patients undergoing bariatric surgery: a meta-analysis. *Surgery for Obesity and Related Disorders* **10**: 725–733.

Kearon C, Akl EA, Comerota AJ, *et al.* (2012). Antithrombotic therapy for VTE disease: Antithrombotic Therapy and Prevention of Thrombosis, 9th ed: American College of Chest Physicians Evidence-Based Clinical Practice Guidelines. *Chest* **141**(2 Suppl): e419S–94S.

Konstantinides S, Torbicki A, Agnelli G, Danchin N, Fitzmaurice D, Galiè N, Gibbs JSR, Huisman M, Humbert M, Kucher N, Lang I, Lankeit M, Lekakis J, Maack C, Mayer E, Meneveau N, Perrier A, Pruszczyk P, Rasmussen LH, Schindler TH, Svitil P, Vonk Noordergraaf A, Zamorano J, Zompatori M (2014). 2014 ESC Guidelines on the diagnosis and management of acute pulmonary embolism. *European Heart Journal* **35**(43): 3033–3073.

Lyman GH, Khorana AA, Falanga A, *et al* (2007). American society of clinical oncology guideline: recommendations for venous thromboembolism prophylaxis and treatment in patients with cancer. *Journal of Clinical Oncology* **25**(34): 5490–5505.

Mismetti P, Laporte S, Pellerin O, *et al.* (2015). Effect of a Retrievable Inferior Vena Cava Filter Plus Anticoagulation vs Anticoagulation Alone on Risk of Recurrent Pulmonary Embolism – A Randomized Clinical Trial. *JAMA* **313**(16): 1627–1635.

PREPIC Study Group (2005). Eight-year follow-up of patients with permanent vena cava filters in the prevention of pulmonary embolism: the PREPIC (Prevention du Risque d'Embolie Pulmonaire par Interruption Cave) randomized study. *Circulation* **112**(3): 416–422.

Rajasekhar A, Streiff MB (2013). Vena cava filters for management of venous thromboembolism: a clinical review. *Blood Reviews* **27**(5): 225–41.

Rogers FB, Cipolle MD, Velmahos G, Rozycki G, Luchette FA (2002). Practice management guidelines for the prevention of venous thromboembolism in trauma patients: the EAST practice management guidelines work group. *Journal of Trauma* **53**(1): 142–164.

Disclosures

A.R. has funding from the American Society of Hematology. She has past involvement on physician advisory boards for Octapharma, Baxter, Bayer and Alexion. She has no other financial interests to disclose. M.W.M. has no financial interests to disclose.

References

Abtahian F, Hawkins BM, Ryan DP *et al.* (2014). Inferior Vena Cava Filter Usage, Complications, and Retrieval Rate in Cancer Patients. *The American Journal of Medicine* **127**: 1111–1117.

Agnelli G, Buller HR, Cohrn A, Curto M, Gallus AS, Johnson M, Masiukiewicz U, Pak R, Thompson J, Raskob GE, Weitz JI (2013). Oral Apixaban for the Treatment of Acute Venous Thromboembolism. *New England Journal of Medicine* **369**: 799–808.

Angel LF, Tapson V, Galgon RE *et al.* (2011). Systematic review of the use of retrievable inferior vena cava filters. *Journal of Vascular and Interventional Radiology* **22**(11): 1522–1530.e3.

Arnesen H, Hoiseth A, Ly B (1982). Streptokinase of heparin in the treatment of deep vein thrombosis. Follow-up results of a prospective study. *Acta Medica Scandinavica* **211**(1–2): 65–68.

Athanasoulis CA, Kaufman JA, Halpern EF *et al.* (2000). Inferior vena cava filters: review of a 26-year single-center clinical experience. *Radiology* **216**: 54–66.

Baglin TP, Brush J, Streiff M, British Committee for Standards in Haematology Writing Group (2006). Guidelines on use of vena cava filters. *British Journal of Haematology* **134**(6): 590–595.

Barba CA, Harrington C, Loewen M (2009). Status of venous thromboembolism prophylaxis among bariatric surgeons: have we changed our practice during the past decade? *Surgery for Obesity and Related Diseases* **5**(3): 352–356.

Barginear MF, Gralla RJ, Bradley TP, Ali SS, Shapira I, Greben C, Nier-Shoulson N, Akerman M, Lesser M, Budman DR (2012). Investigating the benefit if adding a vena cava filter to anticoagulation with fondaparinux sodium in patients with cancer and venous thromboembolism in a prospective randomized clinical trial. *Support Care Cancer* **20**: 2865–2872.

Bass AR, Mattern CJ, Voos JE, Peterson MG, Trost DW (2010). Inferior vena cava filter placement in orthopedic surgery. *American Journal of Orthopedics* **39**(9): 435–439.

Billett HH, Kornblum N, Jacobs L, Gargiulo N, III (2004). A Preliminary Analysis of Inferior Vena Cava Filters with and without Anticoagulation vs Anticoagulation Only: Readmission and Mortality Rates. *ASH Annual Meeting Abstracts* **104**(11): 1776.

Birkmeyer NJ, Share D, Baser O, Carlin AM, Finks JF, Pesta CM *et al.* (2010). Preoperative placement of inferior vena cava filters and outcomes after gastric bypass surgery. *Annals of Surgery* **252**: 313–18.

Browne RJ and Estrada FP (1998). Guidewire entrapment during Greenfield filter deployment. *Journal of Vascular Surgery* **27**(1): 174–176.

Byrne TK (2001). Complications of surgery for obesity. *Surgical Clinics of North America* **81**(5): 1181–93, vii–viii.

Caplin DM, Nikolic B, Kalva SP, Ganguli S, Saad WE, Zuckerman DA (2011). Quality improvement guidelines for the performance of inferior vena cava filter placement for the prevention of pulmonary embolism. *Journal of Vascular and Interventional Radiology* **22**: 1499–506.

Carrier M, Le Gal G, Wells PS, Rodger MA (2010). Systematic review: case-fatality rates of recurrent venous thromboembolism and major bleeding events among patients treated for venous thromboembolism. *Annals of Internal Medicine* **152**(9): 578–589.

Decousus H, Leizorovicz A, Parent F *et al.* (1998). A clinical trial of vena cava filters in the prevention of pulmonary embolism in patients with proximal deep-vein thrombosis. Prevention du Risque d'Embolie Pulmonaire par Interruption Cave Study Group. *New England Journal of Medicine* **38**(7): 409–415.

Deitcher SR, Kessler CM, Merli G *et al.* (2006). Secondary prevention of venous thromboembolic events in patients with active cancer: enoxaparin alone versus initial enoxaparin followed by warfarin for a 180-day period. *Clinical and Applied Thrombosis/Hemostasis* **12**: 389–396.

Durack JC, Wang JH, Schneider DB, Kerlan RK (2012). Vena cava filter scaffold to prevent migration of embolic materials in the treatment of a massive renal arteriovenous malformation. *Journal of Vascular and Interventional Radiology* **23**: 413–16.

EINSTEIN Investigators, Bauersachs R, Berkowitz SD *et al.* (2010). Oral rivaroxaban for symptomatic venous thromboembolism. *New England Journal of Medicine* **363**(26): 2499–2510.

EINSTEIN-PE Investigators, Buller HR, Prins MH *et al.* (2012). Oral rivaroxaban for the treatment of symptomatic pulmonary embolism. *New England Journal of Medicine* **366**(14): 1287–1297.

Elliot MS, Immelman EJ, Jeffery P *et al.* (1979). The role of thrombolytic therapy in the management of phlegmasia caerulea dolens. *British Journal of Surgery* **66**(6): 422–424.

Enden T, Klow NE, Sandvik L *et al.* (2009). Catheter-directed thrombolysis vs. anticoagulant therapy alone in deep vein thrombosis: results of an open randomized, controlled trial reporting on short-term patency. *Journal of Thrombosis and Haemostasis* **7**(8): 1268–1275.

Eriksson S, Backman L, Ljungstrom KG (1997). The incidence of clinical postoperative thrombosis after gastric surgery for obesity during 16 years. *Obesity Surgery* **7**(4): 332–5; discussion 336.

Falck-Ytter Y, Francis CW, Johanson NA *et al.* (2012). Prevention of VTE in orthopedic surgery patients: Antithrombotic Therapy and Prevention of Thrombosis, 9th ed: American College of Chest Physicians Evidence-Based Clinical Practice Guidelines. *Chest* **141**(2 Suppl): e278S–325S.

Farge D, Debourdeau P, Beckers M *et al.* (2013). International clinical practice guidelines for the treatment and prophylaxis of venous thromboembolism in patients with cancer. *Journal of Thrombosis and Haemostasis* **11**(1): 56–70.

Food and Drug Administration (FDA). http://www.fda.gov. Accessed 28 July 2015.

Fox MA, Kahn SR (2008). Postthrombotic Syndrome in Relation to Vena Cava Filter Placement: A Systematic Review. *Journal of Vascular and Interventional Radiology* **19**: 981–985.

Geerts WH, Bergqvist D, Pineo GF *et al.* (2008). Prevention of venous thromboembolism: American College of Chest Physicians Evidence-Based Clinical Practice Guidelines, 8th Edition. *Chest* **133**(6 Suppl): 381S–453S.

Geerts WH, Jay RM, Code KI *et al.* (1996). A comparison of low-dose heparin with low-molecular-weight heparin as prophylaxis against venous thromboembolism after major trauma. *New England Journal of Medicine* **335**(10): 701–707.

Geerts WH, Code KI, Jay RM, Chen E, Szalai JP (1994). A prospective study of venous thromboembolism after major trauma. *New England Journal of Medicine* **331**(24): 1601–1606.

Girard P, Meyer G, Parent F, Mismetti P (2014). Medical Literature, vena cava filters and evidence of efficacy. *Thrombosis and Haemostasis* **111**: 1–9.

Glotzbecker MP, Bono CM, Wood KB, Harris MB (2009). Thromboembolic Disease in Spinal Surgery. *Spine* **34**: 291–303.

Gould MK, Garcia DA, Wren SM *et al.* (2012). Prevention of VTE in nonorthopedic surgical patients: Antithrombotic Therapy and Prevention of Thrombosis, 9th ed: American College of Chest Physicians Evidence-Based Clinical Practice Guidelines. *Chest* **141**(2 Suppl): e227S–77S.

Grossman C and McPherson S (1999). Safety and efficacy of catheter-directed thrombolysis for iliofemoral venous thrombosis. *American Journal of Roentgenology* **172**(3): 667–672.

Haut ER, Garcia LJ, Shihab HM, Brotman DJ, Stevens KA, Sharma R, Chelladurai Y, Akande TO, Shermock KM, Kebede S, Segal JB, Singh S (2014). The Effectiveness of Prophylactic Inferior Vena Cava Filters in Trauma Patients. *JAMA Surgery* **149**(2): 194–202.

Helling TS, Kaswan S, Miller SL *et al.* (2009). Practice patterns in the use of retrievable inferior vena cava filters in a trauma population: a single center experience. *Journal of Trauma* **67**: 1293–1296.

Hokusia-VTE Investigators (2013). Edoxaban versus Warfarin for the Treatment of Symptomatic Venous Thromboembolism. *New England Journal of Medicine* **369**: 1406–1415.

Irwin E, Byrnes M, Schultz S *et al.* (2010). A systematic method for follow-up improves removal rates for retrievable inferior vena cava filters in a trauma patient population. *Journal of Trauma* **69**(4): 866–9.

Ishibashi H, Takashi O, Hosaka M *et al.* (2005). Heparin-induced thrombocytopenia complicated with massive thrombosis of the inferior vena cava after filter placement. *International Angiology* **24**(4): 387–390.

Jaff MR, McMurty S, Archer SL, Cushman M, Goldenberg N, Goldhaber SZ, Jenkins S, Kline JA, Michaels AD, Thistlethwaite P, Vedantham S, Whilte RJ, Zierler BK (2011). Management of Massive and Submassive Pulmonary Embolism, Iliofemoral Deep Vein Thrombosis, and Chronic Thromboembolic Pulmonary Hypertension. *Circulation* **123**: 1788–1830.

Kaufman JA, Rundback JH, Khee ST *et al.* (2009). Development of a Research Agenda for inferior venca cava filters: proceedings from a multidisciplinary research consensus panel. *Journal of Vascular and Interventional Radiology* **20**: 697–707.

Kaufman JA, Kinney TB, Streiff MB, Sing RF, Proctor MC, Becker D, Cipolle M, Comerota AJ, Millward SF, Rogers FB, Sacks D, Venbrux AC (2006). Guidelines for the Use of Retrievable and Convertible Vena Cava Filters: Report from the Society of Interventional Radiology Multidisciplinary Consensus Conference. *Journal of Vascular and Interventional Radiology* **17**: 449–459.

Kearon C (2003). Natural history of venous thromboembolism. *Circulation* **107**(23 Suppl 1): I22–30.

Kearon C and Hirsh J (1997). Management of anticoagulation before and after elective surgery. *New England Journal of Medicine* **336**(21): 1506–1511.

Kearon C, Akl EA, Comerota AJ *et al.* (2012). Antithrombotic therapy for VTE disease: Antithrombotic Therapy and Prevention of Thrombosis, 9th ed: American College of Chest Physicians Evidence-Based Clinical Practice Guidelines. *Chest* **141**(2 Suppl): e419S–94S.

Khamashta MA, Cuadrado MJ, Mujic F, Taub NA, Hunt BJ, Hughes GR (1995). The management of thrombosis in the antiphospholipid-antibody syndrome. *New England Journal of Medicine* **332**(15): 993–997.

Khorana AA (2010). Venous thromboembolism and prognosis in cancer. *Thrombosis Research* **125**(6): 490–493.

Khorana AA, Francis CW, Culakova E, Kuderer NM, Lyman GH (2007). Thromboembolism is a leading cause of death in cancer patients receiving outpatient chemotherapy. *Journal of Thrombosis and Haemostasis* **5**(3): 632–634.

Knudson MM, Ikossi DG, Khaw L, Morabito D, Speetzen LS (2004). Thromboembolism after trauma: an analysis of 1602 episodes from the American College of Surgeons National Trauma Data Bank. *Annals of Surgery* **240**(3): 490–6; discussion 496–8.

Konstantinides S, Torbicki A, Agnelli G, Danchin N, Fitzmaurice D, Galiè N, Gibbs JSR, Huisman M, Humbert M, Kucher N, Lang I, Lankeit M, Lekakis J, Maack C, Mayer E, Meneveau N, Perrier A, Pruszczyk P, Rasmussen

LH, Schindler TH, Svitil P, Vonk Noordergraaf A, Zamorano J, Zompatori M (2014). 2014 ESC Guidelines on the diagnosis and management of acute pulmonary embolism. *European Heart Journal* **35**(43): 3033–3073.

Kucher N, Rossi E, De Rosa M, Goldhaber SZ (2006). Massive pulmonary embolism. *Circulation* **113** (4): 577–582.

Lee AY, Levine MN, Baker RI *et al.* (2003). Low-molecular-weight heparin versus a coumarin for the prevention of recurrent venous thromboembolism in patients with cancer. *New England Journal of Medicine* **349**: 146–153.

Loesberg A, Taylor FC, Awh MH (1993). Dislodgment of inferior vena caval filters during 'blind' insertion of central venous catheters. *American Journal of Roentgenology* **161**(3): 637–638.

Lorio A, Guercini F, Pini M (2003). Low-molecular-weight heparin for the long-term treatment of symptomatic venous thromboembolism: meta-analysis of the randomized comparisons with oral anticoagulants. *Journal of Thrombosis and Haemostasis* **1**: 1906–1913.

Lyman GH, Khorana AA, Kuderer NM *et al.* (2013). Venous Thromboembolism Prophylaxis and Treatment in Patients With Cancer: American Society of Clinical Oncology Clinical Practice Guideline Update. *Journal of Clinical Oncology* **31**: 2189–2204.

Melinek J, Livingston E, Cortina G, Fishbein MC (2002). Autopsy findings following gastric bypass surgery for morbid obesity. *Archives of Pathology & Laboratory Medicine* **126**(9): 1091–1095.

Mewissen MW, Seabrook GR, Meissner MH, Cynamon J, Labropoulos N, Haughton SH (1999). Catheter-directed thrombolysis for lower extremity deep venous thrombosis: report of a national multicenter registry. *Radiology* **211**(1): 39–49.

Mismetti P, Laporte S, Pellerin O *et al.* (2015). Effect of a Retrievable Inferior Vena Cava Filter Plus Anticoagulation vs Anticoagulation Alone on Risk of Recurrent Pulmonary Embolism: A Randomized Clinical Trial. *JAMA* **313**(16): 1627–1635.

Mission JF, Kerlan RK Jr, Tan JH (2010). Rates and predictors of plans for inferior vena cava filter retrieval in hospitalized patients. *Journal of General Internal Medicine* **25**(4): 321–5.

Narayan A, Streiff MB, Hong K, Lee A, Kim H (2009). Anticoagulation does Not Prevent Venous Thromboembolism Following IVC Filter Placement: A Retrospective Study of 702 Patients. *ASH Annual Meeting Abstracts* **114**(22): 2104.

Oh JC, Trerotola SO, Dagli M, Shlansky-Goldberg RD, Soulen MC, Itkin M *et al.* (2011). Removal of retrievable inferior vena cava filters with computed tomography findings indicating tenting or penetration of the inferior vena cava wall. *Journal of Vascular and Interventional Radiology* **22**: 70–4.

Pacouret G, Alison D, Pottier JM, Bertrand P, Charbonnier B (1997). Free-floating thrombus and embolic risk in patients with angiographically confirmed proximal deep venous thrombosis. A prospective study. *Archives of Internal Medicine* **157**(3): 305–308.

Palareti G, Leali N, Coccheri S *et al.* (1996). Bleeding complications of oral anticoagulant treatment: an inception-cohort, prospective collaborative study (ISCOAT). Italian Study on Complications of Oral Anticoagulant Therapy. *Lancet* **348**(9025): 423–428.

Prandoni P, Lensing AW, Piccioli A *et al.* (2002). Recurrent venous thromboembolism and bleeding complications during anticoagulant treatment in patients with cancer and venous thrombosis. *Blood* **100**(10): 3484–3488.

PREPIC Study Group (2005). Eight-year follow-up of patients with permanent vena cava filters in the prevention of pulmonary embolism: the PREPIC (Prevention du Risque d'Embolie Pulmonaire par Interruption Cave) randomized study. *Circulation* **112**(3): 416–422.

Rajasekhar A, Lottenberg R, Lottenberg L, Liu H, Ang D (2011a). Pulmonary embolism prophylaxis with inferior vena cava filters in trauma patients: a systematic review using the meta-analysis of observational studies in epidemiology (MOOSE) guidelines. *Journal of Thrombosis and Thrombolysis* **32**(1): 40–46.

Rajasekhar A, Lottenberg L, Lottenberg R *et al.* (2011b). A pilot study on the randomization of inferior vena cava filer placement for venous thrombomebolism prophylaxis in high-risk trauma patients. *Journal of Trauma* **71**(2): 323–328.

Ray CE, Prochazka A (2008). The need for anticoagulation following inferior vena cava filter placement: a systematic review. *CardioVascular and Interventional Radiology* **31**(2): 316–324.

Rogers FB, Cipolle MD, Velmahos G, Rozycki G, Luchette FA (2002). Practice management guidelines for the prevention of venous thromboembolism in trauma patients: the EAST practice management guidelines work group. *Journal of Trauma* **53**(1): 142–164.

Ruiz-Irastorza G, Cuadrado MJ, Ruiz-Arruza I *et al.* (2011). Evidence-based recommendations for the prevention and long-term management of thrombosis in antiphospholipid antibody-positive patients: report of a task force at the 13th International Congress on antiphospholipid antibodies. *Lupus* **20**(2): 206–218.

Sack GH, Jr, Levin J, Bell WR (1977). Trousseau's syndrome and other manifestations of chronic disseminated coagulopathy in patients with neoplasms: clinical, pathophysiologic, and therapeutic features. *Medicine (Baltimore)* **56**(1): 1–37.

Sapala JA, Wood MH, Schuhknecht MP, Sapala MA (2003). Fatal pulmonary embolism after bariatric operations for morbid obesity: a 24-year retrospective analysis. *Obesity Surgery* **13**(6): 819–825.

Sarosiek S, Crowther M, Sloan M (2013). Indications, Complications, and Management of Inferior Vena Cava Filters. *JAMA Internal Medicine* **173**(7): 513–517.19.

Schulman S, Kearon C, Kakkar AK *et al.* (2009). Dabigatran versus warfarin in the treatment of acute venous thromboembolism. *New England Journal of Medicine* **361**(24): 2342–2352.

Sharifi M, Bay C, Skrocki L *et al.* (2012). Role of IVC filters in endovenous therapy for deep venous thrombosis: the FILTER-PEVI (filter implantation to lower thromboembolic risk in percutaneous endovenous intervention) trial. *CardioVascular and Interventional Radiology* **35**(6): 1408–1413.

Smouse B and Johar A (2010). Is Market Growth of Vena Cava Filters Justified? *Endovascular Today*: 74–77.

Sorensen HT, Mellemkjaer L, Olsen JH, Baron JA (2000). Prognosis of cancers associated with venous thromboembolism. *New England Journal of Medicine* **343**(25): 1846–1850.

Stein PD, Matta F, Hull RD (2011). Increasing use of vena cava filters for prevention of pulmonary embolism. *American Journal of Medicine* **124**: 655–61.

Streib EW and Wagner JW (2000). Complications of vascular access procedures in patients with vena cava filters. *Journal of Trauma* **49**(3): 553–7; discussion 557–8.

Streiff MB (2003). Vena Caval Filters: A Review for Intensive Care Specialists. *Journal of Intensive Care Medicine* **18**(2): 59–79.

Thoung Van Ha (2011). Retrievable Filters: Maximizing Retrieval Rates. *Seminars in Roentgenology* **46**(2): 154–8.

Tschoe M, Kim HS, Brotman DJ *et al.* (2009). Retrievable vena cava filters: a clinical review. *Journal of Hospital Medicine* **4**: 441–448.

Uberoi R, Chalmers N, Kinsman R, Walton P (2011). *The first BSIR inferior vena cava filter registry report.* Oxfordshire, UK: Dendrite Clinical Systems Ltd.

United States Food and Drug Administration. Manufacturer and user facility device experience database. http://www.accessdata.fda.gov/scripost-thromboticsyndrome/cdrh/cfdocs/cfMAUDE/search.cfm.

Usoh F, Hingorani A, Ascher E *et al.* (2010). Prospective randomized study comparing the clinical outcomes between inferior vena cava Greenfield and TrapEase filters. *Journal of Vascular Surgery* **52**: 394–399.

Voet D and Afschrift M (1991). Floating thrombi: diagnosis and follow-up by duplex ultrasound. *British Journal of Radiology* **64**(767): 1010–1014.

Warkentin TE, Greinacher A, Koster A, Lincoff AM, American College of Chest Physicians (2008). Treatment and prevention of heparin-induced thrombocytopenia: American College of Chest Physicians Evidence-Based Clinical Practice Guidelines (8th Edition). *Chest* **133**(6 Suppl): 340S–380S.

Wu EC and Barba CA (2000). Current practices in the prophylaxis of venous thromboembolism in bariatric surgery. *Obesity Surgery* **10**(1): 7–13 discussion 14.

Xiao L, Huang D, Shen J *et al.* (2012). Introducer Curving Technique for the Prevention of Tilting of Transfemoral Günther Tulip Inferior Vena Cava Filter. *Korean Journal of Radiology* **13**(4): 483–491.

Section IV

Special Situations

15

VTE in Pregnancy

Catherine Nelson Piercy

Professor of Obstetric Medicine, Women's Health Academic Centre, Guy's and St Thomas' Foundation Trust, London, UK

Introduction

Venous thromboembolism (VTE) in pregnancy is worthy of special consideration, because it is a significant cause of maternal mortality. There are differences in presentation, diagnostic pathways and management, compared with outside of pregnancy. Clinicians need to be aware that women are given hand-held maternity notes, which they keep throughout their pregnancy, and practitioners (both obstetric and non-obstetric) should document in these notes to facilitate good communication between teams.

Incidence

- Thrombosis and thromboembolism is the leading direct cause of maternal death in the UK.
- Six to ten women die in the UK each year from pulmonary embolism (PE) in pregnancy and the puerperium.
- Though the number of women dying from VTE in pregnancy is relatively small, many of these deaths are preventable.
- The incidence of fatal VTE in pregnancy is between 0.78 and 1.26 per 100 000 maternities in the UK over the last 10 years.
- The risk of antenatal VTE is four to five times higher in pregnant women than in non-pregnant women of the same age.
- VTE occurs in approximately 1 in 1000 pregnancies.
- VTE can occur at any gestation, but the puerperium is the period of highest risk.

Normal Physiological Changes of Pregnancy

- Normal physiological changes of pregnancy and the puerperium result in a relatively pro-thrombotic state, which starts in early pregnancy and persists for at least 12 weeks post partum.
- The elements that contribute to the pro-thrombotic state in pregnancy can be classified according to Virchow's triad (see Figure 15.1).

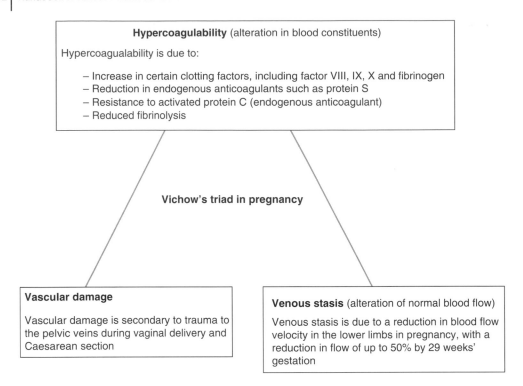

Figure 15.1 Virchow's triad in pregnancy.

Risk Factors

- Risk factors for VTE in pregnancy are outlined in Table 15.1.
- The most important risk factors are personal history of VTE and hospitalization.
- Other risk factors have varying degrees of risk associated with them.
- Risk factors can be divided into pre-existing, obstetric and transient.
- Risk assessment for VTE should begin in early pregnancy, and be repeated if the woman becomes unwell or is admitted to hospital for any reason, as the level of risk may change over the course of the pregnancy.
- In the first trimester, there may be transient risk factors, such as hyperemesis gravidarum and ovarian hyperstimulation syndrome
- Later in the pregnancy, other acquired conditions, such as pre-eclampsia (PET) increase risk of VTE, demonstrating the importance of re-assessing VTE risk through pregnancy.

Thrombophilias

- Thrombophilias are due to deficiencies or abnormalities in the naturally occurring inhibitor proteins of the coagulation system.
- Women with thrombophilias have an increased tendency to form blood clots, and are at increased risk of VTE in pregnancy.
- Thrombophilias can be inherited (antithrombin deficiency, Protein C deficiency, Protein S deficiency, Factor V Leiden, or Prothrombin gene mutation) or acquired later in life (such as antiphospholipid syndrome, including lupus anticoagulant and anticardiolipin antibodies).

Table 15.1 Risk factors for venous thromboembolism in pregnancy and the puerperium (from RCOG Green-top Guideline No. 37a).

Pre-existing	Previous VTE	
	Thrombophilia	*Heritable* Antithrombin deficiency Protein C deficiency Protein S deficiency Factor V Leiden Prothrombin gene mutation
		Acquired Antiphospholipid antibodies Persistent lupus anticoagulant and/or persistent moderate/high titre anticardiolipin antibodies and/or β_2-glycoprotein 1 antibodies
	Medical comorbidities, e.g. cancer; heart failure; active SLE, inflammatory polyarthropathy or IBD; nephrotic syndrome; type I diabetes mellitus with nephropathy; sickle cell disease, current intravenous drug user	
	Age > 35 years	
	Obesity (BMI > 30 kg/m^2) either pre-pregnancy or in early pregnancy	
	Parity ≥ 3 (a woman becomes para 3 after her third delivery)	
	Smoking	
	Gross varicose veins (symptomatic or above knee or with associated phlebitis, oedema/skin changes)	
	Paraplegia	
Obstetric risk factors	Multiple pregnancy Current pre-eclampsia Caesarean section Prolonged labour (>24 hours) Mid-cavity or rotational operative delivery Stillbirth Pre-term birth Post-partum haemorrhage (>1 litre/requiring transfusion)	
New onset/ transient	Any surgical procedure in pregnancy or puerperium except immediate repair of the perineum, e.g. appendicectomy, postpartum sterilisation Bone fracture	
	Hyperemesis, dehydration	
	Ovarian hyperstimulation syndrome (first trimester only)	Assisted reproductive technology (ART), *in vitro* fertilisation (IVF)
	Admission or immobility (≥3 days bed rest)	e.g. pelvic girdle pain restricting mobility
	Current systemic infection (requiring intravenous antibiotics or admission to hospital)	e.g. pneumonia, pyelonephritis, postpartum wound infection
	Long-distance travel (>4 hours)	

Source: Reproduced with permission of Royal College of Obstetricians and Gynaecologists.

- Some pregnant women will have a pre-existing diagnosed thrombophilia.
- Thrombophilia testing is usually prompted by VTE that was unprovoked, at a young age, or in an unusual site.
- Women may also have been screened due to a family member having a thrombophilia.
- The prevalence of various thrombophilias and their associated risk of developing VTE in pregnancy are detailed in Table 15.2.

Table 15.2 Prevalence and pregnancy risk of VTE with different heritable thrombophilias.

	Thrombophilic disorder	% of general population	Relative risk of VTE
Inherited	Antithrombin deficiency	0.07	5–20
	Protein C deficiency	0.3	2–8
	Protein S deficiency	0.2	2–6
	Factor V Leiden (heterozygous)	5–8	4–10
	Factor V Leiden (homozygous)	0.06	10–80
	Prothrombin gene mutation (heterozygous)	2–3	2–10
Acquired	Antiphospholipid antibodies Lupus anticoagulant Anticardiolipin antibodies	2	9
	Acquired APC resistance without Factor V Leiden	8–11	2–4

- Women with thrombophilias who are considering pregnancy need to have an individual VTE risk assessment, taking into consideration their thrombophilia, in addition to other risk factors, and be given VTE prophylaxis where appropriate.

VTE Prophylaxis in Pregnancy

- All women should undergo a VTE risk assessment pre-pregnancy or in early pregnancy (see Figure 15.2).
- Low molecular weight heparin (LWMH) is the main pharmacological agent used in VTE prophylaxis (see Table 15.3).
- Alternatives include:
  - fondaparinux, for women who are heparin-intolerant;
  - unfractionated heparin (UFH);
  - warfarin, which is restricted to situations where LMWH is unsuitable (e.g. some mechanical heart valves).
- Drugs *not* used for VTE prophylaxis in pregnancy are:
  - Aspirin, which, although safe in pregnancy, does not have good evidence of efficacy in VTE prophylaxis;
  - non-vitamin K antagonist oral anticoagulants (NOACS).
- Non-pharmacological interventions include anti-embolic stockings and pneumatic compression devices. These can be used in women with a contraindication to LMWH – for example, major obstetric haemorrhage.
- All pregnant and puerperal women should be advised to stay mobile and well hydrated.

Diagnosis of VTE in pregnancy

- Clinical assessment alone has a low specificity and sensitivity in the diagnosis of VTE in pregnancy, and investigations are needed to make an objective diagnosis.
- Symptoms of normal pregnancy (e.g. breathlessness, leg swelling) may mimic symptoms of VTE.

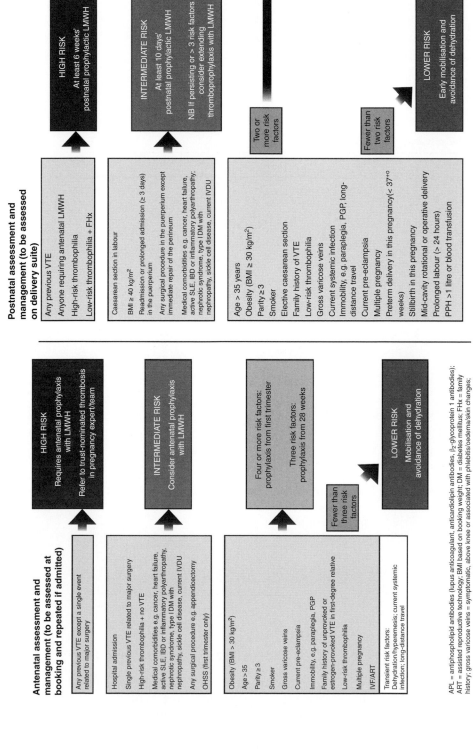

APL = antiphospholipid antibodies (lupus anticoagulant, anticardiolipin antibodies, β₂-glycoprotein 1 antibodies); ART = assisted reproductive technology; BMI based on booking weight; DM = diabetes mellitus; FHx = family history; gross varicose veins = symptomatic, above knee or associated with phlebitis/oedema/skin changes;

Figure 15.2 Obstetric thromboprophylaxis risk assessment and management.

Table 15.3 Suggested LMWH doses for antenatal and postnatal VTE prophylaxis.

Weight	Enoxaparin	Dalteparin	Tinzaparin
<50 kg	20 mg daily	2500 units daily	3500 units daily
50–90 kg	40 mg daily	5000 units daily	4500 units daily
91–130 kg	60 mg daily*	7500 units daily	7000 units daily*
131–170 kg	80 mg daily*	10 000 units daily	9000 units daily*
170 kg	0.6 mg/kg/day*	75 u/kg/day	75 u/kg/day*

* may be given once daily or as two divided doses.

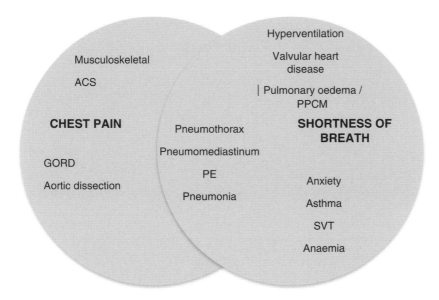

ACS = acute coronary syndrome, GORD = gastro-oesophageal reflux disease,
PPCM = peripartum cardiomyopathy, SVT = supraventricular tachycardia

Figure 15.3 Common and important causes of chest pain and breathlessness in pregnancy.

- The majority of pregnant women with breathlessness and chest pain do not have PE, so clinicians should think broadly about other possible causes (see Figure 15.3).
- Clinical decision scores largely do not apply in the pregnant population.
- The modified Well's score is not validated in pregnancy, and should not be used in this context.
- Women suspected of having VTE in pregnancy should commence treatment with low molecular weight heparin (LMWH) while they await investigations, which should be stopped only if VTE is excluded.

D-dimer in Pregnancy

- D-dimer should not be relied on to risk-stratify pregnant women.
- Physiology of pregnancy causes a progressive rise in D-dimer, and most women will have positive results.
- A negative D-dimer does not exclude VTE in pregnancy.
- The diagnostic pathways for VTE have been developed to exclude PE in low-risk individuals with a negative D-dimer, and should not be extrapolated to include higher-risk individuals, such as those who are pregnant.
- Checking D-dimer in pregnancy can give false positive and false negative results.

DVT in Pregnancy

- DVT can present with:
  - typical features of DVT outside of pregnancy:
    - o unilateral leg pain;
    - o leg erythema;
    - o leg swelling.
  - atypical features:
    - o low grade pyrexia;
    - o leucocytosis;
    - o lower abdominal pain (due to extension of thrombus into pelvic vessels and/or development of a collateral circulation).
- DVT is predominantly left-sided in pregnancy (ratio of 9:1 left : right) due to compression of the left iliac vein by the right iliac artery and the ovarian artery (compared with 55% left-sided outside pregnancy).

Investigations for DVT in Pregnancy

- Duplex ultrasound venography is the investigation of choice. There is no radiation from this test.
- If the initial ultrasound is negative, and clinical suspicion is low, LMWH can be discontinued (see Figure 15.4).
- If the initial ultrasound is negative and clinical suspicion remains high, LMWH should be stopped and the investigation should be repeated (at three and seven days after the initial investigation).
- Magnetic resonance imaging (MRI) is sometimes used, particularly where proximal DVT is suspected. This investigation does not expose the woman and fetus to any radiation.
- Around 10% of people with suspected DVT have the diagnosis confirmed with imaging, and the vast majority of studies are normal.
- Suspect iliac vein thrombosis in the presence of back, iliac fossa or buttock pain, or swelling of the entire leg. In this instance, ultrasound is the appropriate initial investigation, and MRV or conventional venography should be considered if results are negative and clinical suspicion remains high.

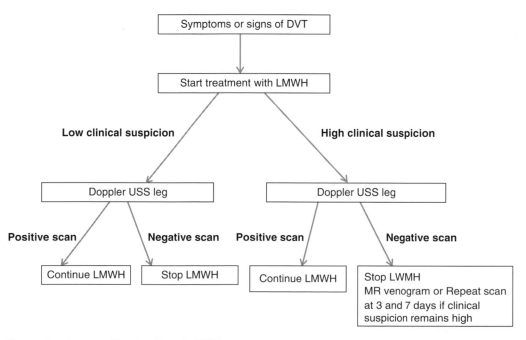

Figure 15.4 Investigation algorithm for DVT in pregnancy.

PE in Pregnancy

- PE typically presents with symptoms such as breathlessness, pleuritic chest pain of sudden onset, or collapse.
- The majority of pregnant women will experience a degree of breathlessness as part of normal pregnancy, particularly in the third trimester, and a thorough clinical assessment is needed to appropriately target investigations.
- A useful bedside test is to check oxygen saturations with a pulse oximeter. It is a reassuring feature if oxygen saturations are normal (≥96%) at rest and do not fall with exercise.
- Clinical assessment alone is not adequate to diagnose PE, and definitive investigations are required (V/Q scan or CTPA).
- Only about 5% of imaging for PE in pregnancy is positive.

Investigations for PE in Pregnancy

- Figure 15.5 outlines the diagnostic algorithm for PE in pregnancy.
- Helpful supporting investigations for PE in pregnancy are CXR, ECG, ABG and routine blood tests (FBC, renal profile, LFTs, CRP). These investigations will not make the diagnosis directly, but will help exclude other causes of symptoms.
- Definitive investigations for PE in pregnancy are perfusion scans (V/Q, Q, or V/Q SPECT) or CTPA scans.
- Pregnant women with suspected PE should have a CXR. This can exclude alternative causes of chest pain and breathlessness, such as pneumothorax, lobar collapse or pneumonia.
- The CXR in women with PE can be abnormal, with features such as atelectasis, pleural effusion, focal opacities or regional oligaemia.
- An ECG is also useful and should be carried out when PE is suspected. It is a quick and easy investigation to perform, and can help exclude other causes of chest pain and breathlessness (for example, ST elevation associated with ST-elevation MI).
- The most common ECG abnormality seen with PE in pregnancy is sinus tachycardia. However, other changes include:
  - Right axis deviation (RAD);
  - Right bundle branch block (RBBB);
  - T wave inversion;
  - Classic S1Q3T3 pattern.
- An arterial blood gas (ABG) may reveal hypoxia and hypocapnia:
  - Those with a normal CXR should proceed to V/Q scan.
  - V/Q SPECT scans are being used increasingly, and offer a greater degree of sensitivity than conventional V/Q scans.
- Advantages of V/Q scanning over CTPA are:
  - less non-diagnostic scans compared with CTPA;
  - less radiation to maternal lung and breast.
- CTPA may be chosen instead of V/Q scanning when:
  - V/Q scanning is not readily available;
  - a woman is haemodynamically unstable;
  - the CXR is abnormal and PE is suspected.
- Women with symptoms suggestive of a DVT (i.e. leg pain/swelling/erythema) *and* a PE (chest pain, breathlessness) may have Doppler US of the legs as an indirect way of diagnosing PE because, if the result is positive, there is no need for V/Q scan or CTPA and the chest pain and breathlessness can be attributed to PE.
- In women with no leg symptoms, Doppler US of the legs can be performed as an investigation to screen for DVT. However, it can delay definitive investigations for PE (i.e. V/Q or CTPA), and the result is very likely to be negative in the absence of leg symptoms.

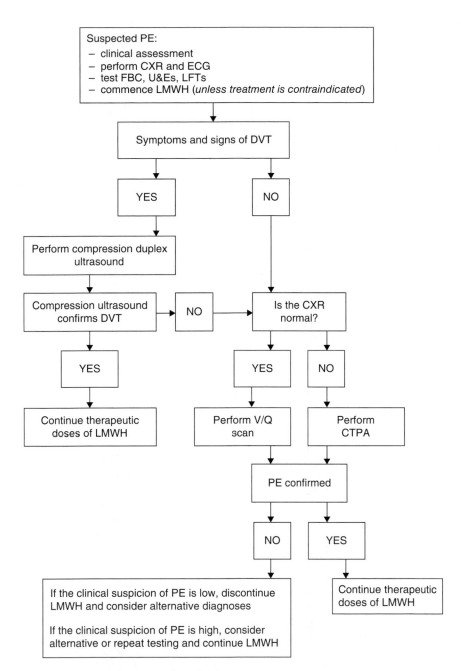

Figure 15.5 RCOG diagnostic algorithm for PE in pregnancy.

- A bedside transthoracic echocardiogram (TTE) is very helpful when massive PE is suspected. In this situation, the echocardiogram may show:
  - raised pulmonary artery pressure;
  - right ventricular dilatation;
  - right ventricular wall hypokinesis.

Radiation from Investigations in Pregnancy

- Women are often concerned about the radiation dose associated with imaging in pregnancy. This can be considered in terms of radiation to the fetus and radiation to the mother
- The estimated radiation dose from investigations for VTE (see Table 15.4a/b) is given as a range, because the dose varies according to local imaging protocols.
- The radiation dose associated with a CXR is very low (equivalent to around nine days' background radiation), and pregnancy is not a reason to withhold this investigation where it is indicated.
- The maximum recommended radiation exposure in pregnancy is 5 rad (50 000 µGy). The radiation dose associated with both CTPA and V/Q scanning is well below this threshold.
- The radiation dose to maternal lung and breast tissue is lower with V/Q scanning, compared with CTPA.
- The fetal radiation dose is lower with CTPA, compared with V/Q scan
- Some centres may perform a 'Q' or perfusion scan alone, reducing the radiation dose further.

Table 15.4 Estimated radiation doses associated with investigations for VTE.

Table 15.4a Estimated foetal radiation doses.

Investigation	Radiation (mGy) 1 rad = 50,000 mGy
CXR	<10
Limited venography	<500
Unilateral venography without abdominal shield	3140
Perfusion lung scan	400
Ventilation lung scan	10–350
CTPA	<10
Pulmonary angiography via brachial route	<500
Pulmonary angiography via femoral route	2210–3740

Table 15.4b Estimated maternal radiation doses from investigations for PE (from Cook and Kyriou, 2005).

	Radiation dose to maternal lung (mGy)	Radiation dose to maternal breast (mGy)
CTPA	39.5	10–60
V/Q	5.7–13.5	0.98–1.07

Reproduced with permission of BMJ Publishing Group Ltd.

Management

Anticoagulation in Pregnancy

- Low molecular weight heparin (LMWH) should be commenced once VTE is suspected or diagnosed (see Table 15.5a/b).
- The dose is based on the woman's booking or early pregnancy weight.
- Women should have blood samples sent for a full blood count, coagulation screen, renal profile and liver function tests, prior to commencing LMWH.

Table 15.5a Therapeutic dose (treatment dose) of enoxaparin.

Booking or early pregnancy weight	Initial dose of enoxaparin
<50 kg	40 mg BD or 60 mg OD
50–69 kg	60 mg BD or 90 mg OD
70–89 kg	80 mg BD or 120 mg OD
90–109 kg	100 mg BD or 150 mg OD
110–125 kg	120 mg BD or 180 mg OD
>125 kg	Discuss with haematologist

Table 15.5b Therapeutic dose (treatment dose) of tinzaparin.

Initial dose of tinzaparin (based on booking or early pregnancy weight)
175 units/kg OD

- LMWH can be given either once daily or twice daily, depending on the preparation, and should be in accordance with local guidelines.
- There is no need to monitor anti-Xa levels for the majority of women. However, for those at extremes of weight (<50 kg or >90 kg), this may be required.
- Women on LMWH for mechanical heart valves require anti-Xa monitoring.
- Vitamin K antagonists (e.g. warfarin) and novel oral anticoagulants (NOACs) are not licensed in pregnancy. Warfarin may be used in lactating women.
- Those diagnosed with DVT should wear graduated elastic compression stockings for two years following the DVT.
- Women should see the obstetric anaesthetist prior to term, to discuss regional anaesthesia and analgesia.
- Clinicians should write a plan for peripartum anticoagulation in the hand-held maternity notes.

Anticoagulation Intrapartum

- If a woman is diagnosed with VTE at term, intravenous unfractionated heparin (UFH) can be used instead of LMWH subcutaneous injections. The benefit of this strategy is that the woman is still receiving treatment for newly diagnosed VTE, but intravenous UFH has a shorter half-life than LMWH. Thus, the infusion can be stopped, should the woman develop bleeding complications or go into labour.
- Women on LMWH should be advised to discontinue their injections as soon as they experience onset of labour. Those who are scheduled for an elective caesarean section or induction of labour should omit their LMWH in the preceding 24 hours. If induction is delayed or prolonged, further doses of LMWH (or UFH) should be administered
- There should be a gap of at least 24 hours between the most recent LMWH injection and regional analgesia or anaesthesia (epidural or spinal), to reduce the risk of epidural haematoma.
- LMWH should not be given for at least four hours after the epidural catheter has been removed, and the cannula should not be removed within 12 hours of the most recent injection.

Anticoagulation Post-partum

- Following delivery, women can be converted to oral anticoagulants (such as warfarin), or choose to remain on LMWH.
- Some will have become accustomed to LMWH and choose to continue taking it, because of the advantage of blood monitoring not being required.

- It is advisable to wait until at least five days after delivery before starting warfarin, and longer in women at risk of post-partum haemorrhage.
- The total period of anticoagulation needs to be assessed on an individual basis, but should be:
  - for a minimum of three months AND
  - for at least six weeks post-partum AND
  - for the remainder of the pregnancy.
- Women should be advised that LMWH and warfarin are both safe for breastfeeding.
- Local guidelines should be followed for warfarin loading.
- NOACs can be used for postnatal anticoagulation in women who are not breastfeeding.

LMWH vs. UFH (Unfractionated Heparin)

- LMWH has several advantages over UFH:
  - It is easy to administer LMWH as a subcutaneous injection at home, and it comes in pre-filled syringes.
  - LMWH does not require platelet monitoring, whereas this is needed for women on UFH, due to the risk of heparin-induced thrombocytopenia (HIT).
  - LMWH is associated with a lower incidence of heparin-induced-osteoporosis and a reduced risk of haemorrhage compared with UFH.
  - LMWH does not require monitoring of APTT ratio.
- The major advantage of UFH is the rapid onset and offset, making it a useful treatment in:
  - women at risk of haemorrhage;
  - the treatment of women with massive life-threatening PE.

IVC Filters

- Inferior vena cava filters (IVC filters) are placed in the inferior vena cava, usually by interventional radiologists, with the aim of reducing PE in people with DVT.
- IVC filters are very rarely necessary in pregnancy.
- Outside of pregnancy, IVC filters reduce PE, increase DVT, and do not change the overall frequency of VTE.
- Their use is generally restricted to:
  - women with proven DVT and ongoing PE despite adequate anticoagulation;
  - women with contraindications to anticoagulation, such as recent or severe haemorrhage.
- The risks associated with IVC filters are hazards of placement, such as filter migration (>20% of patients), filter fracture (5%) and IVC perforation (5%)
- IVC filters should be removed as soon as possible.
- Women who become pregnant and have IVC filters in place that pre-date the pregnancy should be given anticoagulation with LMWH, as pregnancy in addition to IVC filter increases their risk of developing DVT in pregnancy.

VTE in Unusual Sites

- Women can develop VTE in unusual sites, such as upper extremity DVT, and cerebral venous sinus thrombosis (CVT).
- There is a particular association between upper extremity DVT and ovarian hyperstimulation syndrome following IVF.
- Anyone who develops thrombus in unusual sites should be investigated for thrombophilias.

CVT

- CVT presents with symptoms such as headache, seizures and neurological deficit, such as hemiparesis.
- It can occur at any gestation, but is more common in the post-partum period.

- Investigations for CVT are a CT scan initially (to exclude haemorrhage and other acute cerebral disorders) and MRV (magnetic resonance or CT venography).
- CVT is associated with mortality, ranging from 4–36%.
- Management is with rehydration and anticoagulation, with anti-epileptic drugs for control of seizures if necessary.

Thrombophilia Screening

- Almost half of all women who have an episode of VTE in pregnancy will have an underlying heritable or acquired thrombophilia.
- The presence of an acquired or heritable thrombophilia does not alter the acute management of VTE, but it does inform decisions regarding length of period of anticoagulation and management of future pregnancies.
- Thrombophilia screening is not advised at the time of acute VTE, because normal physiological changes of pregnancy (for example, protein S levels falling,) can affect results.
- Acute VTE itself can also give misleading results. Levels of protein C, protein S and antithrombin can fall, particularly if the clot is extensive.
- Genetic testing – for example, for Factor V Leiden, can be done at any time.

Massive PE/thrombolysis

- Massive, life-threatening PE can be defined as embolus associated with haemodynamic compromise (systolic blood pressure < 90 mm Hg or a drop in systolic blood pressure of ≥ 40 mm Hg from baseline for a period of 15 minutes, with no other explanation, such as hypovolaemia, sepsis or arrhythmia).
- In women diagnosed with massive PE in pregnancy, the first line treatment of choice is intravenous unfractionated heparin.
- In some women, thrombolysis is a therapeutic option.

Thrombolysis for PE in Pregnancy

- In those with massive PE associated with circulatory collapse and risk of imminent arrest, thrombolysis should be considered.
- It is potentially life-saving, and pregnancy is not a reason to withhold this treatment.
- Thrombolysis is sometimes used for sub-massive PE with high clot burden, to reduce the risk of chronic pulmonary hypertension. There is no increased risk of haemorrhage compared with outside pregnancy.
- The approach to thrombolysing a pregnant woman should be multidisciplinary, with involvement of obstetrics, intensivists, experienced physicians and radiologists.
- Alternative therapeutic options used successfully in pregnancy include catheter-directed thrombolytic therapy, or thoracotomy and surgical embolectomy.

Post-thrombotic Syndrome

- Post-thrombotic syndrome (PTS) is characterized by leg pain, swelling, abnormal pigmentation, varicose veins, eczema and, sometimes, ulcers following DVT.
- Those affected by DVT are advised to wear graduated elastic compression stockings (class two) on the affected leg for two years, to reduce the risk of PTS.
- The evidence to support graduated elastic compression stockings is not conclusive, and the main benefit is relief from symptoms.

Follow-up

- Women diagnosed with VTE in pregnancy should receive specialist follow-up, ideally from obstetric medicine or joint obstetric haematology clinics.
- Thrombophilia screening should only be carried out if it will influence future management and once anticoagulants have been stopped, as concurrent anticoagulant therapy will affect results.
- The need for VTE prophylaxis in future pregnancies should be discussed, so that women know to start LMWH early in their next pregnancy.

Key Points

- VTE remains the leading direct cause of maternal death in the UK.
- Previous VTE is a major risk factor for VTE in pregnancy
- Women should undergo VTE risk assessment in early pregnancy, and receive individualized advice and prophylaxis.
- In diagnosing VTE in pregnancy, D-dimer rises in normal pregnancy, and should not be tested, as false positive and false negative results are misleading.
- The symptoms and signs of DVT and PE are difficult to differentiate from those of normal pregnancy, and objective testing is required if the history is suggestive.
- The radiation exposure from both V/Q and CTPA scans is well below the maximum recommended radiation exposure in pregnancy.
- V/Q scans expose the maternal lung and breast to less radiation than CTPA, and have a lower incidence of non-diagnostic scans than CTPA in pregnancy.
- NOACs are not currently licensed for use in pregnant and lactating women.
- Thrombolysis should be considered for massive life-threatening PE, and this should be a multidisciplinary team decision.
- Women diagnosed with VTE in pregnancy should receive specialist follow-up.

Further Reading

Cook JV, Kyriou J (2005). Radiation from CT and perfusion scanning in pregnancy. *BMJ* **331**: 350.

Goodacre S, Nelson-Piercy C, Hunt B *et al.* (2015). When should we use diagnostic imaging to investigate for pulmonary embolism in pregnant and postpartum women? *Emergency Medicine Journal* **32**:78–82.

Greer IA (2012). Thrombosis in pregnancy: updates in diagnosis and management. *American Society of Haematology Education Book* **1**: 203–20.

Knight M, Kenyon S, Brocklehurst P *et al.* (2014). *Saving lives, improving mothers' care: lessons learned to inform future maternity care from the UK and Ireland confidential enquiries into maternal deaths and morbidity 2009–2012.* Oxford: National Perinatal Epidemiology Unit, University of Oxford.

Nelson-Piercy C (2015). *Handbook of obstetric medicine*, 5th edition. Boca Raton, FL: CRC Press.

Neuberger F, Nelson-Piercy C (2015). Acute presentation of the pregnant patient. *Clinical Medicine* **15**(4): 1–5.

Pavford S, Hunt B (2010). *The obstetric haematology manual.* Cambridge University Press.

Royal College of Obstetricians and Gynaecologists (2015). *Reducing the risk of venous thromboembolism during pregnancy and the puerperium.* Green Top Guideline 37a. London: RCOG.

Royal College of Obstetricians and Gynaecologists (2015). *Thromboembolic disease in pregnancy and the puerperium: acute management.* Green Top Guideline 37b. London: RCOG.

16

Paediatric Venous Thromboembolism

Paul Monagle[1] and Rebecca Barton[2]

[1] *Department of Clinical Haematology & Department of Paediatrics, University of Melbourne Royal Children's Hospital, Victoria, Australia*
[2] *Department of Clinical Haematology, Royal Children's Hospital, Melbourne, Australia*

Paediatric venous thromboembolism (VTE) is considered a severe problem, because of the potential for associated mortality and significant complications, including pulmonary embolism and cerebrovascular events, as well as post-thrombotic syndrome. VTE occurs when one or more components of Virchow's triad are activated: stasis of blood flow; injury to the endothelial lining; or hypercoagulability of blood components. This is the most useful pathophysiological construct for thinking about thromboembolism in children.

Over recent years, there has been a dramatic increase in available information, knowledge and expertise in relation to appropriate diagnosis, prevention and clinical management of VTE in neonates and children. However, there remain many unknowns, and large data registries and ongoing studies will hopefully continue to improve our knowledge.

For the purpose of this chapter, 'paediatric patients' refers to neonates and children (birth to 18 years), and neonates refers to infants from birth to 28 days (corrected for gestational age). Children specifically refers to the age from 28 days to 18 years, with adolescence being from 13 years until 18 years.

The age of the patient can have an effect on natural history of the VTE, treatment options, response to treatment and also monitoring of treatment.

Incidence

Patient registries from Canada, the United States and the Netherlands have reported anywhere from 0.07 to 0.49 per 10 000 children aged between 1 month and 18 years, with a peak less than one year of age, and a second peak in the adolescent group (Andrew, 1994).

In contrast to adults, the majority of paediatric venous thromboembolisms occur in the setting of an associated risk factor or condition. If one considers hospitalised children, the rate is 100-1000 times the population rate, increased to at least 58 per 10 000 admissions. Thus, despite some exceptions, venous thrombosis should be considered a disease of sick children. The commonest age groups for VTE are neonates and teenagers, and this reflects the pattern of associated underlying diseases and interventions. Within the adolescence age group, there appears to be a further increase in the incidence in females compared with males, which is thought to be secondary to the oral contraceptive pill and pregnancy.

The majority of studies report that the number of venous thromboembolisms is increasing. However, it is unclear from the data obtained whether this is a true increase in the incidence of venous thromboembolism, or whether improved vigilance, detection and diagnosis is the reason.

Handbook of Venous Thromboembolism, First Edition. Edited by Jecko Thachil and Catherine Bagot.
© 2018 John Wiley & Sons Ltd. Published 2018 by John Wiley & Sons Ltd.

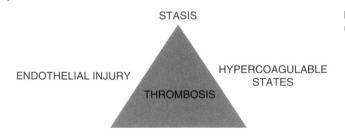

STASIS

ENDOTHELIAL INJURY

HYPERCOAGULABLE STATES

THROMBOSIS

Figure 16.1 Virchow's triad explains the pathophysiology underlying the majority of thrombosis in children.

Paediatric Pathophysiology

Pathological thrombus occurs both as a result of local coagulation activation, as well as of an imbalance between anti-coagulant and pro-coagulant states. In 1855, Rudolf Virchow postulated that abnormalities in blood flow, hypercoagulability of the blood and endothelial injury/dysfunction were all causally linked to thrombus formation which, as a concept, demonstrates the multifactorial nature of thrombosis (Figure 16.1).

'Developmental Haemostasis', a concept introduced by Dr Maureen Andrews and colleagues in the late 1980s, describes that, from birth to adulthood, a child's coagulation system is developing and, overall, favours a reduced incidence of thrombosis without an increased risk of bleeding.

Within the newborn period, the vitamin K-dependent factors (Factors II, VII, IX, X) are at a lower level within the plasma, at almost 50% of adult values, with similar values obtained in both the term and premature neonatal populations. Furthermore, these levels remain reduced by 10–20% throughout childhood. With the administration of vitamin K at birth, and subsequent development of the coagulation system, the levels of the vitamin K-dependent factors increase rapidly within the first few weeks of life.

In addition, the anticoagulant proteins, Protein C and S, and also anti-thrombin, are low in neonates and remain decreased, compared to adults, throughout childhood. As a result of both of these elements, a neonate, and a child to a lesser extent, has a reduced ability to generate thrombin – to almost 50% of adults. Levels of many coagulation proteins appear to approach 50% of adult values by six months of age, although there remains differences with both respect to a normal reference range and mean values, which may have further implications in diagnosis of inherited hypercoagulable states (Andrew, 1992; Monagle, 2006).

Animal studies have suggested that the structure of specific anticoagulation proteins are substantially different in the newborn period.

Despite the haemostatic system being different in children compared with adults, there is currently no evidence to suggest that children are at a greater risk of thrombosis or haemorrhage (Andrew, 1992; Monagle, 2006).

Risk Factors

Risk factors of venous thromboembolism include anything that causes vascular disruption, a protein-losing state or an inflammatory state. More than 90% of paediatric venous thromboembolisms have more than one risk factor, with venous access devices being the most common single risk factor, accounting for greater than 90% of neonatal and greater 50% of paediatric venous thromboembolisms.

A list of common paediatric risk factors is shown in Table 16.1.

Central Venous Access Devices (CVADs)

Central venous access devices account for two-thirds of venous thromboembolism in children, the majority of which occur in the upper venous system – notably, the jugular vein and subclavian vein. The mechanism

Table 16.1 A list of common paediatric risk factors for thrombosis.

Causes	
Acquired	**Congenital**
Central Venous Access Device	Nephrotic syndrome
Malignancy	Congenital heart disease
Infection	
Surgery – particularly cardiothoracic	Inherited hypercoagulable states
Trauma	
Systemic lupus erythematosus/ antiphospholipid syndrome	
High BMI	
Medication	
Inflammatory bowel disease	
Hormonal therapy/pregnancy	
Immobilisation	

by which indwelling catheters cause thrombosis is not only from the presence of a foreign body within the vessel, but also from this foreign body then causing disruption to laminar flow and damage to vessel wall.

The risk is highest within the first four days, and continues to decrease thereafter, but does not return to baseline. The use of larger bore and external catheters appears to be associated with a higher risk of VTE, which has important implications in the neonatal population, where the lines are proportionately larger within the vessel size.

Inherited Hypercoagulable States

Inherited thrombophilias such as antithrombin-, protein C- or protein S deficiencies and pro-thrombotic mutations of Factor II & V, as well as acquired thrombophilias such as antiphospholipid syndrome and lupus anticoagulant, have been found to be additional risk factors for VTE in the adult population. However, there is currently limited evidence to suggest this in a paediatric population, with the results to date being both contradictory and or inconclusive (Kenet, 2012).

Paediatric patients who are diagnosed with inherited hypercoagulable states do not usually present with thrombosis until later in the adolescent period or, in fact, through to adulthood. As such, it is not recommended to screen otherwise healthy children with a family history of thrombophilia (Tormene, 2002).

Risk Factor Stratification

A number of retrospective case-control studies have emerged which focus on the development of risk scores for sub-groups of hospitalised children. For example, in critically ill children, studies suggest that the presence of a central venous access device (CVAD), length of stay (within a Paediatric Intensive Care Unit) of greater than or equal to four days and significant infection, as being the only independent statistically significant risk factors.

Of note, age, when either examined as a continuous variable or by stratification into age groups, was not a statistically significant independent risk factor for the development of venous thromboembolism. In addition, there currently exists similarly designed paediatric studies which have focused on risk stratification within other subgroups, such as non-critical patients, patients with cardiac disease, trauma, and neonates.

From the stratification data in these studies, clinicians can, hopefully, determine the need for either pharmacological or mechanical thromboprophylaxis. However, prospective studies using the aforementioned risk scores for validation are required.

Clinical Manifestations

The clinical manifestations of venous thromboembolism vary, depending upon the location and duration of the thrombus. The majority of paediatric venous thromboembolisms occur in the upper limb venous system, and are related to venous access devices.

Central Venous Access Device (CVAD)-related Thrombosis

The majority of venous access device thromboses are asymptomatic, and manifest through either loss of patency of the venous device, development of prominent collaterals in the superficial venous system, or device-related infection or sepsis. Over half of the CVAD-related thromboses occur in the upper limb, and may be symptomatic, presenting with swelling and or discolouration of the arm, swelling of the neck (which may be unilateral) and face, pulmonary embolism, chylothorax and superior vena cava syndrome.

The use of CVADs thus require a risk-benefit analyses, and it is necessary that they are removed as soon as practically and clinically possible.

Intracardiac Thrombosis

Patients undergoing cardiopulmonary bypass are at an increased risk of VTE, as exposure of the patients' blood to large synthetic surfaces causes activation of platelets, coagulation factors and the fibrinolytic system, as well as activation of an overall inflammatory response peri-and post-operatively. When this environment is then combined with areas of turbulent blood flow or stasis at the site of cardiac surgery, prosthetic valves/shunts and sutures, the risk of intracardiac thrombosis is increased further (Manlhiot, 2011).

Renal Vein Thrombosis

Although rare, renal vein thrombosis is the second most common venous thrombotic event in the neonatal age group, with an incidence of two per 100 000 births, and appears to be more common in males.

Risk factors include: maternal diabetes mellitus; neonatal shock; dehydration; perinatal hypoxia; polycythaemia; sepsis; cyanotic heart disease; and umbilical cord catheterisation.

The clinical features of renal vein thrombosis are variable, but can include: haematuria; oliguria-anuria; vomiting; renal mass; hypertension; thrombocytopenia; and decreased renal function (especially if bilateral renal vein thrombosis). Extension of the thrombus into the inferior vena cava may produce symptoms of a DVT, such as lower limb oedema, decreased temperature and capillary return.

Pulmonary Embolism (PE)

Pulmonary embolism results in acute obstruction of the pulmonary outflow tract and subsequent right ventricular decompensation. Although less common in children, it can also cause sudden collapse and death, and a majority of cases are asymptomatic. The current incidence of pulmonary embolism in children is unknown and likely under-diagnosed, with the majority of studies suggesting it is uncommon, with the incidence highest in infants, children under two years of age and in teenage girls (Chan, 2003; Biss, 2008). CVAD-related VTE remains the most common source of PE in the paediatric population. Presentation of PE in the paediatric population is similar to adults, with cough, chest pain, tachycardia, tachypnoea, dyspnoea and collapse being the most common symptoms and signs and, unfortunately, too many cases being diagnosed at autopsy (Chan, 2003).

Cerebro-sinovenous thrombosis (CSVT)

The incidence of childhood CSVT is higher in children than neonates, and Canadian studies report 0.67 per 100 000 per children per year. Clinical features can be subtle, with signs of raised intracranial pressure developing over hours to days. The most frequent neurological signs include headache, decreased consciousness and seizures, with hemiplegia and visual changes being less common (Chan, 2003). The majority of cases are attributed to underlying illnesses or prothrombotic medications and, in contrast to adults, idiopathic cases remain rare.

Portal Vein Thrombosis

Portal vein thrombosis is most commonly seen in the neonatal period, and is usually as a result of umbilical catheterisation or sepsis. However, in the older paediatric population, it can be seen secondary to liver transplantation, splenectomy, in sickle cell disease, infection, chemotherapy, or in the presence of phospholipid antibodies.

Diagnosis

Imaging methods for diagnosis of venous thromboembolism in children include ultrasonography, computed tomography (CT), magnetic resonance imaging (MRI), echocardiography or angiography, as well as direct identification via surgical techniques or at autopsy (Manlhiot, 2011).

Venography remains the gold standard for diagnosis of DVT, but less invasive methods, such as ultrasonography (compression and duplex), are preferred in the paediatric population, because of bedside availability and non-invasive technique. Sensitivity of ultrasound remains dependent on the experience of the technician and site of examination; for example, upper versus lower limbs, and popliteal and femoral veins, as opposed to calf veins

CT, with the addition of intravenous contrast in certain populations, is used to diagnosis VTE in the upper venous system, abdominal and pelvic venous systems. CT pulmonary angiogram (CTPA) and ventilation perfusion lung scans are used to diagnose pulmonary embolism, and MRI with venography is the most sensitive and specific modality for evaluation of the intracranial venous system and superior vena cava system and specific diagnosis of CSVT.

Treatment

Treatment of venous thromboembolic events in children is different from that in adults, mostly because of the aetiology of the VTE itself, 'developmental haemostasis', pharmacokinetics and pharmacodynamics of the medications used, as well as co-morbidities.

Anticoagulant treatment options in children include unfractionated heparin (UFH) at dose adjusted levels, low molecular weight heparin (LMWH) and vitamin K antagonists (VKA). The choice of these is largely dependent upon clinical situation, age, bleeding risk, ease of administration and monitoring of dose. Novel oral anticoagulant medications are not currently used in the paediatric population and, until there is further evidence around dosing, monitoring and efficacy, this is unlikely to change. In addition, the lack of reversal agent is problematic.

Pharmacokinetic studies have shown that the distribution, binding and subsequent clearance of anticoagulants is age-, weight- and disease-related, and further influenced by diet and medications. In addition, the administration, testing and monitoring of these medications can be troublesome in children, due to limited vascular access and concerns regarding painful procedures. Long-term use of anticoagulants (heparinoids and vitamin K antagonists) have been associated with an increased risk of osteoporosis, which can potentiate the already limited bone health in unwell children.

Treatment Recommendations

The following recommendations are based upon the American College of Chest Physicians (ACCP) guidelines, and evidence is largely based on systematic reviews or observational studies (Monagle, 2012).

Children with First Provoked VTE (Venous Access Device Related or Non-venous Access Device Related)

Commence anticoagulant therapy with either UFH or LMWH, for at least five days, and then continue LMWH or Vitamin K antagonist for three months, presuming resolution of causative risk factor. If risk factor is ongoing, then consider continuation of prophylactic anticoagulant therapy until the risk factor has resolved. The question of whether a CVAD should be removed depends on the ongoing need for central venous access for management of the primary disorder, whether the CVAD is still functioning, and whether the CVAD related thrombosis is life- or limb-threatening.

Idiopathic VTE

Commence of anticoagulant therapy with either UFH or LMWH, for at least five days, and then continue LMWH or Vitamin K antagonist for at least 6–12 months.

Recurrent Idiopathic VTE

Anticoagulant therapy for an indefinite period of time with VKA.

Thrombolysis

Thrombolytic treatment in the paediatric population remains controversial, with a largely unknown risk/benefit ratio, with evidence regarding safety and efficacy coming largely from paediatric case reports. Retrospective studies in children have reported bleeding complications, both major and minor, in 68% of patients, with 39% requiring a red cell transfusion (Gupta, 2001). The ACCP guidelines recommend that thrombolysis be used only for life- or limb-threatening thrombosis.

Thrombectomy

Thrombectomy is recommended in children with life-threatening VTE, which should be followed by anticoagulant therapy.

Thromboprophylaxis

There is currently no data to support the recommendation of anti-coagulation in children with short- or medium-term CVADs. However, for children who receive long-term TPN, it is recommended that thromboprophylaxis be achieved with VKAs.

Monitoring of Anticoagulant

Monitoring is largely dependent upon the choice of anticoagulant. However, this must be considered in context of the child and the current medical situation. Point of care testing is frequently being used to monitor vitamin K antagonists, and has been validated in the paediatric age group for INRs less than 5.

Immune heparin-induced thrombocytopenia is rare in the paediatric population, so other causes of thrombocytopenia should be investigated in these cases.

Complications

Complications of venous thromboembolism are both acute and chronic, with some sequelae being experienced life-long for children. Studies from cardiac patients have shown that patients with established thrombosis are at increased risk of severe complications such as; pulmonary embolism, strokes, haemorrhage and cardiac failure, with an overall increased mortality rate (Manlhiot, 2011). Furthermore occlusive and symptomatic thrombi have been found to have a higher risk of complications, with suboptimal clinical outcomes (Manlhiot, 2011). Recent reports have suggested that over half of children treated for a VTE will have residual thrombus following completion of treatment, which is an important consideration for diagnosis of recurrence (Revel-Vilk, 2004).

Post-thrombotic Syndrome (PTS)

Post-thrombotic syndrome is an important chronic consequence of venous thromboembolism, and can cause significant morbidity to children and their families. Manifestations of post-thrombotic syndrome can vary from mild to severe, with symptoms and signs including: oedema; chronic pain; sensory changes; ulceration; and subsequent loss of mobility and activity. These symptoms can be either intermittent or persistent in their nature. Post-thrombotic syndrome can have significant effects of quality of life and productivity, with substantial community costs from health care utilisation and disability funding, particularly in children who may potentially suffer these sequelae for longer periods.

The incidence of post-thrombotic syndrome in children is unknown, but a recent systematic literature review performed by Goldenberg and colleagues has suggested a mean frequency of 26% (confidence interval 95%), from a total of nearly 1000 events. Interestingly, this figure is within the stated incidence range for adult post-thrombotic syndrome (Goldenberg, 2010).

Post-thrombotic syndrome develops as a result of chronic venous insufficiency, and involves both the early inflammatory process and vessel damage, as well as obstruction of venous outflow system, subsequent destruction of valves and, ultimately, the development of venous reflux (Goldenberg, 2010).

Diagnosis of post-thrombotic syndrome is made on clinical symptoms and signs, with no routine imaging required. The absence of documented venous congestion, reflux and persistent thrombosis on imaging does not preclude a diagnosis. As such, a number of clinical tools have been designed to standardise the diagnosis of post-thrombotic syndrome and, subsequently, provide objective measures of burden of disease. The two main scoring systems for measuring post-thrombotic syndrome in children are the modified Villalta and the Manco-Johnson instrument but, to date, only the latter has published validation data for use in children. The Manco-Johnson instrument evaluates pain symptoms by combining a basic classification system, CEAP (Clinical-Etiologic-Anatomic-Pathophysiologic), with the Wong-Baker faces scale.

Follow-up

The current recommendation is for children to be followed up throughout childhood, at least annually, to allow for early identification and management of post-thrombotic syndrome, as well as recognising future risk factors for patients as they move through adolescence into adulthood. In addition, ongoing education is required, particularly in adolescent girls, to guide and counsel around the commencement of oral contraception or, indeed, pregnancy.

Further Reading

Andrew M, David M, Adams M, Ali K, Anderson R, Barnard D, Bernstein M, Brisson L, Cairney B, DeSai D, Grant R, Israels S, Jardine L, Luke B, Massicotte P, Silva M (1994). Venous Thromboembolic Complications (VTE) in Children: First Analyses of the Canadian Registry of VTE. *Blood* **83**(5): 1251–1257.

Andrew, M, Vegh, P, Johnston, M, Bowker, J, Ofosu, F, Mitchell, L. (1992). Maturation of the Hemostatic System During Childhood. *Blood* **80**(8): 1998–2005.

Biss, TT, Brandao, LR, Kahr, WH, Chan, AK, Williams S (2008). Clinical features and outcome of pulmonary embolism in children. *British Journal of Haematology* **142**: 808–818.

Chan AK, Deveber G, Monagle P, Brookers LA, Massocittes PM (2003). Venous thrombosis in children. *Journal of Thrombosis & Haemostasis* **1**: 1443–1455.

Goldenberg NA, Donadini MP, Kahn SR, Crowther M, Kenet G, Nowak-Gottl U, Manco-Johnson MJ (2010). Post-thrombotic syndrome in children: a systematic review of frequency of occurrence, validity of outcome measures, and prognostic factors. *Haematologica* **95**(11): 1952–1959.

Gupta AA, Leaker M, Andrew M, Massicotte P, Liu L, Benson LN, McCrindle BW (2001). Safety and outcomes of thrombolysis with tissue plasminogen activator for treatment of intravascular thrombosis in children. *Journal of Pediatrics* **139**(5): 682–688.

Kenet G (2012). Venous thromboembolism in neonates and children. *Best Practice & Research Clinical Haematology* **25**: 333–344.

Manlhiot C, Menjak IB, Brandao LR, Gruenwald CE, Schwartz SM, Ben Sivarajan V, Yoon H, Maratta R, Carew CL, McMullen JA, Clarizia NA, Holtby HM, Williams S, Caldarone CA, Van Arsdell GS, Chan AK, McCrindle BW (2011). Risk, Clinical Features, and Outcomes of Thrombosis Associated with Pediatric Cardiac Surgery. *Circulation* **124**: 1511–1519.

Monagle P, Barnes C, Ignjatovic V, Furmedge J, Newall F, Chan A, De Rosa L, Hamilton S, Ragg P, Robinson S, Auldist A, Crock C, Roy N, Rowlands S (2006). Developmental haemostasis: Impact for clinical haemostasis laboratories. *Thrombosis & Haemostasis* **95**: 362–372.

Monagle P, Chan AK, Goldenberg NA, Ichord RN, Journeycake JM, Nowak-Gottl U, Vesely SK (2012). AntiThrombotic Therapy in Neonates. *Chest* **141**(2): 737s –801s.

Revel-Vilk S, Sharathkumar A, Massicotte P, Marzinotto V, Daneman A, Dix D, Chan A (2004). Natural history of arterial and venous thrombosis in children treated with low molecular weight heparin: a longitudinal study by ultrasound. *Journal of Thrombosis & Haemostasis* **2**: 42–46.

Tormene D, Simioni P, Prandoni P, Franz F, Zerbinati P, Tognin G, Girolami A (2002). The incidence of venous thromboembolism in thrombophilic children: a propsective cohort study. *Blood* **100**(7): 2403–2405.

17

Cancer-associated Thrombosis

Simon Noble

Division of Population Medicine, Cardiff University, Cardiff, Wales

Introduction

The association between cancer and venous thromboembolism (VTE) has been recognised for over 150 years. Its first description is attributed to the Parisian Physician Armand Trousseau who, in the 1860s, published a series of lectures in his famous text *Clinique Medale de l'Hotel-Dieu*. It is in this compilation of lectures that he described what later was to be known as Trousseau's syndrome: thrombophlebitis as a presenting sign of visceral malignancy. Ironically, on January 1, 1867, he diagnosed in himself a deep vein thrombosis of the left arm, and told one of his colleagues: 'I am lost; I have no doubt about the nature of my disease'. He died six months later of gastric cancer.

Pathophysiology of Cancer-associated Thrombosis

Virchow's triad of stasis, endothelial perturbation and hypercoagulability encompasses all risk factors associated with the development of VTE. For the non-cancer patient, VTE typically follows exposure to a temporary increase in one or more risk factors, after which the provoking factor subsides and the ongoing thrombotic tendency diminishes. The cancer patient may, however, face a succession of varying risk factors throughout the cancer journey, thereby being exposed to a waxing and waning background of thrombogenicity. As such, the cancer patient should always be considered high risk for VTE.

Figure 17.1 illustrates the various risk factors associated with cancer-associated thrombosis (CAT). Cancer itself induces a hypercoaguable state through the direct and indirect release of procoagulants (i.e. tissue factor) and inflammatory mediators (e.g. IL-1). However, not all cancers are the same, and the VTE risk varies according to primary tumour types and histology. It is highest in lung, ovary, brain and upper gastrointestinal cancers, and lowest in breast and prostate. This is not to say that CAT is rare in clinical practice for these cancers; for example, 2% of stage I/II breast cancer patients will develop CAT during adjuvant chemotherapy, and 8% of those with stage IV during palliative chemotherapy. Since breast cancer is so common, VTE is frequently seen, due to the sheer numbers of new diagnoses. The VTE risk also increases with disease progression, and the presence of distant metastases increases the VTE rate up to 19 fold.

Over 50% of CAT cases will occur in the first three months after the cancer diagnosis. This coincides with exposure to extrinsic risk factors, such as chemotherapy, surgery and central venous access.

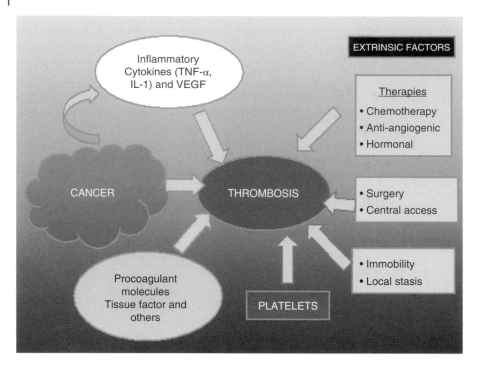

Figure 17.1 Risk factors for cancer-associated thrombosis.

The Psychological Impact of CAT

The experience and diagnosis of a VTE is a distressing one. Studies have identified that some patients will develop a chronic anxiety state after their VTE, with a proportion of these experiencing post-traumatic stress disorder. Interestingly, the severity of the long-term psychological distress is unrelated to the symptom burden conferred by the VTE. As stated before, the majority of CATs occur within three months of the cancer diagnosis, the majority associated with chemotherapy. As such, the thrombosis and its implications must not be treated in isolation, since most patients will still be coming to terms with this devastating diagnosis. A diagnosis of CAT will often be seen as a further life-threatening event and complication of their cancer journey. For many, the symptoms attributed to CAT are more distressing than those of the cancer, at the time of diagnosis.

Diagnosis of CAT

The investigations for deep vein thrombosis (DVT) and pulmonary emboli (PE) are Doppler ultrasound and computer tomography pulmonary angiography (CTPA), respectively, regardless of whether the patient has cancer or not. However, it is important to acknowledge several differences when considering VTE in the cancer setting.

Firstly, it is often inadequately considered as a cause of symptoms when they could be explained by other pathologies. Breathlessness is more likely to be attributed to anaemia, pneumonia, pleural effusion, heart failure, or pulmonary metastases, before considering a PE. Similarly, swollen legs may be managed as cellulitis, hypoalbuminaemia or lymphoedema, rather than DVT. Furthermore, such diagnoses are commonly seen in oncology, and may mask the symptoms of VTE if occurring concurrently.

Secondly, tools embedded in clinical practice for the assessment of suspected VTE might not be helpful in the context of cancer. The Wells score, a commonly used clinical prediction tool for the presence of DVT or PE, has a limited utility with cancer patients. With one point attributed to the presence of active cancer (as defined by treatment within six months or palliative), only one more is required to support a 28% chance of VTE. As such, it is unlikely to be helpful as an exclusory prediction model. Similarly, elevated D-dimer levels are commonplace with cancer, and only of use as an exclusory test. As such, they are not recommended in the routine work-up of suspected CAT.

The identification of pulmonary emboli on CT scans performed for indications other than investigation of suspected VTE is a growing clinical problem. Most commonly identified on staging scans, or those undertaken to evaluate response to treatment, incidental pulmonary emboli (IPE) occur in 3.1% of all cancer patients. Describing them as 'asymptomatic PE' is generally incorrect, since a careful history will usually identify symptoms that have not previously been volunteered. Current guidelines recommend using the same approach to type and duration of anticoagulation as is used for symptomatic cancer-associated PE, particularly those as far down as segmental branches, or the pulmonary vasculature. However, data regarding the significance of subsegmental PE (SSPE) in the oncology setting are unclear, although survival data suggests that there is no advantage in anticoagulating an isolated incidental SSPE. Therefore, in the absence of any radiological evidence of leg DVT, many clinicians opt not to anticoagulate.

Challenges in the Management of CAT

Not only is VTE more prevalent in the cancer population, recent studies have demonstrated that the incipient clot microstructure is considerably denser and potentially more resistant to lysis. Particular issues that make the treatment of CAT such a challenge include:

- Greater risk of VTE recurrence – up to 17% with warfarin and 9% with LMWH.
- Greater risk of bleeding on anticogulation – up to 11% at 3.5 months and 19.8% at 12 months.
- Ongoing and varying risk of VTE – due to extrinsic factors such as chemotherapy and surgery, or intrinsic factors such as disease progression or regression.
- Receiving on going cancer treatments – not only may these alter thrombogenicity but, also, chemotherapy-induced thrombocytopenia may make anticoagulation hazardous during a cytopenic nadir.

Initial Treatment

The mainstay of VTE treatment in the general population comprises of five days of weight-adjusted low molecular weight heparin (LMWH), followed by three to six months of anticoagulant with a vitamin K antagonist (i.e. warfarin). More recently, the direct-acting oral anticoagulants (DOACs) have demonstrated non-inferiority with warfarin for the treatment of VTE, and a superior safety profile with respect to major bleeding. Requiring no monitoring or dose adjustments, and with significantly fewer drug-drug interactions, the NOACs are an attractive alternative to current standard practice.

The management of VTE in patients with cancer is less straightforward, with a higher rate of bleeding and recurrent VTE than that seen in patients without cancer. Furthermore, both bleeding and thrombotic risks are likely to fluctuate over time, especially in patients receiving chemotherapy or those with progressive disease. Current clinical guidelines recommend LMWH as the first-line treatment of CAT, since it has demonstrated superiority over warfarin with respect to preventing recurrent VTE, without an increase in bleeding complications. In addition, the use of warfarin is particularly challenging in many patients receiving chemotherapy, due to drug-drug interactions rendering the INR unstable. Conversely, LMWH has fewer drug-drug interactions and rarely requires monitoring. Table 17.1 summarises the LMWH available for the treatment of CAT and their recommended dosing schedule.

Table 17.1 Dosing schedules of different LMWHs in treatment and secondary prevention of CAT.

LMWH	Dose first month	Dose months 2–6
Dalteparin	200 IU/kg s/c o.d.	150 IU s/c o.d.
Tinzaparin	175 IU/kg s/c o.d.	175 IU s/c o.d.
Enoxaparin	1.5 mg/kg s/c o.d.	1.5 mg/kg s/c o.d.

Since LMWH is administered as a daily subcutaneous injection, there are concerns that this form of administration may have a negative impact on patients' quality of life, and be a less acceptable intervention than oral alternatives. Qualitative studies suggest that patients find LMWH acceptable within the context of their cancer journey, and quickly adapt to the daily routine of self-injection. Compliance with LMWH can be optimised with sufficient information and support when commencing anticoagulation. Key information should include:

- Why they got CAT.
- Importance of treating CAT.
- Why LMWH, rather than an oral medicine.
- Injection technique advice.
- Education of signs and symptoms which would necessitate medical review (e.g. haemorrhage or recurrent VTE).

Currently, there is insufficient data to recommend the use of DOACs as first line in the treatment of CAT. However, the DOACS have demonstrated non-inferiority over warfarin in the treatment of VTE in studies which contained a small proportion of cancer patients and, by inference, they offer an additional alternative to LMWH, should patients be intolerant or unable to receive injections. While an oral agent may seem more appealing than the injectable LMWH, even if the data is not as strong in the cancer population, it appears that most patients would still opt for LMWH.

A recent study evaluated patient's preferences of different anticoagulants, based on the characteristics they considered most important. CAT patient responses from two countries were strongly concordant: they considered the most important attributes to be lack of interference with cancer treatments, efficacy and safety. Other attributes considered less important were the mode of administration, the number of times to be taken and monitoring requirements.

Long-term Anticoagulation

While the standard treatment of CAT with weight-adjusted LMWH for 3–6 months is based on data from several RCTs, the data for the management beyond six months is considerably lacking in comparison. To date, only a few observational studies in heterogeneous populations have been published.

For CAT patients in whom there remains active cancer, the thrombotic risk is arguably ongoing and, intuitively, indefinite anticoagulation seems justified. However, the data on VTE recurrence, with or without continued anticoagulation, is limited, and it is impossible to advise with accuracy whether a patient's risk of VTE recurrence exceeds the bleeding risk of ongoing anticoagulation.

International guidelines recommend, therefore, that each patient is evaluated individually, and the decision to continue anticoagulation should be based on weighing up the following factors:

- Perceived bleeding risk:
  - Ongoing risk of 0.7% major bleeding for every month of anticoagulation beyond six months.
  - Risk increased in presence of thrombocytopenia/marrow failure/liver failure.

- Ongoing thrombotic risk
  - Risk greater in upper GI, gynae, lung cancers.
  - Risk increased in presence of distant metastases.
- Patient wishes:
  - Patients with distressing VTE symptoms at diagnosis will wish to continue anticoagulation.
  - Those with incidental PE often do not wish to continue anticoagulation.

Until now, clinicians have usually continued patients on LMWH, since data has supported its use for the first six months of treatment. However, it is readily acknowledged that continuing LMWH beyond six months may be problematic for some patients. While many patents develop daily routines for self-injection, other patients find the injections problematical over time, especially those with little body fat to inject into.

As well as there being little data to inform the management of CAT beyond six months, there is even less data supporting any particular anticoagulant of choice. For those wishing to avoid further LMWH, the options remaining are warfarin or a choice of the DOACs. The challenges of using warfarin in CAT have been described previously. Interestingly, a recent observational study suggested that warfarin could be used safely and effectively beyond six months, although strict INR monitoring may be required. Since there is no convincing data to support any particular anticoagulant, there has been a move amongst some clinicians towards using a DOAC after six months of LMWH, the rationale being that it is a preferable alternative to warfarin for a patient who no longer wishes to continue LMWH.

Challenging Cases

Clinical guidelines are only as helpful as the data that informs them. As such, the more complex CAT patient is unlikely to be addressed, since their characteristics will have made them ineligible for participation in the studies.

Fortunately, 80% of CAT patients will be straightforward to manage with weight-adjusted LMWH. However, approximately 20% will fall outside the guidelines by nature of having recurrent VTE, thrombocytopenia or bleeding. The International Society for Thrombosis and Haemostasis Scientific Sub Committee (ISTH SCC) for Haemostasis and Malignancy published guidance on such challenging cases. It must be stressed that the purpose of such guidance documents are to provide pragmatic advice in clinical scenarios where robust evidence is lacking. As such, the recommendations will often be for the use of anticoagulants outside of their licensed indications. The recommendations of the ISTH SCC are summarised in Table 17.2.

Use of Inferior Vena Cava Filters

The rationale for using inferior vena cava (IVC) filters is to reduce the risk of a fatal or clinically significant PE from a large embolus arising from the limb or pelvic veins. It is consequently used in the setting of recurrent PE or DVT extension despite anticoagulation, and in patients with contraindications to anticoagulation. Currently, the data does not demonstrate a reduction in fatal PE, but does show a reduction in non-fatal PE at the expense of an increase in recurrent DVT. Data in the cancer patient are limited to a small clinical trial, which showed no benefit and retrospective studies showing high rates of lower limb DVT.

In practice, the use of filters should be considered carefully on an individual patient basis and, wherever possible, a retrievable filter should be used and removed at the earliest opportunity. As such, it should be used for patients at high risk of fatal PE, in whom anticoagulation is contraindicated.

Table 17.2 Summary of ISTH SCC haemostasis and malignancy guidance for challenging cases.

Recurrent VTE despite anticoagulation

1) If on warfarin, switch to therapeutic LMWH.
2) If already on LMWH, increase dose by 25% or increase back up to therapeutic weight-adjusted dose if they are receiving non-therapeutic dosing.
3) If no symptomatic improvement, use peak anti-Xa level to estimate next dose escalation.

Management of CAT in thrombocytopenia

1) For platelet count $> 50 \times 10^9 l^{-1}$, give full therapeutic dose LMWH.
2) For acute CAT and platelet count $< 50 \times 10^9 l^{-1}$:
   a) Full anticoagulation with platelet transfusion to maintain platelet count $> 50 \times 10^9 l^{-1}$.
   b) If platelet transfusion not possible, consider retrievable IVC filter.
3) For subacute or chronic CAT and thrombocytopenia (platelet count $< 50 \times 10^9 l^{-1}$):
   a) Reduce therapeutic dose by 50% or use prophylactic dose for platelet count $25 - 50 \times 10^9 l^{-1}$.
   b) Omit LMWH if platelet count $< 25 \times 10^9 l^{-1}$.

Bleeding while anticoagulated

1) Assess each bleeding episode to identify bleeding source, severity, impact and reversibility.
2) Provide supportive measures to stop bleeding including transfusion where indicated.
3) For a major or life-threatening bleeding episode: withhold anticoagulation
   a) Consider IVC filter insertion in patients with acute or subacute CAT with a major or life-threatening bleeding episode.
   b) Do not consider IVC filter insertion in patients with chronic CAT.
   c) Once bleeding resolves, remove retrievable filter (if inserted) and resume/ initiate anticoagulation.

Thromboprophylaxis in Hospitalised Cancer Patients

VTE is a largely preventable illness, and multiple anticoagulants are available and used in a variety of settings as primary prophylaxis. Thromboprophylaxis with LMWH is currently recommended for cancer inpatients without contraindications. These recommendations are based on extrapolation from large trials conducted in the medically ill population, which included a minority of patients with malignancy. Unfortunately, no cancer-specific studies have been conducted, which remains a major knowledge gap in the field.

Thromboprophylaxis in Ambulant Cancer Patients Receiving Chemotherapy

Chemotherapy is recognised as an independent risk factor for VTE, and the majority is administered in an outpatient setting. Consequently, 80% of CAT occurs in the non-hospitalised patients. Several studies have looked at using thromboprophylaxis for ambulant patients receiving chemotherapy but, while demonstrating a statistically significant reduction in VTE, the results did not support a change in clinical practice. This was largely due to the study population being too heterogeneous with respect to cancer types.

To date, the only data supporting primary thromboprophylaxis for chemotherapy outpatients lies with the treatment of pancreatic cancer and myeloma. LMWH is recommended for pancreatic cancer patients, while current recommendations for myeloma patients suggest either aspirin or LMWH.

Recent attention has been towards identifying characteristics, which might identify those at particular risk of CAT during chemotherapy. One risk assessment tool, known as the Khorana Score (see Table 17.3) has been developed, based on cancer site, full blood count parameters and body mass index.

Table 17.3 Khorana score for risk of developing VTE during chemotherapy.

Patient characteristics	Score
Site of cancer	
Very high risk (stomach, pancreas)	2
High risk (lung, lymphoma, gynae, GU excluding prostate)	3
Platelet count > 350 000/mm^3	1
Hb < 10 g/dl or use of erythropoiesis stimulating agents	1
Leukocyte count > 11 000/mm^3	1
Body mass index > 35	1

High risk ≥ 3, intermediate risk 1–2; low risk 0.

Whilst the Khorana Score is useful in highlighting high risk patients, its it is likely to require additional biomarkers to tighten its positive predicative value before it is used routinely in clinical practice. Such biomarkers that are currently being evaluated are listed below, although it should be noted that many are not freely available in clinical practice.

- D-dimer
- Tissue factor (antigen expression, circulating microparticles, antigen or activity)*
- Soluble P-selectin (>53.1 ng/ml)*
- Factor VII*
- Prothrombin fragment F1 + 2 (>358 pmol/l)*

Since primary thromboprophylaxis is not routinely used during chemotherapy, the best approach to CAT management would be to alert patients to the red-flag symptoms of VTE that would require medical attention. Most cancer hospitals will have a specific pathway for managing febrile neutropenia, and patients are well informed of what signs to recognise and how to act on them. However, this is rarely the case for CAT. One study has suggested that patients are ill informed about CAT prior to chemotherapy, and are late to act on symptoms suggestive of VTE, because they assume they are associated with the cancer or chemotherapy. Consequently, patients may present later and more unwell with CAT.

Conclusion

Cancer-associated thrombosis is a problem which is unlikely to go away. As people live longer, and more oncological therapies emerge, cancer patients are living longer with metastatic disease and receiving more chemotherapy. In America, the increase in chemotherapy usage has seen a parallel increase in CAT diagnosis.

The differences between the management of CAT and VTE in the non-cancer patient cannot be underestimated, and the management of CAT is rapidly becoming a sub-specialty within thrombosis and haemostasis. The field is rapidly developing, with new clinical research and laboratory data emerging all the time. In the future, clinicians are less likely to manage CAT as a single pathology but, rather, take a more individualised approach, similar to the personalised medicine approach adopted for oncological treatments. Likewise, as further research is conducted, a greater understanding of the newer anticoagulants in the cancer setting may offer further alternatives for patient-centred treatment.

---

*Denotes the test is not routinely available in clinical practice.

Further Reading

Noble S, Pasi J (2010). Pathophysiology of cancer associated thrombosis. *British Journal of Cancer* **102**: S2–S9.

Farge-Bancel D, Debourdeau P, Beckers, M, Baglin C, Bauersachs R, Brenner B, Brilhante D, Falanga A, Gerotziafas G, Haim N, Kakkar AK, Khorana A, Lecumberri R, Mandala M, Marty M, Monreal M, Mousa S, Noble S, Pabinger I, Prins M, Qari M, Streiff M, Zervas K, Bounameaux H, Buller H (2013). International clinical practice guidelines for the treatment and prophylaxis of thrombosis associated in patients with cancer. *Journal of Thrombosis and Haemostasis* **11**(1): 56–70.

Carrier M, Khorana AA, Zwicker JI, Noble S, Lee AYY (2013). Management of challenging cases of patients with cancer-associated thrombosis including recurrent thrombosis and bleeding: guidance from the SSC of the ISTH. *Journal of Thrombosis and Haemostasis* **11**(9): 1760–65.

18

Venous Thromboembolism Management in Obese Patients

Kathryn Lang[1] and Jignesh Patel[1,2]

[1] King's Thrombosis Centre, Department of Haematological Medicine, King's College Hospital Foundation NHS Trust, London
[2] Institute of Pharmaceutical Science, Faculty of Life Sciences and Medicine, King's College, London

Obesity is a common clinical problem. The World Health Organisation defines obesity as a body mass index (BMI) equal to or greater than $30 \, kg/m^2$ (sub-classified as: obese class I, BMI $30–34.9 \, kg/m^2$; class II, BMI $35–39.9 \, kg/m^2$; and, class III, BMI $>40 \, kg/m^2$). Both the diagnosis of venous thromboembolism (VTE) and its subsequent management present clinicians with challenges.

Challenges of VTE Diagnosis

Whether there exists a causal relationship between excess weight and VTE risk remains controversial: US registry data has found a relative risk of 2.50 in obese individuals, compared with those whose BMI is less than $30 \, kg/m^2$. The greatest risk pertains to patients of any gender under 40 years of age. Obese females are known to have a higher risk of DVT than obese males.

Clinical assessment at presentation is made more challenging due to overlap between the clinical features of DVT/PE, the physiological adaptations of high BMI, and the cardiovascular and respiratory co morbidities of obesity. Features typically found in VTE are more common in obese individuals (without demonstrable underlying pathology other than excess weight), including limb swelling, skin changes, dyspnoea, tachypnoea, chest pain and exertional breathlessness. Moreover, while most VTE prophylaxis risk assessment scores include obesity as a risk factor, none of the commonly used VTE treatment clinical decision rules specifically take obesity into account.

D-dimers are used to exclude VTE in those with low clinical probability, but this can be problematic in the setting of obesity, as D-dimer values are often elevated in this population, and some studies show a positive correlation between D-dimer elevation and waist circumference. Heterogeneous alterations to coagulation factor concentrations (increases in all of: fibrinogen; factor VIII; factor XII; von Willebrand factor; factor VII; protein C; and tissue plasminogen activator) in obesity have been considered as contributory to the observed increased incidence in this population, but must be interpreted cautiously and may add little clinical value to initial diagnosis.

Perhaps the most important consideration in the diagnosis of the obese patient with suspected VTE is the access to and accuracy of imaging techniques. Both compression ultrasonography (CUS) and CT pulmonary angiography (CTPA) are limited by body habitus. CUS is operator-dependent and, in the largest limbs, technical quality is often poor, making it difficult to confidently exclude DVT. CT scanning equipment is limited by table weight limitations, with 220 kg the upper limit of operation for most standard tables in the UK. Chest circumference must also be taken into account for pulmonary angiography. Beyond this threshold, options

Handbook of Venous Thromboembolism, First Edition. Edited by Jecko Thachil and Catherine Bagot.
© 2018 John Wiley & Sons Ltd. Published 2018 by John Wiley & Sons Ltd.

include locating a scanner with higher weight limits, use of veterinary equipment, and alternative modality scanning, including so-called 'open' MRI scans, where evidence for diagnostic value exists, though is not considered gold standard. Any of these approaches clearly present both logistical and temporal challenges and add to the complexity of managing an acutely unwell patient.

Treatment of VTE

Once diagnosis is made, the optimal anticoagulant dose to prescribe remains a challenge, in terms of whether the anticoagulant dose needs to be increased in line with increasing body weight, or whether the dose should be capped.

In order to understand the dosing of anticoagulants to prescribe for this population, it is important to understand how obesity affects some key pharmacokinetic principles – namely, drug absorption, volume of distribution (V_d) and clearance.

In the obese, oral drug absorption is not thought to be significantly altered. Evidence suggests that, with the administration of subcutaneous injections, although absorption takes longer in the obese than in their normally weighted counterparts, total bioavailability is unaffected.

The V_d of a drug provides an estimate of the extent to which it distributes into extravascular tissues. The V_d is largely dependent on the physiochemical attributes of the drug – namely, molecular size, degree of ionisation, lipid solubility and its ability to cross biological membranes. Any pharmacokinetic alterations in the V_d of a particular drug in the obese population will be drug-specific and needs to be considered on an individual drug basis.

Clearance describes the relationship between concentration and the rate of elimination of drug from the body, and is inversely related to the steady-state plasma concentration of a drug. Clearance is largely influenced by the liver and kidneys, the principal organs involved in the removal of drugs and their metabolites. Limited information exists on the effects of obesity on the cytochrome P450 pathway and on glomerular filtration, tubular secretion and tubular re-absorption. Research has found that, in non-diabetic obese patients, obesity is associated with functional and structural renal changes and glomerular hyperfiltration, which increases glomerular filtration and renal plasma flow by up to 51% and 31%, respectively. This potentially has implications for drugs which are renally cleared.

Han and colleagues have stipulated three hypotheses on the relationship between drug clearance and obesity (Figure 18.1), namely:

1) Obese individuals exhibit higher *absolute* drug clearances than their normally weighted counterparts.
2) Clearance does not increase linearly with total body weight.
3) Clearance and lean body weight are linearly correlated.

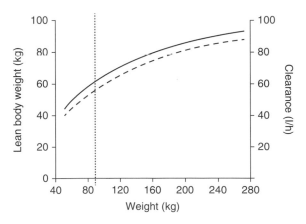

Figure 18.1 Relationship between lean body weight (LBW) and drug clearance, as stipulated by Han *et al*. (2007). Patients to the right of the vertical dashed line are obese (>30 kg/m²). The linear relationship between clearance and LBW is shown by the LBW (solid curve) and clearance graphs (dotted curve) running parallel to each other. Reprinted by permission from Macmillan Publishers Ltd © 2007 and the American Society for Clinical Pharmacology and Therapeutics.

Evaluating these pharmacokinetic principles means that no single rule will fit all anticoagulant drugs used for the management of VTE in the obese, as any pharmacokinetic changes will be drug-specific.

Published clinical studies suggest that, when obese patients are prescribed anticoagulant therapy for the management of VTE, they are often under-dosed. This may, in part, be due to a perceived increased risk of bleeding when increasing the dose in line with weight, but it could also be related to obtaining an accurate weight for the patient in question. Data published by the National Patient Safety Agency in the UK found that patients are not commonly weighed in UK hospitals, and that clinicians are poor at estimating patients' weights and are more likely to underestimate an obese patient's actual weight.

Drugs Where Recognised Therapeutic Drug Monitoring Overcomes the Challenges of any Changes That Obesity May Have on Drug Pharmacokinetic Profiles

Anticoagulants such as warfarin and unfractionated heparin have a long tradition of close therapeutic drug monitoring and adjustment of the drug dose, in order to achieve a recognised therapeutic range. The role of therapeutic drug monitoring has evolved, due to the inter-patient and intra-patient variability observed with these agents. For warfarin, this variability is explained by factors such as age, nutritional status, other medications, and the presence of genetic polymorphisms. For unfractionated heparin, its binding to plasma proteins, macrophages and endothelial cells complicates its pharmacokinetic profile, leading to the variability seen.

Therefore, when prescribing either of these agents for the obese population for the management of VTE, close monitoring and dose adjustment is recommended in order to reach the desired therapeutic range. Indeed, VKA therapy has the most experience of being prescribed in the very obese population and currently remains the first line oral agent of choice, until further clinical experience emerges with the use of the direct oral anticoagulants (DOACs). Following the availability of low molecular weight heparin in clinical practice in the 1990s, unfractionated heparin (UFH) is rarely used for the management of VTE. However, when prescribed, research demonstrates that weight-based nanograms for unfractionated heparin perform much better, with weight reported to be the single best predictor of an individual's dose requirements of UFH.

Low Molecular Weight Heparins (LMWH)

Current practice in the UK would be to prescribe LMWH as the first line agent for a very obese patient being managed for VTE, alongside a VKA. Since their introduction into clinical practice in the 1990s, LMWH have become the preferred agents when an immediately acting anticoagulant is required, given their favourable pharmacokinetic profile relative to UFH, meaning that dosing in normally weighted patients with a *normal* renal function does not require routine monitoring when dosed on a mg/kg or IU/kg basis.

In brief, the pharmacokinetic profile of LMWH following subcutaneous injection is as follows; C_{max} 3–4 hours, the area under the plasma concentration (AUC) versus time curve for the different LMWH increases with rising doses, with repeated doses of LMWH also increasing the AUC. LMWH are largely confined to the intra-vascular space, and their apparent V_d corresponds to the plasma volume. The elimination of LMWH is primarily through a non-saturable renal route. Given that the dosing of LMWH is based on a mg/kg or IU/kg basis, is there a dose cap that should be applied for the LMWHs when treating VTE in the obese?

In the UK, three LMWH are commonly prescribed: dalteparin, enoxaparin and tinzaparin. The manufacturers of dalteparin recommend a dose cap of 18 000 IU per day, while the other two have no dose cap listed in their summary of product characteristics for the management of VTE.

Small-scale studies from clinical practice, where anti-Xa activity has been measured as a proxy for LMWH pharmacokinetic profile, suggests that supra-therapeutic concentrations are not reached, assuming a normal renal function, when LMWH is dosed on actual body weight. Indeed, for the management of unstable angina

Table 18.1 Summary of key points for the treatment of VTE with anticoagulant therapy.

Indication	Agents	Manufacturers' recommendations	Comments
VTE treatment	LMWH	Doses are based on an IU/kg basis, with dose banding considered best practice in the UK. Manufacturers of dalteparin suggest a dose cap at 18 000 IU daily.	Dose capping is not justified, and dose can be increased with increasing weight. Information in Class III (BMI > 40 kg/m^2) obese patients is still lacking when dosed on actual body weight. In all cases, monitoring of anti-Xa activity and subsequent dose adjustment would seem prudent. At our centre, assuming normal renal function, we prescribe enoxaparin 1.5 mg/kg daily, based on actual body weight for patients weighing up to 130 kg, For patients >130 kg, depending on patient factors, an individualised decision is made on whether to prescribe 1.5 mg/kg daily or 0.75 mg/kg bd.
	Fondaparinux	Dose banding already exists, with a suggested dose of 10 mg once daily for patients weighing > 100 kg.	Published data demonstrates that, as weight increases, so does the clearance of fondaparinux. Data is lacking for Class II (BMI 35–39.9 kg/m^2) and Class III (BMI ≥ 40 kg/m^2) obese patients, so uncertainty exists whether 10 mg once daily is sufficient.
	Oral direct thrombin and direct Xa inhibitors	Dosing is fixed according to the specific agent. Manufacturers do not suggest that the dose needs altering in the obese population	Further clinical experience and research required before any firm recommendations can be made.

or ST elevation myocardial infarction (STEMI), the manufacturers of enoxaparin suggest a dose of 1 mg/kg twice a day, with 150 mg twice a day appearing as the highest dose in their dosing tables. The dose for the treatment of VTE in the UK is lower, at 1.5 mg/kg once a day, so it would not be unreasonable to prescribe a 200 kg patient either the 1.5 mg/kg dose (i.e. 300 mg once a day), or split the dose to 150 mg every 12 hours, as any dose of enoxaparin for a patient > 150 kg would require patients to administer two injections per day.

For tinzaparin, a small-scale pharmacokinetic study suggested that anti-Xa activity was consistent over the weight ranges, and concluded that weight-adjusted tinzaparin produces a predictable response and that the dose does not need to be capped. It is well tolerated, although injection site bruising may be more common.

The manufacturers of dalteparin recommend that the maximum dose for the management of VTE is 18 000 IU daily. This would see all significantly obese patients receiving a dose cap. Clinical studies where patients have been treated with dalteparin 200 IU/kg once daily, based on actual body weight (range: 56–190 kg and range 91–182 kg), report no thromboembolic or bleeding complications and suggest, like other LMWH, that dosing should be on actual weight, assuming a *normal* renal function.

For LMWH, from the information published to date, dosing should be based on actual body weight, and dose capping is not justified. However, this data is largely based on obese class I (BMI 30–34.9 kg/m^2) and II (BMI 35–39.9 kg/m^2) patients. Data on morbidly obese class III (BMI > 40 kg/m^2) patients is still lacking. In all cases, it would seem prudent to monitor anti-Xa activity and adjust doses as necessary. Table 18.1 summarises the main points for LMWH, along with other agents for the treatment of VTE and the practice at our centre when prescribing enoxaparin to obese patients.

Fondaparinux

Though not commonly prescribed in UK practice for the management VTE, in some circumstances (e.g. allergy to LMWH), there may be a requirement to prescribe fondaparinux. This synthetic pentasaccharide, which has a high affinity for antithrombin following subcutaneous injection, reaches a peak plasma concentration around two hours. Its V_d is reported to be 8.2 l, and it largely resides in the intravascular space. It is found to be highly protein-bound to antithrombin (>94%) in the plasma, with complete (100%) absorption following subcutaneous injection. Its elimination half-life is around 17 hours, and it is excreted largely through the renal route as an unchanged compound.

The dosing of fondaparinux for the treatment of VTE for normally weighted patients is weight-based, and the manufacturers themselves acknowledge that plasma clearance of fondaparinux increases with body weight (9% increase per 10 kg). The information on fondaparinux dosing in the obese is largely derived from sub-group analysis from clinical trial data. For the treatment of VTE, the MATISSE trials compared once-daily fondaparinux (5 mg if < 50 kg, 7.5 mg if 50–100 kg and 10 mg if > 100 kg) to LMWH (enoxaparin 1 mg/kg bd) for the initial treatment of DVT and to IV UFH (APTR 1.5–2.5) in the initial treatment of PE.

Fondaparinux was found to be just as effective as its comparators in both trials, and obese patients were found to be relatively well represented in both trials, with 11.4% of patients weighing > 100 kg (100.5–175.5) and 27% having a BMI > 30 kg/m² (30–80.3) in the fondaparinux arms. No significant differences were reported between treatment groups in any of the weight or BMI subgroups. This suggests that increasing the dose with increasing weight is required for fondaparinux for the management of VTE, confirming a relationship between clearance and weight. What is not known is by how much to increase the dose, due to the limited experience that exists. It would seem prudent to monitor anti-Xa activity, if this agent were to be prescribed in a morbidly obese patient.

Direct Oral Anticoagulants (DOACs)

More recently, the direct oral anticoagulants have become available for clinicians to prescribe for the management of VTE, with apixaban, dabigatran, edoxaban and rivaroxaban all licensed for use for this indication in the UK. These agents overcome many of the practical disadvantages that VKA and LMWH therapy possess, and are redefining how VTE is managed, both acutely and long-term, in clinical practice. Perhaps surprisingly, the agents have been licensed at fixed doses, despite other anticoagulants (even those with predictable pharmacokinetic profiles) requiring a *discriminating* factor for determining a patient's dose (e.g. weight for LMWH). The pharmacokinetic properties of the four DOACs available in the UK are compared to LMWH in Table 18.2.

Dabigatran

There is limited published information on dabigatran use in the obese population. The current summary of product characteristics states that the available clinical and pharmacokinetic data suggests that no dose adjustment is necessary, but close clinical surveillance is recommended in patients with a body weight < 50 kg.

The RE-COVER study formed the basis for dabigatran's license for the acute management of venous thromboembolism. In this study, the mean weight in the dabigatran arm was 85.5 kg (range 38–175 kg), with a mean BMI of 28.9 kg/m². The pre-specified analysis of evaluating BMI was not found to influence the observed treatment effect, but the number of patients in the very high weight category would have been small, so it is difficult to draw any robust conclusions from this data.

Though a different indication, in the RE-LY study, evaluating dabigatran versus warfarin in patients with atrial fibrillation, the overall mean weight of patients was 82.6 kg (32–222 kg); 17.1% of patients weighed above 100 kg. Sub-group analysis from this trial showed a tendency of increasing dabigatran concentrations with decreasing body weight; geometric mean values of dose normalised trough concentrations were reported as 0.998, 0.824 and 0.652 ng/ml/mg in < 50 kg, 50–100 kg and > 100 kg patients, respectively. This suggests a relationship of increasing weight leading to a decrease in overall dabigatran exposure.

Table 18.2 The pharmacokinetic profiles of the newer anticoagulant agents compared to enoxaparin.

	Apixaban	Dabigatran	Edoxaban	Rivaroxaban	Enoxaparin
Mode of action	Direct Xa inhibitor	Direct IIa inhibitor	Direct Xa inhibitor	Direct Xa inhibitor	Indirect Xa inhibitor
Protein binding	≈87%	≈35%	≈50%	>90%	≈80%
Cmax (hrs)	1–3	0.5–2	1–2	2.5–4	3–4
Volume of distribution (l)	21	60–70	107	50	6
Dialyzable	Not expected to be effective	Yes	Not expected to be effective	Not expected to be effective	No
Half life (hours)	8–15	12–14	10–14	5–9	4–5
Activation	No	Yes – prodrug dabigatran etexilate converted to dabigatran via hydrolysis	No	No	No
Metabolism	Oxidation (via CYP 3A4) and conjugation	Conjugation	Oxidation, hydrolysis and conjugation (via CYP3A4/5)	Oxidation (via CYP 3A4) and CYP2J2 and hydrolysis	–
Interactions	Potent CYP 3A4 inhibitors	P-gp inhibitors	P-gp inhibitors	Combined P-gp inhibitors and CYP 3A4 inhibitors	–
Renal excretion of unchanged drug	25%	80%	35%	36%	10%

Until further data is available, particularly on outcomes in morbidly obese patients prescribed dabigatran, caution is warranted in prescribing fixed doses of dabigatran for the acute management of VTE.

Rivaroxaban

The current summary of product characteristics for rivaroxaban states that extremes of body weight (<50 kg or >120 kg) have only a small influence on rivaroxaban plasma concentrations (<25%). In both the DVT and PE studies for rivaroxaban, approximately 14% of the trial population weighed > 100 kg, but further data, including subgroup analysis for patients in different weight categories, is not available. Until further outcome information is available with the use of rivaroxaban in the morbidly obese population, caution is required with its use for the acute management of VTE.

Apixaban

In a study to specifically assess the effect of body weight on apixaban pharmacokinetics, 18 healthy subjects were enrolled into each of three weight groups: < 50 kg; reference 65–85 kg; and 120 kg or more. Following a single 10 mg dose, the PK and PD profile was determined. Those in the > 120 kg group had a 30% and 20% lower apixaban Cmax and AUC, and those weighing < 50 kg had a 30% and 20% higher apixaban Cmax and AUC, compared with the reference group. The authors of the study also report that anti-Xa activity was well correlated with apixaban plasma concentrations, regardless of body weight, and they conclude that the effect of body weight on apixaban exposure is modest and that dose adjustment is not required at the extremes of body weight. This data from healthy subjects clearly shows that, as weight increases, Cmax and AUC decreases. Although for obese patients the change might be insignificant, the effectiveness of the licensed apixaban doses for morbidly obese patients remains unknown.

The current summary of product characteristics for apixaban states that no dose adjustment is required for body weight for the treatment of VTE. The data from the AMPLIFY and AMPLIFY-EXT trials demonstrated primary efficacy and safety outcomes in patients, regardless of weight or body mass index. In the AMPLIFY study, the mean weight in the apixaban arm was 84.6 kg (±19.8), of which 522 patients (19.4%) were > 100 kg, although the number in the very obese category is not published. The published data with the use of apixaban in the morbidly obese is lacking and, once again, caution is warranted with its use.

Edoxaban

The standard dose of edoxaban for the management of VTE (and stroke prevention in the context of AF) is 60 mg once a day. The manufacturers of this agent, however, do recommend a dose reduction to 30 mg once daily if one of the following factors is present: renal impairment (15–50 ml/min); low body weight (<60 kg); or the presence of P-gp inhibitors (e.g. ciclosporin, dronedarone, erythromycin, ketaconazole). Weight being a factor for dose reduction suggests over-exposure of edoxaban in those with a low body weight. Indeed, in the phase III clinical studies (both NVAF and VTE indications), patients with body weight ≤ 60 kg had a 50% edoxaban dose reduction, and had similar efficacy and less bleeding when compared to warfarin. Furthermore, in a population pharmacokinetic analysis of the ENGAGE AF-TIMI 48 study in the non-valvular AF population, C_{max} and AUC in patients with median low body weight (55 kg) were increased by 40% and 13%, respectively, compared with patients with median high body weight (84 kg).

Information on the impact of obesity with edoxaban is scarce. In the Hokusai-VTE study, the median weight of subjects in the edoxaban arm was 80.5 (60, 108 (10th, 90th percentile)). Therefore, it is fair to conclude that practical experience of using this agent in an obese population is very limited, similar to the other DOACs.

For all the DOACs, the manufacturers of these agents give mixed messages about their compounds. Some of the manufacturers suggest that no dose adjustments are necessary for patients at the extremes of body weight, while others suggest that dose adjustments are required, particularly for those of low body weight. In our opinion, based on the information currently available on the obese population, it seems too early to draw such a conclusion. All four drugs demonstrate that, at lower body weights, a higher exposure of the drug is seen, and the opposite occurs with increasing weight. Therefore, for a 181 kg patient presenting with an acute PE, we cannot be confident that the manufacturer's fixed dose will be as efficacious as in a *normally* weighted individual.

Further use and research will determine whether their suggested fixed dose is truly efficacious in the morbidly obese sub-population, and there is an urgent need for studies evaluating outcomes in the very obese with the use of these agents. Currently, if any of the DOACs were to be prescribed in a morbidly obese patient, it would be prudent to monitor the respective plasma concentration of the drug prescribed, to ensure adequate response.

Key Points

- Obesity is a recognised risk factor for VTE.
- Objectively diagnosing VTE in a morbidly obese patient remains challenging and, in some circumstances, alternative imaging modalities to usual methods may need to be explored, including the use of high weight limit or open MRI scanners.

- Obese patients have been consistently under-represented in studies evaluating anticoagulants for the management of VTE.
- Small-scale studies on LMWH and fondaparinux suggest that, as weight increases, so does their clearance and, thus, higher doses reflecting increased body weight are warranted.
- For DOACs, the studies to date evaluating these drugs in the obese population are limited so, until further evidence is available, LMWH combined with VKA remains the treatment of choice for the morbidly obese patient.

Further Reading

Abernethy DR, Greenblatt DJ (1986). Drug disposition in obese humans: an update. *Clinical Pharmacokinetics* **11**: 199–213.

Cheymol G (2000). Effects of obesity on pharmacokinetics implications for drug therapy. *Clinical Pharmacokinetics*; **39**: 215–231.

Green B, Duffull SB (2003). Developing a dosing strategy for enoxaparin in obese patients. *British Journal of Clinical Pharmacology* **56**: 96–103.

Han PY, Duffull SB, Kirkpatrick CMJ, Green B (2007). Dosing in obesity: A simple solution to a big problem. *Clinical Pharmacology and Therapeutics* **82**: 505–508.

Hanley MJ, Abernethy DR, Greenblatt DJ (2010). Effect of obesity on the pharmacokinetics of drugs in humans. *Clinical Pharmacokinetics* **49**(2): 71–87.

Hawley PC, Hawley MP (2011). Difficulties in diagnosing pulmonary embolism in the obese patient: a literature review. *Vascular Medicine* **16**(6): 444–51.

Patel JP, Roberts LN, Arya R (2011). Anticoagulating obese patients in the modern era. *British Journal of Haematology* **155**: 137–149.

Raschke RA, Reilly BM, Guidry JR, Fontana JR, Srinivas S (1993). The Weight-based Heparin Dosing Nomogram Compared with a 'Standard Care' Nomogram – A Randomized Controlled Trial. *Archives of Internal Medicine* **119**: 874–881.

19

Venous Thromboembolism in Intensive Care

Gill Parmilan[1] and Jecko Thachil[2]

[1] Core Trainee, Manchester Royal Infirmary, Manchester, UK
[2] Department of Haematology, Manchester Royal Infirmary, Manchester, UK

Introduction

Critically ill patients are at high risk of venous thromboembolism (VTE), and they often have a number of risk factors which are commonly associated with heightened risk of VTE. However, the diagnosis of VTE may not be easy in these patients. First of all, the patient may not be able to explain the classical symptoms of deep vein thrombosis (DVT) or pulmonary embolism (PE). In addition, the underlying clinical state of respiratory illness or generalised oedema means that the diagnosis of DVT or PE respectively may be overlooked. Diagnostic tests may be difficult, due to transportation issues and technical difficulties in delineating the cause of the underlying abnormalities. Treatments can also have issues, in that anticoagulant medications are often required by parenteral methods, and there may be issues with monitoring.

Incidence

PE is one of the frequently under-diagnosed illnesses identified during autopsies. When specifically looking at critically ill patients, up to one-third of the autopsies has PE as the cause of death, with it not having been clinically suspected in most of the cases. The incidence can vary depending on the type of ICU – whether they predominantly deal with trauma or surgical patients, when the likelihood is higher, compared with predominantly medical patients. Also, the incidence can vary, compared to historical studies, since thromboprophylaxis, pharmacological or otherwise is standard in most ICUs in the current era.

   Reports have shown an incidence of DVT of up to 30% in the absence of thromboprophylaxis. In a prospective cohort study, Minet *et al.* (2012) analysed all mechanically ventilated patients requiring a thoracic computed tomography (CT) scan for any medical reason. Of 176 included patients, 33 (18.7%) had PE diagnosed although, in 20 of these patients, there was no clinical suspicion. In the pivotal PROTECT Investigators trial, proximal lower limb DVT occurred in 96 patients (5.1%) receiving dalteparin, and 109 (5.8%) receiving unfractionated heparin, of a total of 1087 patients. The proportion of patients with PE was 24 (1.3%) and 43 (2.3%) with dalteparin and unfractionated heparin, respectively.

Diagnosis

Diagnosis of VTE in the non-critically ill is well established, with clear clinical algorithms (e.g. Wells rule) and exclusion tests such as D-dimer. The clinical prediction scores have, however, been not validated for use in the critical care setting and, thus, cannot be used as standard. Also, there is no role for D-dimer in the exclusion of VTE in the critically ill. It is well-known that the several co-morbid conditions in the ICU patient would make the D-dimer test unhelpful.

As would be the case in non-ICU patients, diagnosis of DVT is primarily using Doppler ultrasonography in the upper or lower limb thromboses. Portable ultrasound machines may make diagnosis easier. CT pulmonary angiogram is preferred for the evaluation of PE over ventilation perfusion scan, because changes in the pulmonary fields affect result interpretation in the latter case. In patients who cannot have CTPA for various reasons, including renal impairment or contrast allergy, ultrasound Doppler of the lower limbs might help to diagnose DVT, which would mean a PE is likely to be present as well. Echocardiography can be used to demonstrate acute right ventricular strain which, in the absence of alternate explanations, may be attributable to a new PE. However, it does need to be remembered that echocardiography can be normal in many cases of CTPA-confirmed PE and, thus, cannot be used as an exclusion modality.

Thromboprophylaxis or Not?

The American College of Chest Physicians (ACCP) gives a grade 1a (strong) recommendation for thromboprophylaxis for prevention of VTE in critical care patients. Also, there is definite evidence that mortality in patients who did not receive thromboprophylaxis within 24 hours of ICU admission was higher than those who were treated with early thromboprophylaxis (7.6% vs 6.3%, $P = .001$). This association between lack of early thromboprophylaxis and mortality is significant, even after adjusting for variables. It would seem logical to think thromboprophylaxis should be the norm in the critical care units, but there are several reasons why this may not be the case. Some of these exclusion criteria for pharmacological thromboprophylaxis include heightened bleeding risk, avoiding drugs which can accumulate in renal impairment, coexisting thrombocytopenia or abnormal coagulation screen.

Abnormal clotting screen should probably be never considered as an absolute contraindication for pharmacological thromboprophlyaxis, since the former, by itself, does not constitute a risk factor for bleeding. There is now enough evidence in the medical literature on liver disease that abnormal coagulation screen (extremely common in these patients) does not provide an autoanticoagulated state, and such patients can still develop thrombosis, including DVT and PE. This is due to the fact that clotting screens only measure the procoagulant pathway, which is always counterbalanced by the mechanisms provided by the natural anticoagulants, protein C, protein S and antithrombin.

Critically ill patients may also form a similar cohort to patients with liver disease, wherein there is a balance between the procoagulant and anticoagulant mechanisms, which means they are not at an increased risk of bleeding from the point of view of an abnormal laboratory clotting screen. Thrombocytopenia, however, does provide some dilemma. There is no evidence-based threshold for platelet count above which pharmacological thromboprophylaxis is safe. It is generally accepted that a platelet count above $25–30 \times 10^9/l$ may be acceptable for administering low molecular weight heparin at a prophylactic dose, in the absence of additional bleeding risks.

There is always a worry regarding bleeding in patients undergoing thromboprophylaxis. A prospective cohort study in 2007 found that up to 80% of ICU patients receiving thromboprophylaxis will have at least one minor episode of bleeding. The same study also found that major bleeding occurred in 5.6% of ICU patients, regardless of whether or not they received thromboprophylaxis. Taking into account all this information, the National Institute for Health and Care Excellence guidelines advise physicians to follow local protocols for prevention of VTE, and state that it is important to understand each individual patient's physiological status before making the decision of thromboprophylaxis or not.

The PROTECT trial has given us confidence in deciding which may be the best agent if pharmacological thromboprophylaxis is chosen. In this randomised trial, which compared unfractionated heparin with low molecular weight heparin as VTE prophylaxis in the ICU, there was no significant difference between the group randomly allocated to receive 5000 units of subcutaneous dalteparin once daily and the cohort which received 5000 units subcutaneous unfractionated heparin twice daily. The proximal DVT incidence within 48 hours after admission was 5.1 % DVT in the dalteparin group versus 5.8 % in the UFH group, while the rate of PE was significantly lower in the dalteparin group (1.3 % vs 2.3 %; $P = 0.01$).

Mechanical Thromboprophylaxis

Mechanical thromboprophylaxis (using compression stockings or intermittent pneumatic compression) alone is recommended for ICU patients at high risk of bleeding, in whom thromboprophylaxis with antico-agulant agents is contraindicated. Compression stockings provide continuous stimulation of linear blood flow, prevent venous dilatation, and can stimulate endothelial fibrinolytic activity. Intermittent pneumatic compression empties blood from behind the valve cusps, thereby preventing venous stasis, and increases the velocity of blood flow.

However, both of the above are contraindicated in the following conditions:

- Local leg conditions or extreme deformity.
- Marked leg oedema or pulmonary oedema from congestive heart failure.
- Ischaemic vascular disease, diabetic neuropathy or arteriosclerosis.
- Lack of patient co-operation.

Despite there being copious amounts of evidence and guidelines from various bodies supporting the use of pharmacological and mechanical thromboprophylaxis, the ENDORSE multinational study, which enrolled more than 60 000 patients in more than 30 countries, concluded that recommended VTE prophylaxis is only prescribed to 50% of at-risk patients around the world.

Treatment of Venous Thromboembolism in the Critically Ill

Pharmacological treatment of a newly diagnosed DVT or PE in the ICU is no different from a non-ICU patient. However, in general, low molecular weight heparin is the drug of choice, for various reasons. Unfractionated heparin has the disadvantage of needing frequent monitoring using the APTT method, and can be a problem if the patient has a prolonged APTT prior to its commencement. The other theoretical issue is the problem of acute phase reactants and activated endothelium, which can bind to the unfractionated version of heparin more readily than the low molecular weight formulation. However, unfractionated heparin is certainly attractive in patients with severe renal impairment and those with extremely high bleeding risk, where easy reversibility is advantageous. For the same reason, in patients who may need major surgery or procedures, unfractionated heparin may be a better choice.

In all other cases, low molecular weight heparin at therapeutic dose is ideal, due to very low risk of heparin-induced thrombocytopenia, predictable pharmacokinetics, and easy administration. There is controversy regarding the measurement of anti-factor Xa activity in patients receiving the low molecular weight heparins. The proponents of measurement explain the possibility of patient-dependent factors influencing the anti-factor Xa activity, such as decreased bioavailability from generalised oedema, and vasoconstrictive treatment, even in the absence of renal failure. They suggest that impaired peripheral circulation may make the systemic bioavailability of the anticoagulant inadequate, although not all reports concur with this finding. It is reasonable to consider the measurement of anti-factor Xa in patients with moderate to severe renal impairment, and those with high risk of bleeding, where marinating the drug level at the lower end of the therapeutic range may be useful.

The relatively new direct oral anticoagulants may seem attractive in the critical care setting, but there have been no randomised trials in this group and, thus, the use of these drugs will be unlicensed. Although the lack of monitoring is an advantage with these oral anticoagulants, the unpredictability of absorption in critically ill patients may mean inadequate bioavailability without being obvious.

In patients who may have an absolute contraindication for pharmacological thromboprophylaxis, mechanical thromboprophylaxis should be ensured, and an inferior vena cava filter may be inserted. However, the filters should be considered as a temporary measure, and should be removed as soon as adequate anticoagulation can be resumed.

Conclusion

VTE is a common and overlooked complication in the ICU. It is imperative to understand the interplay of the plethora of general and ICU-specific risk factors that can lead to a VTE. This is especially so since the diagnosis is not often considered. Even when suspected, the diagnosis can be arduous, as critically ill patients are usually mechanically ventilated and sedated, which can lead to practical issues with radiological imaging. Despite increasing evidence for the use of thromboprophylaxis to decrease the rate of VTE-related mortality, its uptake has not been universal, probably due to the perceived fear of bleeding. In such cases, mechanical thromboprophylaxis can be used, and may provide some protection from thrombosis. An individual risk/benefit assessment should be made for each patient prior to commencing pharmacological thromboprophlayxis, while monitoring of anti-factor Xa should be considered in selected patients who require treatment of thromboembolic episode.

Further Reading

Arnold DM, Donahoe L, Clarke FJ, Tkacyzyk AJ, Heels-Ansdell D, Zytaruk N *et al.* (2007). Bleeding during critical illness: a prospective cohort study using a new measurement tool. *Clinical and Investigative Medicine* **30**: E93–102.

Attia J, Ray JG, Cook DJ, Douketis J, Ginsberg JS, Geerts WH (2001). Deep vein thrombosis and its prevention in critically ill adults. *Archives of Internal Medicine* **161**: 1268–79.

Cook D, Meade M, Guyatt G, Walter S, Heels-Ansdell D, Warkentin TE *et al.* (2011). Dalteparin versus unfractionated heparin in critically ill patients. *New England Journal of Medicine* **364**: 1305–14.

Dorffler-Melly J, de Jonge E, Pont AC, Meijers J, Vroom MB, Buller HR *et al.* (2002). Bioavailability of subcutaneous low molecular weight heparin to patients on vasopressors. *Lancet* **359**: 849–50.

Geerts WH, Bergqvist d, Pineo GF, Heit JA, Samama CM, Lassen MR *et al.* (2008). Prevention of venous thromboembolism: American College of Chest Physicians Evidence Based Clinical Practice Guidelines (8th edition). *Chest* **133**: 381S–453S.

Ho KM, Chavan S, Pilcher D (2011). Omission of early thromboprophylaxis and mortality in critically ill patients: a multicentre registry study. *Chest* **140**: 1436–46.

Ibrahim EH, Iregui M, Prentice D, Sherman G, Kollef MH, Shannon W (2002). Deep vein thrombosis during prolonged mechanical ventilation despite prophylaxis. *Critical Care Medicine* **30**: 771–4.

McLeod AG, Geerts W (2011). Venous Thromboembolism prophylaxis in critically ill patients. *Critical Care Clinics* **27**: 765–80.

Minet C, Lugosi M, Savoye PY, Menez C, Ruckly S, Bonadona A *et al.* (2012). Pulmonary embolism in mechanically ventilated patients requiring computed tomography: Prevalence, risk factors and outcome. *Critical Care Medicine* **40**: 3202–8.

Minet C, Potton L, Bonadona A *et al.* (2015). Venous thromboembolism in the ICU:main characteristics, diagnosis and thromboprophylaxis. *Critical Care* **19**: 287–94.

National Institute for Health and Clinical Excellence (2010). *Venous Thromboembolism: reducing the risk*. NICE clinical guideline 92: reducing the risk of venous thrombolism (deep vein thrombosis and pulmonary embolism) in patients admitted to hospital. NICE. Available at: https://www.nice.org.uk/guidance/cg92.

Thachil J (2013). Is coagulopathy a contraindication for thromboprophylaxis? *QJM* **106**(12): 1155–6.

20

Venous Thromboembolism; a Primary Care Perspective

David Fitzmaurice

Professor of Cardiorespiratory Primary Care, University of Warwick, Coventry, UK

Introduction

This chapter looks at the diagnosis and management of venous thromboembolic (VTE) disease from a primary care perspective. VTE covers the clinical conditions of deep vein thrombosis and pulmonary embolism. While these are considered a spectrum of the same disease process, for convenience they will be considered separately.

Deep Vein Thrombosis (DVT)

In primary care, the classical presentation of DVT is as an acutely painful, red, swollen calf. Diagnosis needs to be confirmed radiologically, and is defined as a radiologically confirmed partial or total occlusion of the deep venous system of the legs sufficient, to produce symptoms of pain or swelling (Fitzmaurice and Hobbs, 1999). DVT is associated with pregnancy, contraceptive pill use, immobility, surgery, malignancy, advancing age, smoking and certain clotting disorders (Hirsh and Hoak, 1996). Both proximal and isolated calf vein thromboses can cause post-thrombotic syndrome, recurrent venous thrombosis and pulmonary embolus, with associated morbidity and mortality.

From a primary care perspective, the principle dilemma is how to distinguish clinically between potential VTE, which may need referral for further investigation, and other causes of leg swelling. As always, a balance needs to be struck between over-referral to diagnostic services (in this case, radiology) and missing a potentially life-threatening illness. Care pathways utilising clinical assessment and biomarkers are evolving all the time, with less dependence on secondary care.

Diagnosis and Investigation

The clinical diagnosis of deep venous thrombosis (DVT) was historically made on the basis of pain, swelling, venous distension, and pain on forced dorsiflexion of the foot (Homan's sign), but this is notoriously unreliable (Weinman and Salzman, 1994; Wells *et al.*, 1995), with many conditions mimicking it – for example, cellulitis, muscular sprain, and popliteal inflammatory cysts (Baker's cysts) (Weinman and Salzman, 1994). The predominant diagnostic test for DVT is now ultrasonography, with venography rarely used, as this is an invasive test which is inconvenient, painful, and can be associated with allergic and other side-effects (Wells *et al.*, 1995). The sensitivity and specificity of ultrasound has been reported as 78% and 98% respectively

(Wells *et al.*, 1995). Light reflection rheography is also an effective non-invasive technique for screening patients with suspected DVT (Thomas *et al.*, 1991).

For all clinicians, but especially within a community environment, it is important to decide whether or not to refer for a diagnostic investigation, so it is important to determine whether the diagnosis is likely or not (pre-test probability). In primary care, there are currently two pieces of information which can help guide this decision – the Well's score and D-dimer testing. These are best used in combination and within a pre-defined diagnostic pathway. The National Institute for Health and Care Excellence (NICE) have published guidelines which recommend for DVT an initial clinical assessment, followed by a two-level Wells DVT probability score (NICE, 2012a).

The Well's score is a simple scoring system which aims to discriminate between patients with a high risk of DVT, who require imaging, and those with low risk, in whom an alternative diagnosis should be sought.

In order to calculate the Well's score of an individual, it is necessary to score one point for each of the following:

- Active cancer (treatment ongoing or within the previous six months, or palliative).
- Paralysis, paresis or recent plaster immobilisation of the legs.
- Recently bedridden for three days or more, or major surgery within the previous 12 weeks, requiring general or regional anaesthesia.
- Localised tenderness along the distribution of the deep venous system (such as the back of the calf).
- Entire leg is swollen.
- Calf swelling by more than 3 cm, compared with the asymptomatic leg (measured 10 cm below the tibial tuberosity).
- Pitting oedema confined to the symptomatic leg.
- Collateral superficial veins (non-varicose).
- Previously documented DVT.

It is also necessary to subtract two points if an alternative cause is considered at least as likely as DVT. This is perhaps the most important component of the score.

The risk of DVT is likely if the score is 2 or more, and unlikely if the score is 1 or less.

In many environments, the Well's score is used on its own, in order to identify those patients who require further investigation. It is possible to improve the diagnostic pathway, however, by combining the Well's score with a particular biomarker – the D-dimer. It is important, however, that anyone utilising a D-dimer measurement understands what the test is measuring, and the implications of high and low values. It remains the case that many radiology departments insist on D-dimer measurements, even with a positive Well's score. This has proved useful in determining whether patients with a negative scan require repeat scanning.

D-dimer levels are elevated in plasma in the presence of acute thrombosis, because of simultaneous activation of coagulation and fibrinolysis, The negative predictive value of D-dimer testing is high, and a normal D-dimer level renders acute VTE unlikely. On the other hand, fibrin is also produced in a wide variety of conditions, such as cancer, inflammation, bleeding, trauma, surgery and necrosis. Accordingly, the positive predictive value of elevated D-dimer levels is low, and D-dimer testing is not useful for confirmation of VTE. Thus, the diagnostic utility of D-dimer testing is in excluding disease, rather than confirming it. From a clinical perspective, in a situation where a Well's score is 2 or more, conferring high risk, a D-dimer test is unhelpful, as the patient will require diagnostic imaging anyway. If, though, a patient has a low Well's score, a negative D-dimer would confirm that the patient has a very low likelihood of VTE, and would not require further investigation.

It is important, however, to understand that not all tests are the same. A number of D-dimer assays are available. The quantitative enzyme-linked immunosorbent assay (ELISA) or ELISA-derived assays report diagnostic sensitivity of 95% or more and can, therefore, be used to exclude VTE in patients with a low pre-test probability using the Well's score. Point-of-care tests generally have moderate sensitivity, and it is important that primary care users are aware of the strengths and limitations of the test they are using.

In summary, D-dimer tests indicate active fibrinolysis and, hence, provide a screening technique for DVT. While not specific to DVT, D-dimer has a high (>95%) negative predictive value, and is a reliable method for the exclusion of DVT in symptomatic patients, in combination with a clinical risk assessment tool such as the Well's score (Turkstra *et al.*, 1998).

By combining clinical assessment and including a D-dimer test within the diagnostic pathway, it is possible to avoid hospitalisation for the majority of patients with suspected DVT, with the only hospital contact being the diagnostic procedure – usually ultrasound. As we will see, in combining these diagnostic pathways with new treatment options, DVT becomes much more a primary care issue than previously, with full primary care management now possible.

As a rule of thumb, patients require two negatives from the Well's score, D-dimer and ultrasound scan to confidently rule out a DVT. Thus, patients with a high Well's score and a positive D-dimer will require a follow-up scan if the initial scan is negative. This is because below-knee DVTs may not be picked up on initial scan, although a proportion of these will develop into above-knee DVTs. Thus, it would be good practice to re-scan after one week.

Treatment

Goals of treatment of DVT are prevention of pulmonary embolism, restoration of venous patency and valvular function, and prevention of post-thrombotic syndrome (Lagerstedt *et al.*, 1985; Kakkar *et al.*, 1969). Standard management for these patients was, until relatively recently, emergency referral to hospital for diagnostic confirmation, bed rest and commencement of anticoagulation. Anticoagulation typically involves a hospital in-patient stay of around seven days for intravenous heparin administration, with daily Partial Thromboplastin Time (PTT) estimation, together with warfarin for approximately three months (with monitoring) (Weinman and Salzman, 1994).

It is now clear that subcutaneous administration of low-molecular weight heparin (LMWH) is as safe and effective as traditional intravenous therapy, with fewer complications and the advantage that PTT monitoring is not required (Hull *et al.*, 1992). Dosing schedules for LMWH are based solely on body weight. Secondary care data has suggested that LMWH can be cost-effective due to the reduced cost of monitoring and reduced hospital stay (Gould *et al.*, 1999). These studies have also highlighted the possibility of home treatment, with patients either self-dosing or receiving injections from a nurse or a relative (Wells *et al.*, 1998).

There is now an alternative to both of these treatment pathways, with new agents available for the treatment of both DVT and PE. The first of these licensed in Europe was rivaroxaban (NICE, 2012b). This is an oral factor Xa inhibitor, which is given without the need for parenteral medication such as warfarin, and affords the possibility of community management for patients with either DVT of sub-massive PE, where the only contact with secondary care would be for a diagnostic procedure. Other agents now licensed include: dabigatran, an oral direct thrombin inhibitor, which still requires heparin and is used in the same way as warfarin; and apixaban, an oral factor Xa inhibitor which works in the same way as rivaroxaban.

While oral anticoagulation is established in the treatment of patients with deep vein thrombosis, the duration of therapy remains debatable. Two prospective randomised studies for treatment of proximal deep vein thrombosis, comparing four weeks with three months (Levine *et al.*, 1995) and six weeks with six months warfarin therapy (Schulman *et al.*, 1995), have gone some way to resolving the issue. Although there are problems in comparing studies, due to difficulties in standardising diagnostic criteria, these studies showed recurrence rates after two years of 8.6% in the four-week group, compared with 0.9% in the three-month group (odds ratio = 10.1, 95% confidence interval 1.3–81.4), and 18.1% in the six-week group, compared with 9.5% in the six-month group (odds ratio = 2.1, 95% confidence interval 1.4–3.1).

Debate continues over the treatment of distal deep vein thrombosis, where thrombus is limited to the calf veins only. However, evidence for treatment is strong. Untreated symptomatic calf vein thrombosis in non-surgical patients has a recurrence rate of over 25%, with an attendant risk of proximal extension and pulmonary embolisation. This risk is reduced to 7.6% with treatment aiming for an INR of 2.0–3.0 for three months, which compares with rates of 12.4% with four weeks, 11.8% with six weeks, and 5.8% with six months oral anticoagulant therapy (Schulman *et al.*, 1995).

Future Developments

As we have seen above, it is now possible for diagnosis and treatment of DVT to be almost completely undertaken in primary care. This has the potential to improve the patient experience, while reducing the costs of hospital admission. There remain some contentious areas, however, such as the role of thrombophilia testing and the need for cancer screening. The current NICE guidelines essentially exclude thrombophilia testing in patients other than those with unusual presentations, but do recommend cancer screening for most patients. It is recommended to offer all patients diagnosed with unprovoked DVT or PE, who are not already known to have cancer, the following investigations for cancer: a physical examination (guided by the patient's full history), CXR, blood tests (FBC, serum calcium and LFTs) and urinalysis (NICE, 2012a).

Pulmonary Embolism

Pulmonary emboli usually arise from veins in the pelvis and leg. The risk factors are the same as for DVT. Up to 50% of those with fatal PE have no warning signs. The clinical presentation depends upon the size of the emboli, with small emboli remaining asymptomatic. Large, non-fatal emboli cause acute pleuritic chest pain, associated with shortness of breath, tachycardia and pyrexia. Associated features include haemoptysis, pleural effusion, hypotension, cyanosis and shock.

In primary care, any suspicion of pulmonary embolism (PE) should be treated as an acute medical emergency, with admission to hospital arranged urgently. The mainstay of diagnosis remains the ventilation/perfusion scan, although spiral CT scan is now regarded as the gold standard for diagnosis.

As seen within the section on DVT, there is scope for the management of sub-massive PE out of hospital; however, this needs carefully defined diagnostic and treatment pathways, which may evolve over the next few years.

Diagnosis

NICE recommend that the initial investigation for anyone with a suspected PE should be a chest X-ray. Thus, from a primary care perspective, any suspicion of a PE will require an emergency referral. If there is an abnormal chest X-ray and PE is still suspected, it is recommended that a two-level PE Well's score is undertaken. If the Well's score is 'unlikely', a D-dimer test is required. If the D-dimer test is negative, PE can be excluded. If the Well's score is positive, imaging is required.

Treatment

The traditional management of pulmonary embolism has been to stabilise the patient medically, and then anticoagulate in exactly the same manner as for DVT. This remains essentially the same today, but advances in the use of LMWH for DVT have seen investigation into the use of LMWH for the home management of PE (Simonneau *et al.*, 1997). Newer agents, including rivaroxaban, dabigatran and apixaban, are now available for treatment of PE (NICE, 2012b). While home management may be suitable for a small number of low-risk stable patients, the main priority from a primary care perspective is to arrange for hospital admission for assessment, stabilisation and confirmation of diagnosis.

No studies have looked specifically at the intensity of oral anticoagulation therapy for the treatment of pulmonary embolus. The current UK recommendation for patients diagnosed with a first pulmonary embolus is to aim for an INR of 2.5. These recommendations are based on results of studies primarily investigating the treatment of proximal deep vein thrombosis, where the occurrence of a pulmonary embolus was taken as an endpoint in interventional studies (Carson *et al.*, 1992; Hull *et al.*, 1982).

Future Developments

It is likely that, with the advent of oral anticoagulants which can replace the heparin/warfarin combination and require no monitoring, more patients with PE will be treated in the community, following either a short admission to hospital, or even no admission following a diagnostic procedure. These developments will require safe diagnostic and treatment pathways which suit the requirement of patients, primary care, and secondary care.

Prevention

One of the most useful advances in the area of thromboembolic disease has been preventative therapy, particularly with regard to hospital admissions. For patients who are at high risk due to their medical condition, or who are having high-risk operations, there are various options to reduce the incidence of DVT. These include formal anticoagulation, use of compression stockings, intra-operative pressure devices, and use of low molecular weight heparin. Newer agents, such as oral factor Xa inhibitors, are as effective as warfarin in both treatment and prevention of thromboembolism (NICE, 2012b).

The biggest single population risk factor for DVT is the use of female hormones, either as hormone replacement (HRT) or as oral contraception. The increased individual risk is very small, however and, particularly in the case of oral contraception, the overall health risk of not taking therapy is outweighed by the risk of taking it. The absolute risk of venous thrombosis in healthy young women is around 1 per 10 000 person years, rising to 3–4 per 10 000 person years during the time oral contraceptives are being used (Vandenbroucke *et al.*, 2001). Pregnancy, however, is itself is a risk factor for DVT. Pregnant patients at high risk, or with a previous history of thrombosis, should be treated with low-molecular weight heparin. Warfarin is contra-indicated in pregnancy, as it is teratogenic.

There are various conditions which may predispose to a clotting tendency. These are generally congenital (e.g. Factor V Leiden, protein C deficiency), but may be acquired (e.g. lupus anticoagulant). They are generally not problematic, and are only investigated if a patient presents with an unusual thrombotic history. If thrombophilia is suspected, this should prompt a referral, rather than investigation in primary care.

An increasing problem encountered in primary care is what to do with patients who have a history of thrombosis and wish to travel by air. The risk of thrombosis appears to be greatest when there is travel of over six hours, where the patient is confined to a particular position (usually sitting). Traveller's thrombosis has been reported from air, car and bus travel. If there is any suggestion of an association between long-distance travel and thrombosis, or there is a strong family history of thrombosis, then specialist referral is indicated. The risk of prolonged travel, either by air or other means, is probably overstated, with patients suffering an event being pre-disposed to thromboembolism anyway. The principal risk factor for traveller's thrombosis appears to be previous history of a clot. The main preventive measures are the use of full-length graduated compression stockings (Scurr *et al.*, 2001), or prophylactic low molecular weight heparin.

References

Carson J, Kelley M, Duff A, Weg J, Fulkerson W, Palevsky H *et al.* (1992). The clinical course of pulmonary embolism. *New England Journal of Medicine* **326**: 1240–1245.

Fitzmaurice D, Hobbs F (1999). Thromboembolism. *Clinical Evidence* **2**: 130–135.

Gould MK, Dembitzer AD, Sanders GD, Garber AM (1999). Low-molecular-weight heparins compared with unfractionated heparin for treatment of acute deep venous thrombosis. A cost-effectiveness analysis. *Annals of Internal Medicine* **130**(10): 789–99.

Hirsh J, Hoak J (1996). Management of deep vein thrombosis and pulmonary embolism. *Circulation* **93**: 2212–2245.

Hull R Raskob GE Pineo GF *et al.* (1992). Subcutaneous low-molecular-weight heparin compared with continuous intravenous heparin in the treatment of proximal vein thrombosis. *NEJM* **326**: 975–82.

Hull R, Hirsh J, Jay R (1982). Different intensities of oral anticoagulation therapy in the treatment of proximal vein thrombosis. *New England Journal of Medicine* **307**: 1676–1681.

Kakkar VV, Howe CT, Flanc C *et al.* (1969). Natural history of post-operative deep-vein thrombosis. *Lancet* **2**(7614): 230–232.

Lagerstedt CI Olsson CG Fagher BO Oqvist BW Albrechtsson P (1985). Need for long term anticoagulant treatment in symptomatic calf vein thrombosis. *Lancet* **2**(8454): 515–518.

Levine MN, Hirsh J, Gent M, Turpie AG, Weitz J, Ginsberg J *et al.* (1995). Optimal duration of oral anticoagulant therapy: a randomized trial comparing four weeks with three months of warfarin in patients with proximal deep vein thrombosis. *Thrombosis and Haemostasis* **74**: 606–611.

National Institute for Health and Care Excellence (NICE) (2012a). Clinical Guideline 144: *Venous thromboembolic diseases: the management of venous thromboembolic diseases and the role of thrombophilia testing.* http://guidance.nice.org.uk/CG144.

National Institute for Health and Care Excellence (NICE) (2012b). Technology Appraisal Guidance 261: *Rivaroxaban for the treatment of deep vein thrombosis and prevention of recurrent deep vein thrombosis and pulmonary embolism.* http://guidance.nice.org.uk/TA261.

Schulman S, Rhedin A, Lindmarker P, Carlsson A, Larfars G, Nicol P *et al.* (1995). A comparison of six weeks with six months of oral anticoagulant therapy after a first episode of venous thromboembolism. *New England Journal of Medicine* **332**: 1661–1665.

Scurr JH. Machin SJ. Bailey-King S. Mackie IJ. McDonald S. Smith PD (2001). Frequency and prevention of symptomless deep-vein thrombosis in long-haul flights: a randomised trial. *Lancet* **357**: 1485–9.

Simonneau G, Sors H, Charbonnier B, Page Y, Laaban JP, Azarian R *et al.* (1997). A comparison of low-molecular-weight heparin with unfractionated heparin for acute pulmonary embolism. The THESEE Study Group. Tinzaparine ou Heparine Standard: Evaluations dans l'Embolie Pulmonaire. *New England Journal of Medicine* **337**: 663–9.

Thomas PRS, Butler CM, Bowman J, Grieve NWT, Bennett CE, Taylor RS, Thomas MH (1991). Light reflection rheography: an effective non-invasive technique for screening patients with suspected deep venous thrombosis. *British Journal of Surgery* **78**: 207–209.

Turkstra F, van Beek JR, ten Cate JW, Buller HR (1998). Reliable rapid blood test for the exclusion of venous thromboembolism in symptomatic outpatients. *Thrombosis and Haemostasis* **79**: 32–37.

Vandenbroucke JP, Rosing J, Blomenkamp KWM, Middeldorp S, Helmerhorst FM, Bouma BN, Rosendaal FR (2001). Oral contraceptives and risk of venous thrombosis. *New England Journal of Medicine* **344**: 1527–1535.

Weinman EE, Salzman EW (1994). Deep-Vein Thrombosis. *New England Journal of Medicine* **331**: 1630–1644.

Wells PS Hirsh J Anderson DR *et al.* (1995). Accuracy of clinical assessment of deep-vein thrombosis. *Lancet* **345**(8961):1326–1330.

Wells PS, Kovacs MJ, Bormanis J, Forgie MA, Goudie D, Morrow B, Kovacs J (1998). Expanding eligibility for outpatient treatment of deep venous thrombosis and pulmonary embolism with low-molecular-weight heparin: a comparison of patient self-injection with homecare injection. *Archives of Internal Medicine* **158**(16): 1809–12.

Section V

Unusual Site Thrombosis

21

Cerebral Venous Thrombosis

Christian Weimar

Department of Neurology and Stroke Center, University Duisburg-Essen, Germany

Although a rare cause of stroke, cerebral venous thrombosis (CVT) is increasingly diagnosed because of greater clinical awareness, more sensitive neuroimaging techniques, and the survival of patients with previously lethal diseases that confer a predisposition to CVT. The incidence of CVT in adults was investigated in two Dutch provinces, serving 3.1 million people, and was found to be 1.32 per 100 000 person years (95% CI 1.06–1.61) with an incidence of 2.78 (95% CI 1.98–3.82) among women between the ages of 31 and 50 years (Coutinho *et al.*, 2012). The most common condition associated with CVT in women is pregnancy/puerperium, with an incidence of around 10 in 100 000 deliveries in high-income countries, accounting for 5–20% of all CVT (Bousser and Crassard, 2012). The incidence in Canadian children was estimated at 0.67 per 100 000 (95% CI 0.55–0.76), but is likely higher in developing countries due to infective diseases (deVeber *et al.*, 2001).

Aetiology

There are multiple predisposing factors of CVT, which are very similar to those causing extracerebral venous thrombosis, except for a number of local causes. In about 15% of patients, no cause of CVT can be found, but follow-up may detect an underlying disease up to several months later (Ferro *et al.*, 2004). Oral hormonal contraception remains the sole predisposing factor in about 10%, but is also frequently found in combination with coagulation disorders. Coagulation disorders are common causes of CVT, in particular the Factor-V-Leiden mutation, with APC resistance accounting for 10–25% of cases (Dentali *et al.*, 2006; Pai *et al.*, 2012).

Other coagulopathies associated with CVT include: prothrombin mutation G 20210 A; antithrombin III deficiency; protein C and protein S deficiency; antiphospholipid antibody syndrome; plasminogen deficiency; hyperhomocysteinaemia; dysfibrinogenaemia; disseminated intravasal coagulation; heparin-induced thrombocytopenia type 2 (Kenet *et al.*, 2010; Saposnik *et al.*, 2011). Additional causes include malignancies (meningeoma, carcinoma, lymphoma, carcinoid, leukaemia), haematological disorders (polycythaemia, sickle cell disease, paroxysmal nocturnal haemoglobinuria, immune-mediated haemolytic diseases, thrombocytaemia), collagenosis (systemic lupus erythematodes, Sjögren's syndrome) and vasculitis (Behcet's disease, Wegener's granulomatosis, sarcoidosis) (Saposnik *et al.*, 2011).

Other rare causes of CVT include: intracranial hypotension; cerebral concussion; neurosurgical interventions; obstructive hydrocephalus; impaired venous drainage (central venous catheter, dural arteriovenous malformation, strangulation); medication poisoning (asparaginase, other chemotherapeutics, steroids, erythropoietin, drugs, vitamin A overdose); metabolic disorders (diabetes, thyrotoxicosis, uraemia, nephrotic syndrome); gastrointestinal disorders (liver cirrhosis, chronic inflammatory bowel disease); and heart disease (heart failure, cardiomyopathy). Septic CVT can be found in up to 18% of all cases in developing countries

Handbook of Venous Thromboembolism, First Edition. Edited by Jecko Thachil and Catherine Bagot.
© 2018 John Wiley & Sons Ltd. Published 2018 by John Wiley & Sons Ltd.

(Khealani *et al.*, 2008), and is associated with localised infections such as mastoiditis, otitis media, sinusitis, tonsillitis, retropharyngeal abscess with thrombosis of adjacent jugular vein, oral or cerebral abscess, and meningitis. Potential generalised infectious causes include bacterial septicaemia, endocarditis, hepatitis, encephalitis, measles, tuberculosis, typhus, malaria, and aspergillosis.

Pathophysiology

Two separate pathophysiological mechanisms need to be distinguished: thrombosis of cortical veins and thrombosis of the major sinus. The latter are needed for the clearance of cerebrospinal fluid (CSF). This process is mediated by so-called Pacchioni's granulations, which constitute arachnoid protrusions into the cerebral sinus, and enable transport of CSF from the subarachnoid space into the blood. Thrombosis of the cerebral sinus thus results in intracranial hypertension (Brunori *et al.*, 1993). Occlusion of a cerebral vein obstructs the drainage of blood from brain tissue, causing an increase in venous and capillary pressure and breakdown of the blood-brain barrier, which results in parenchymal damage (Ungersbock *et al.*, 1993).

Clinical Presentation

CVT may often remain asymptomatic, due to numerous ways of venous drainage and reversal of venous flow. Headache is the initial symptom in more than 70%, and remains the only symptom in about 16% (Gameiro *et al.*, 2012). It can be associated with other common symptoms, such as nausea/vomiting, seizures, reduced consciousness or confusional state and focal neurological deficits (Ferro *et al.*, 2004). Papilledema can be found in about 40%, mainly in patients with a chronic course or delayed diagnosis. Initial presentation with focal or generalised epileptic seizures occurs in 30–40% of cases. Other less frequent symptoms include thunderclap headache, subarachnoid haemorrhage, cranial nerve palsy, transient ischemic attacks, migraine with aura, psychiatric disturbances and tinnitus.

Neurological findings and type of focal seizures are determined by the localisation of CVT and the associated lesions. The common thrombosis of the superior sagittal sinus (60% of cases) causes headache, papilledema, seizures, motor deficits and impaired consciousness, whereas thrombosis of the cavernosus sinus is associated with ocular nerve palsies and ipsilateral ocular affection (chemosis, proptosis, papilledema). Patients with isolated thrombosis of the lateral sinus present mostly as isolated intracranial hypertension or aphasia, if the left transverse sinus is occluded. Occlusion of the deep cerebral venous system more likely causes coma, motor deficits or aphasia. Bilateral venous congestion of the thalamic region causes decreased consciousness as a major finding, and minor transient cognitive impairment, rather than a severe amnestic syndrome.

Diagnosis

Reliable identification of CVT can be achieved with the enhancement of dynamic venous CT angiography using slices of 1–1.5 mm size. With application of multiplanar reconstruction, sensitivity thereby reaches 95% and specificity 91%, compared with digital subtraction angiography (Wetzel *et al.*, 1999). MR angiography allows more advanced conclusions, and is superior in the detection of cortical venous thrombosis, compared with CT angiography.

Thrombosis of the sinus does not induce signal loss in the axial and sagittal T1- and T2-sequences, but may appear hyperintense because of its content of methaemoglobin. Depending on the structure and localisation of the thrombus, T1- or T2*-weighted sequences and susceptibility-weighted imaging (SWI) are highly sensitive for direct detection of the thrombus (Selim *et al.*, 2002; Leach *et al.*, 2006). Contrast-enhanced 3D gradient recalled echo (GRE) T1-weighted imaging is superior to spin echo (SE) T1-weighted imaging for the detection of dural sinus thrombosis (Saindane *et al.*, 2013). Thus, besides the thrombosed sinus, even single thrombosed veins can be detected as hypointense structures. However, these must be differentiated from localised subarachnoid or subpial haemorrhages, which may also appear as hypointense on T2*-weighted imaging.

Subarachnoid haemorrhage localised along a sulcus may be indicative of a single cortical vein thrombosis (Urban and Muller-Forell, 2005). Following contrast enhancement, contrast is spared in the thrombosed sinus on MRI, like on CT. In a thrombus with a high methaemoglobin level, there may be a hyperintense signal in the time-of-flight angiography (TOF), which should not be confounded with a flow signal. Presence of normal structures in the intracranial dural sinus (arachnoid granulations, intrasinus fibrotic bands) should not be misinterpreted as CVT, leading to unnecessary anticoagulation (Liang *et al.*, 2002; Alper *et al.*, 2004). Also, a hypoplastic left lateral sinus is common, and must be differentiated from CVT. Asymmetry of the sigmoid notches on plain brain CT is a sensitive and specific measure for differentiating an atretic transverse sinus from transverse sinus thrombosis, when absence of transverse sinus flow is visualised on venous angiography (Chik *et al.*, 2012).

Various parenchymal lesions can be visualised on cerebral imaging. Intracerebral haemorrhage (ICH) can be seen in about 30–40%, whereas subdural or subarachnoid haemorrhage is less common (Ferro *et al.*, 2004). Thrombosis of Labbé's vein can cause a large temporal haemorrhage, which must not be confused with aneurysmal haemorrhage. Most ICH present as patchy haemorrhages in an area of brain oedema, which is also called venous haemorrhagic infarct, although the oedema is still reversible (Leach *et al.*, 2006). Small juxtacortical haemorrhages localised at the border zone between the superficial and deep venous drainage system, with little or no surrounding oedema, are very specific for sagittal sinus thrombosis (Coutinho *et al.*, 2014). Isolated cerebral brain oedema, especially of the basal ganglia and thalami in thrombosis of the deep venous system, can be better visualised on MRI.

Acute CVT, presenting with neurological deficits, is strongly associated with D-dimer levels of > 500 ng/ml (Kosinski *et al.*, 2004). On the other hand, D-dimer levels < 500 ng/ml do not rule out CVT, especially when presenting with isolated headache only. A systematic meta-analysis found a mean sensitivity of 93.9% and specificity of 89.7% (Dentali *et al.*, 2012a). False negative D-dimer results were more frequent in patients with isolated headache, longer duration of symptoms and limited sinus involvement. Therefore, although normal D-dimer levels make the presence of CVT unlikely, exclusion of CVT should not be based on D-dimer measurement only.

Treatment

In line with the guidelines for deep venous thrombosis (DVT), anticoagulation is also the treatment of choice for CVT. Initial anticoagulation with heparin is thought to stop the progression of thrombosis, to reduce the risk of pulmonary embolism and to prevent re-occlusion of those vessels which have already been recanalised by internally produced fibrinolytics. Confirmed CVT should, therefore, be treated with heparin, even in the presence of an associated intracranial haemorrhage.

Septic or infectious CVT are treated with antibiotics, according to the underlying infectious agent and focus. In certain cases, surgical treatment can be necessary to control the focus of infection. Despite anti-infective treatment, mortality is higher, compared with non-infectious CVT, and treatment with anticoagulation is justified, even in the absence of evidence from controlled trials.

Heparin

The current guidelines for the diagnosis and treatment of CVT published by the American Heart and Stroke Association, as well as the European Stroke Organization, provide recommendations on anticoagulation for

CVT (Ferro *et al.*, 2017; Saposnik *et al.*, 2011). Evidence for efficacy of treatment with heparin in acute CVT comes from two randomised placebo-controlled studies which, together, included 79 patients.

Einhäupl *et al.* compared dose-adapted PTT-controlled IV treatment with unfractioned heparin versus placebo in 20 patients with CVT. In the heparin group, eight patients showed complete restitution, and all patients survived with no further bleeding complications observed whereas, in the placebo group, only one patient showed full recovery, three patients died and two patients developed new intracerebral haemorrhages (Einhäupl *et al.*, 1991).

De Bruijn *et al.* investigated efficacy and safety of treatment with nadroparin 2 × 90 mg/kg/d for three weeks in subcutaneous application, versus placebo in 59 CVT patients (de Bruijn and Stam, 1999). There was a non-significant trend in favour of treatment with LMWH, and neither new ICH, nor an increase in ICH size, were observed. A meta-analysis of both studies showed a 54% relative risk reduction in mortality and severe disability with heparin treatment (Stam *et al.*, 2008a). Although this meta-analysis was not significant either, results of both studies indicate that treatment with heparin for CVT is safe, and reduces the risk of unfavourable progression.

It is not known whether intravenous dose-adapted treatment with unfractioned heparin (UFH) and weight-adapted treatment with low-molecular weight heparin (LMWH) are equivalent. A small randomised trial from India evaluated the efficacy and safety of LMWH versus UFH in 66 consecutive patients (Misra *et al.*, 2012). Six patients in the UFH group died, and an insignificantly higher number of patients (30 versus 20) in the LMWH group fully recovered. A non-randomised prospective observational study in patients with CVT found treatment with LMWH to be more effective, and associated with fewer bleeding complications (Coutinho *et al.*, 2010). In particular, patients with haemorrhagic infarctions seemed to benefit from treatment with LMWH. Except for patients who may need rapid reversal of anticoagulation because of a neurosurgical intervention, LMWH, therefore, is generally preferable due to a better safety profile.

Pregnancy is not a contraindication for treatment with LMWH or UFH, but peri- and post-partal attenuation of anticoagulation should be considered individually, as risks of both bleeding and thromboembolism are increased during the peripartal phase. Anticoagulation during the acute phase of CVT is also recommended in children (Lebas *et al.*, 2012).

Endovascular Treatment

Endovascular treatment can be attempted by either local application of rt-plasminogen activator or urokinase within the thrombosed sinuses, mechanical thrombosuction, or both. A systematic review that included 169 patients treated with local thrombolysis showed a possible benefit in patients with severe CVT (Canhao *et al.*, 2003). The Thrombolyis or Anticoagulation for Cerebral Venous Thrombosis (To-ACT) trial randomising CVT patients with a high probability of poor outcome (defined by presence of at least one risk factor: mental status disorder, coma, intracranial haemorrhagic lesion, or thrombosis of the deep cerebral venous system) to receive either endovascular thrombolysis or therapeutic doses of heparin was stopped prematurely after inclusion of 65 patients (Coutinho *et al.*, 2013).

Patients with large space-occupying haemorrhagic infarcts particularly do not benefit from thrombolytic therapy, because an increase in haemorrhage size accelerates the imminent herniation (Stam *et al.*, 2008b). Nevertheless, in patients with thrombosis of the inner cranial veins, or extensive CVT without associated haemorrhage, locally applied thrombolysis may be an option, and can be considered individually after failure of conventional heparin treatment. Probably, the major indication for local thrombolysis is multiple sinus occlusions, including the jugular veins with no egress of blood, because these patients have very poor outcomes and markedly increased ICP.

Elevated Intracranial Pressure

Increased intracranial pressure (ICP) can be managed best with sufficient anticoagulation, by optimising the venous drainage, which results in a reduction of ICP. In patients with symptomatic intracranial hypertension and imminent loss of vision, repeated lumbar punctures may be needed, to drain cerebrospinal fluid (CSF) before anticoagulation can be started. If clinical symptoms progress despite repeated CSF drainage, permanent CSF drainage may be necessary.

Specific ICP-lowering treatment is indicated in fewer than 20% of all patients. General rules of ICP-lowering treatment should be applied (upper body elevation, hyperventilation, IV administration of osmo-therapeutic agents). However, these procedures have limited duration of action and are of little effect. The largest uncontrolled case series showed favourable outcome in 26 out of 34 patients after decompressive craniotomy, despite clinical and radiological findings of herniation (Rajan Vivakaran *et al.*, 2012). In particular, patients presenting with large haemorrhagic infarctions and imminent lateral herniation should be offered prompt surgical decompression without removal of the haematoma or infarcted area (Ferro *et al.*, 2017). Anticoagulation should be continued within 12–24 hours after surgical treatment. Volume restrictions should be avoided. Because of its prothrombotic activity and no proven benefit, treatment with steroids is not recommended.

Oral Anticoagulation

MR-based follow-up studies indicate that recanalisation occurs within three months, irrespective of continu-ation of oral anticoagulation (Baumgartner *et al.*, 2003). However, the recanalisation rate has not been found to correlate with the risk of CVT recurrence. Despite the lack of evidence, several guidelines recommend an average duration of 3–12 months for treatment with dose-adapted vitamin K antagonists, whereas long term anticoagulation beyond 12 months is advised only in patients with severe coagulopathies or recurrent CVT (Albers *et al.*, 2008; Saposnik *et al.*, 2011). In addition, children and adolescents below the age of 18 who have heterozygote prothrombin G20210A mutation may benefit from long-term anticoagulation (Kenet *et al.*, 2007). To date, there is not enough clinical experience and evidence for the use of novel anticoagulants (apixa-ban, dabigatran, edoxaban, rivaroxaban) for the treatment of CVT, but a randomised clinical trial (RESPECT-CVT, NCT02913326) is expected to provide results in 2018.

Secondary Prevention in Patients at Risk

The recurrence rate of CVT was investigated in a multicenter retrospective study, including 706 patients with a first episode with CVT (Dentali *et al.*, 2012b). After a median follow-up of 40 months (range 6–29 months), CVT recurred in 31 patients (4.4%), while 46 patients (6.5%) had a VTE in a different site, arriving to an overall incidence of recurrence of 2.36 events per 100 patient-years; 95% confidence interval (CI) 1.78–2.87. Due to this relatively benign prognosis, the use of long-term anticoagulant therapy should be reserved only for patients at high risk of recurrence. Results of screening for thrombophilia rarely change the acute manage-ment (Lauw *et al.*, 2013).

Prophylaxis with weight-adapted LMWH should be given in risk situations (e.g. immobilisation for more than four days, steroid therapy, flight of over four hours) in adults, as well as in infants and adolescents with a history of CVT (Monagle *et al.*, 2008). One retrospective study included 62 women ≤ 40 years with CVT and a mean follow-up of 7.5 years (Ciron *et al.*, 2013). Four patients (6.7%) had a non-cerebral venous thrombosis, but none during a subsequent pregnancy. There were 45 pregnancies in 24 women, most of whom were on preventive antithrombotic medication. Only one woman, with sickle cell disease, had a recurrent CVT during pregnancy.

Results from several case reports also indicate that the risk of recurrence during pregnancy is not increased, unless an inherited or acquired thrombophilia is present (Miranda *et al.*, 2010; Furie *et al.*, 2011). Because the post-partum period carries the greatest day-by-day risk of developing DVT and CVT, anticoagulation with weight-adapted LMWH for six weeks after delivery is recommended in patients with a history of CVT, in line with recommendations from the guidelines for prevention of DVT.

Prognosis

With the help of MR and CT angiography, CVT is increasingly diagnosed in oligosymptomatic patients (i.e. with headache or papilledema only). Therefore, and presumably due to anticoagulation in the acute phase, the rate of death or dependency has declined from about 50% 30 years ago, to about 15% in recent case series (Bousser and Ferro, 2007). Nevertheless, cognitive impairment persists in up to a third of patients hospitalised for CVT, and is more frequent in patients with deep CVT and persistent parenchymal lesions (Bugnicourt *et al.*, 2013). About 10% of patients continue to have seizures, and about 50% complain of various types of headache and/or feel depressed or anxious (Saposnik *et al.*, 2011).

Key Points

- Headache is the initial symptom in more than 70%, and the predominant symptom in up to 90%, of patients with CVT.
- Initial presentation with focal or generalised epileptic seizures can be found in 30–40% of cases.
- There are no pathognomonic symptoms for CVT. Therefore, immediate cerebral imaging, including angiography, is required if CVT is suspected. Both CT and MR venous angiography are suitable for the detection of CVT, while MR angiography is more sensitive to detect small cortical venous thrombosis.
- Although normal D-dimer levels make the presence of CVT unlikely, exclusion of CVT should not be based on D-dimer measurement only.
- Confirmed CVT should be treated with intravenous or low molecular weight heparin, even in the presence of intracranial haemorrhage. Immediate anticoagulation is thought to stop the progression of thrombosis and prevent vessels from closing up again, which already have been recanalised by internally produced fibrinolytics.
- Following the acute phase, treatment with oral anticoagulation is recommended for 3 to 12 months after CVT. Long-term anticoagulation is recommended only in patients suffering from a severe coagulopathy or recurrent CVT.

Suggested Further Reading

Ferro JM, Bousser MG, Canhão P, Coutinho JM, Crassard I, Dentali F, di Minno M, Maino A, Martinelli I, Masuhr F, Aguiar de Sousa D, Stam J (2017). European Stroke Organization guideline for the diagnosis and treatment of cerebral venous thrombosis – endorsed by the European Academy of Neurology European Journal of Neurology 2017 Aug 20. doi: 10.1111/ene.13381. [Epub ahead of print].

Ferro JM, Canhao P, Stam J, Bousser MG, Barinagarrementeria F (2004). Prognosis of cerebral vein and dural sinus thrombosis: results of the International Study on Cerebral Vein and Dural Sinus Thrombosis (ISCVT). *Stroke* **35**(3): 664–70.

Lebas A, Chabrier S, Fluss J, Gordon K, Kossorotoff M, Nowak-Gottl U, de Vries LS, Tardieu M (2012). EPNS/SFNP guideline on the anticoagulant treatment of cerebral sinovenous thrombosis in children and neonates. *European Journal of Paediatric Neurology* **16**(3): 219–28.

Kenet G, Lutkhoff LK, Albisetti M, Bernard T, Bonduel M, Brandao L, Chabrier S, Chan A, deVeber G, Fiedler B, Fullerton HJ, Goldenberg NA, Grabowski E, Gunther G, Heller C, Holzhauer S, Iorio A, Journeycake J, Junker R, Kirkham FJ, Kurnik K, Lynch JK, Male C, Manco-Johnson M, Mesters R, Monagle P, van Ommen CH, Raffini L, Rostasy K, Simioni P, Strater RD, Young G, Nowak-Gottl U (2010). Impact of thrombophilia on risk of arterial ischemic stroke or cerebral sinovenous thrombosis in neonates and children: a systematic review and meta-analysis of observational studies. *Circulation* **121**(16): 1838–47.

Saposnik G, Barinagarrementeria F, Brown RD, Jr., Bushnell CD, Cucchiara B, Cushman M, Deveber G, Ferro JM, Tsai FY (2011). Diagnosis and Management of Cerebral Venous Thrombosis: A Statement for Healthcare Professionals From the American Heart Association/American Stroke Association. *Stroke* **42**(4): 1158–92.

Financial Disclosure

Prof. Dr. C. Weimar received honoraria for participation in clinical trials, contribution to advisory boards or oral presentations from: Alexion, Bayer Pharma, Biogen-Idec, Boehringer Ingelheim, Bristol-Myers Squibb, Daiichi Asubio, Sanofi-Aventis.

References

Albers GW, Amarenco P, Easton JD, Sacco RL, Teal P (2008). Antithrombotic and thrombolytic therapy for ischemic stroke: American College of Chest Physicians Evidence-Based Clinical Practice Guidelines (8th Edition). *Chest* **133**(6 Suppl): 630S–669S.

Alper F, Kantarci M, Dane S, Gumustekin K, Onbas O, Durur I (2004). Importance of anatomical asymmetries of transverse sinuses: an MR venographic study. *Cerebrovascular Diseases* **18**(3): 236–239.

Baumgartner RW, Studer A, Arnold M, Georgiadis D (2003). Recanalisation of cerebral venous thrombosis. *Journal of Neurology, Neurosurgery, and Psychiatry* **74**(4): 459–461.

Bousser MG, Crassard I (2012). Cerebral venous thrombosis, pregnancy and oral contraceptives. *Thrombosis Research* **130**(Suppl 1): S19–22.

Bousser MG, Ferro JM (2007). Cerebral venous thrombosis: an update. *The Lancet Neurology* **6**(2): 162–170.

Brunori A, Vagnozzi R, Giuffre R (1993). Antonio Pacchioni (1665–1726): early studies of the dura mater. *Journal of Neurosurgery* **78**(3): 515–518.

Bugnicourt JM, Guegan-Massardier E, Roussel M, Martinaud O, Canaple S, Triquenot-Bagan A, Wallon D, Lamy C, Leclercq C, Hannequin D, Godefroy O (2013). Cognitive impairment after cerebral venous thrombosis: a two-center study. *Journal of Neurology* **260**(5): 1324–1331.

Canhao P, Falcao F, Ferro JM (2003). Thrombolytics for cerebral sinus thrombosis: a systematic review. *Cerebrovascular Diseases* **15**(3): 159–166.

Chik Y, Gottesman RF, Zeiler SR, Rosenberg J, Llinas RH (2012). Differentiation of transverse sinus thrombosis from congenitally atretic cerebral transverse sinus with CT. *Stroke* **43**(7): 1968–1970.

Ciron J, Godeneche G, Vandamme X, Rosier MP, Sharov I, Mathis S, Larrieu D, Neau JP (2013). Obstetrical Outcome of Young Women with a Past History of Cerebral Venous Thrombosis. *Cerebrovascular Diseases* **36**(1): 55–61.

Coutinho JM, Ferro JM, Canhao P, Barinagarrementeria F, Bousser MG, Stam J (2010). Unfractionated or low-molecular weight heparin for the treatment of cerebral venous thrombosis. *Stroke* **41**(11): 2575–2580.

Coutinho JM, Zuurbier SM, Aramideh M, Stam J (2012). The incidence of cerebral venous thrombosis: a cross-sectional study. *Stroke* **43**(12): 3375–3377.

Coutinho JM, Ferro JM, Zuurbier SM, Mink MS, Canhao P, Crassard I, Majoie CB, Reekers JA, Houdart E, de Haan RJ, Bousser MG, Stam J (2013). Thrombolysis or anticoagulation for cerebral venous thrombosis: rationale and design of the TO-ACT trial. *International Journal of Stroke* **8**(2): 135–140.

Coutinho JM, van den Berg R, Zuurbier SM, VanBavel E, Troost D, Majoie CB, Stam J (2014). Small juxtacortical hemorrhages in cerebral venous thrombosis. *Annals of Neurology* **75**(6): 908–916.

de Bruijn SF, Stam J (1999). Randomized, placebo-controlled trial of anticoagulant treatment with low-molecular-weight heparin for cerebral sinus thrombosis. *Stroke* **30**(3): 484–488.

Dentali F, Crowther M, Ageno W (2006). Thrombophilic abnormalities, oral contraceptives, and risk of cerebral vein thrombosis: a meta-analysis. *Blood* **107**(7): 2766–2773.

Dentali F, Squizzato A, Marchesi C, Bonzini M, Ferro JM, Ageno W (2012a). D-dimer testing in the diagnosis of cerebral vein thrombosis: a systematic review and a meta-analysis of the literature. *Journal of Thrombosis and Haemostasis* **10**(4): 582–589.

Dentali F, Poli D, Scoditti U, Di Minno MN, De Stefano V, Siragusa S, Kostal M, Palareti G, Sartori MT, Grandone E, Vedovati MC, Ageno W, Falanga A, Lerede T, Bianchi M, Testa S, Witt D, McCool K, Bucherini E, Grifoni E, Coalizzo D, Benedetti R, Marietta M, Sessa M, Guaschino C, di Minno G, Tufano A, Barbar S, Malato A, Pini M, Castellini P, Barco S, Barone M, Paciaroni M, Alberti A, Agnelli G, Pierfranceschi MG, Dulicek P, Silingardi M, Federica L, Ghirarduzzi A, Tiraferri E, di Lazzaro V, Rossi E, Ciminello A, Pasca S, Barillari G, Rezoagli E, Galli M, Squizzato A, Tosetto A (2012b). Long-term outcomes of patients with cerebral vein thrombosis: a multicenter study. *Journal of Thrombosis and Haemostasis* **10**(7): 1297–1302.

deVeber G, Andrew M, Adams C, Bjornson B, Booth F, Buckley DJ, Camfield CS, David M, Humphreys P, Langevin P, MacDonald EA, Gillett J, Meaney B, Shevell M, Sinclair DB, Yager J, Canadian Pediatric Ischemic Stroke Study (2001). Cerebral sinovenous thrombosis in children. *New England Journal of Medicine* **345**(6): 417–423.

Einhäupl KM, Villringer A, Meister W, Mehraein S, Garner C, Pellkofer M, Haberl RL, Pfister HW, Schmiedek P (1991). Heparin treatment in sinus venous thrombosis. *Lancet* **338**(8767): 597–600.

Ferro JM, Bousser MG, Canhão P, Coutinho JM, Crassard I, Dentali F, di Minno M, Maino A, Martinelli I, Masuhr F, Aguiar de Sousa D, Stam J (2017). European Stroke Organization guideline for the diagnosis and treatment of cerebral venous thrombosis – endorsed by the European Academy of Neurology European Journal of Neurology 2017 Aug 20. doi: 10.1111/ene.13381. [Epub ahead of print].

Ferro JM, Canhao P, Stam J, Bousser MG, Barinagarrementeria F (2004). Prognosis of cerebral vein and dural sinus thrombosis: results of the International Study on Cerebral Vein and Dural Sinus Thrombosis (ISCVT). *Stroke* **35**(3): 664–670.

Furie KL, Kasner SE, Adams RJ, Albers GW, Bush RL, Fagan SC, Halperin JL, Johnston SC, Katzan I, Kernan WN, Mitchell PH, Ovbiagele B, Palesch YY, Sacco RL, Schwamm LH, Wasserteil-Smoller S, Turan TN, Wentworth D (2011). Guidelines for the prevention of stroke in patients with stroke or transient ischemic attack: a guideline for healthcare professionals from the american heart association/american stroke association. *Stroke* **42**(1): 227–276.

Gameiro J, Ferro JM, Canhao P, Stam J, Barinagarrementeria F, Lindgren A (2012). Prognosis of cerebral vein thrombosis presenting as isolated headache: early vs. late diagnosis. *Cephalalgia* **32**(5): 407–412.

Kenet G, Kirkham F, Niederstadt T, Heinecke A, Saunders D, Stoll M, Brenner B, Bidlingmaier C, Heller C, Knofler R, Schobess R, Zieger B, Sebire G, Nowak-Gottl U (2007). Risk factors for recurrent venous thromboembolism in the European collaborative paediatric database on cerebral venous thrombosis: a multicentre cohort study. *The Lancet Neurology* **6**(7): 595–603.

Kenet G, Lutkhoff LK, Albisetti M, Bernard T, Bonduel M, Brandao L, Chabrier S, Chan A, deVeber G, Fiedler B, Fullerton HJ, Goldenberg NA, Grabowski E, Gunther G, Heller C, Holzhauer S, Iorio A, Journeycake J, Junker R, Kirkham FJ, Kurnik K, Lynch JK, Male C, Manco-Johnson M, Mesters R, Monagle P, van Ommen CH, Raffini L, Rostasy K, Simioni P, Strater RD, Young G, Nowak-Gottl U (2010). Impact of thrombophilia on risk of arterial ischemic stroke or cerebral sinovenous thrombosis in neonates and children: a systematic review and meta-analysis of observational studies. *Circulation* **121**(16): 1838–1847.

Khealani BA, Wasay M, Saadah M, Sultana E, Mustafa S, Khan FS, Kamal AK (2008). Cerebral venous thrombosis: a descriptive multicenter study of patients in Pakistan and Middle East. *Stroke* **39**(10): 2707–2711.

Kosinski CM, Mull M, Schwarz M, Koch B, Biniek R, Schlafer J, Milkereit E, Willmes K, Schiefer J (2004). Do normal D-dimer levels reliably exclude cerebral sinus thrombosis? *Stroke* **35**(12): 2820–2825.

Lauw MN, Barco S, Coutinho JM, Middeldorp S (2013). Cerebral venous thrombosis and thrombophilia: a systematic review and meta-analysis. *Seminars in Thrombosis and Hemostasis* **39**(8): 913–927.

Leach JL, Fortuna RB, Jones BV, Gaskill-Shipley MF (2006). Imaging of cerebral venous thrombosis: current techniques, spectrum of findings, and diagnostic pitfalls. *Radiographics* **26**(Suppl 1): S19–41; discussion S42–13.

Lebas A, Chabrier S, Fluss J, Gordon K, Kossorotoff M, Nowak-Gottl U, de Vries LS, Tardieu M (2012). EPNS/ SFNP guideline on the anticoagulant treatment of cerebral sinovenous thrombosis in children and neonates. *European Journal of Paediatric Neurology* **16**(3): 219–228.

Liang L, Korogi Y, Sugahara T, Ikushima I, Shigematsu Y, Takahashi M, Provenzale JM (2002). Normal structures in the intracranial dural sinuses: delineation with 3D contrast-enhanced magnetization prepared rapid acquisition gradient-echo imaging sequence. *American Journal of Neuroradiology* **23**(10): 1739–1746.

Miranda B, Ferro JM, Canhao P, Stam J, Bousser MG, Barinagarrementeria F, Scoditti U (2010). Venous thromboembolic events after cerebral vein thrombosis. *Stroke* **41**(9): 1901–1906.

Misra UK, Kalita J, Chandra S, Kumar B, Bansal V (2012). Low molecular weight heparin versus unfractionated heparin in cerebral venous sinus thrombosis: a randomized controlled trial. *European Journal of Neurology* **19**(7): 1030–1036.

Monagle P, Chalmers E, Chan A, DeVeber G, Kirkham F, Massicotte P, Michelson AD (2008). Antithrombotic therapy in neonates and children: American College of Chest Physicians Evidence-Based Clinical Practice Guidelines (8th Edition). *Chest* **133**(6 Suppl): 887S–968S.

Pai N, Ghosh K, Shetty S (2012). Hereditary thrombophilia in cerebral venous thrombosis: a study from India. *Blood Coagulation & Fibrinolysis* **24**(5): 540–543.

Rajan Vivakaran TT, Srinivas D, Kulkarni GB, Somanna S (2012). The role of decompressive craniectomy in cerebral venous sinus thrombosis. *Journal of Neurosurgery* **117**(4): 738–744.

Saindane AM, Mitchell BC, Kang J, Desai NK, Dehkharghani S (2013). Performance of spin-echo and gradient-echo t1-weighted sequences for evaluation of dural venous sinus thrombosis and stenosis. *American Journal of Roentgenology* **201**(1): 162–169.

Saposnik G, Barinagarrementeria F, Brown, Jr. RD, Bushnell CD, Cucchiara B, Cushman M, Deveber G, Ferro JM, Tsai FY (2011). Diagnosis and Management of Cerebral Venous Thrombosis: A Statement for Healthcare Professionals From the American Heart Association/American Stroke Association. *Stroke* **42**(4): 1158–1192.

Selim M, Fink J, Linfante I, Kumar S, Schlaug G, Caplan LR (2002). Diagnosis of cerebral venous thrombosis with echo-planar T2*-weighted magnetic resonance imaging. *Archives of Neurology* **59**(6): 1021–1026.

Stam J, de Bruijn S, deVeber G (2008a). Anticoagulation for cerebral sinus thrombosis. *Cochrane Database of Systematic Reviews* (**4**): CD002005.

Stam J, Majoie CB, van Delden OM, van Lienden KP, Reekers JA (2008b). Endovascular thrombectomy and thrombolysis for severe cerebral sinus thrombosis: a prospective study. *Stroke* **39**(5): 1487–1490.

Ungersbock K, Heimann A, Kempski O (1993). Cerebral blood flow alterations in a rat model of cerebral sinus thrombosis. *Stroke* **24**(4): 563–569; discussion 569–570.

Urban PP, Muller-Forell W (2005). Clinical and neuroradiological spectrum of isolated cortical vein thrombosis. *Journal of Neurology* **252**(12): 1476–1481.

Wetzel SG, Kirsch E, Stock KW, Kolbe M, Kaim A, Radue EW (1999). Cerebral veins: comparative study of CT venography with intraarterial digital subtraction angiography. *American Journal of Neuroradiology* **20**(2): 249–255.

22

Upper Extremity Thrombosis

Scott M. Stevens and Scott C. Woller

Department of Medicine, Intermountain Medical Center, Murray, Utah, and Department of Medicine, University of Utah School of Medicine, Salt Lake City, Utah, USA

Overview

Upper extremity deep vein thrombosis is the most common unusual site thrombosis, and can cause complications, including pulmonary embolism and post-thrombotic syndrome. More frequent use of central venous catheters, especially peripherally inserted central catheters, has been associated with an increasing rate of this disorder. There is less evidence regarding the use of preventive measures for upper extremity than for lower extremity deep vein thrombosis, but judicious use of central venous catheters and selection of smaller diameter devices is likely to prevent thrombosis. Accurate diagnosis is essential to guide management, and recent studies have substantially improved the evidence base for the diagnostic approach. Anticoagulation is the mainstay of therapy, but direct-acting oral anticoagulants have yet to be studied for treatment of upper extremity thrombosis. Interventional treatments may be considered is select situations.

Background and Classification

Upper extremity deep vein thrombosis (UEDVT) refers to pathological thrombus within the deep veins of the arm. These can be classified as proximal (usually defined as the subclavian and axillary veins) and distal (from the brachial vein distally). There is some disagreement regarding this classification, and the implications of vein location on treatment decisions (Kearon *et al.*, 2008; Kearon *et al.*, 2012). Two proximal superficial veins – the basilic and cephalic – have anastomoses with the deep veins, and can be the location of superficial venous thrombosis.

Primary UEDVT refers to thrombosis without apparent precipitant, or in the setting of anatomic variants. Secondary UEDVT refers to thrombosis occurring in the setting of a central venous catheter, including peripherally-inserted central catheters (CVC/PICC), malignancy, pregnancy, recent surgery or trauma (Kucher, 2011). CVC/PICC is the most common secondary cause (Grant *et al.*, 2012). UEDVT may be asymptomatic, or may cause pain, swelling, skin discoloration and, occasionally, numbness. An UEDVT may cause a CVC/PICC to dysfunction.

Epidemiology and Risk Factors

The annual incidence of UEDVT is approximately 0.4 to one case per 10 000 persons, and is increasing (Kucher, 2011). About 10% of all DVT occurs in the upper extremities.

Handbook of Venous Thromboembolism, First Edition. Edited by Jecko Thachil and Catherine Bagot.
© 2018 John Wiley & Sons Ltd. Published 2018 by John Wiley & Sons Ltd.

Primary UEDVT

Primary UEDVT comprises about 20–30% of cases (Hingorani *et al.*, 1997). The majority of primary UEDVTs are caused by abnormalities of the costo-clavicular junction – especially thoracic outlet syndrome, a disorder in which the nerves, artery or veins are compressed in the costo-clavicular space (Linnemann *et al.*, 2008). Effort thrombosis, also known by the eponym Paget-Schroetter syndrome (PSS), results from repetitive injury to the vein in a tight thoracic outlet induced by arm movements – especially frequent use of arms above shoulder level (Joffe *et al.*, 2002). Use of assisted reproductive technology, especially when associated with ovarian hyperstimulation syndrome, has a particularly strong association with UEDVT (Chan and Ginsberg, 2006). UEDVT can also be idiopathic.

Secondary UEDVT

CVC/PICCs are the most significant cause of secondary UEDVT, and are present in about half of all cases (Owens *et al.*, 2010; Spencer *et al.*, 2007; Joffe *et al.*, 2004). The rising incidence of UEDVT is likely to be attributable to increasing use of these devices. The incidence of symptomatic and asymptomatic UEDVT following CVC/PICC placement varies by report, with rates ranging from 2% to nearly 30% (Luciani *et al.*, 2001; Martin *et al.*, 1999; De Cicco *et al.*, 1997; Chopra *et al.*, 2015).

Risk factors for CVC/PICC-associated UEDVT include patient characteristics, issues related to catheter insertion and characteristics of the devices (Table 22.1). Of these, perhaps the most important and modifiable factor is catheter diameter. Larger diameter catheters may increase the risk of UEDVT by 10–20 fold, compared with smaller diameter devices (Chopra *et al.*, 2015; Evans *et al.*, 2010). Diameter, rather than number of lumens, seems to predict thrombosis risk (Evans *et al.*, 2013). PICCs are likely to confer a higher risk than surgically tunnelled catheters (Luciani *et al.*, 2001; van Rooden *et al.*, 2005; Saber *et al.*, 2011). Cardiac pacemaker systems with intravenous leads have also been associated with UEDVT (Korkeil *et al.*, 2008).

Malignancy is a risk factor for UEDVT and is present in about one-third of cases (Owens *et al.*, 2010; Isma *et al.*, 2010). CVC/PICCs are often used in patients with cancer, and the risk may be additive (Joffe *et al.*, 2004; Anderson *et al.*, 1989). As with lower extremity DVT (LEDVT), UEDVT may be the initial manifestation of an undiagnosed cancer. A case series found a 23.7% rate of occult malignancy in apparently unprovoked UEDVT – higher than that found in unprovoked LEDVT (Girolami *et al.*, 1999). However, the yield of additional screening for malignancy in patients presenting with unprovoked UEDVT is uncertain (see Chapter 28).

Hereditary and acquired thrombophilia are associated with UEDVT, but the magnitude of risk conferred by these disorders is uncertain. As identifying a thrombophilia does not clearly impact management decisions (Kearon *et al.*, 2012), the utility of screening for thrombophilia is controversial (See Chapter 2c) (Linnemann *et al.*, 2008; Ellis *et al.*, 2000; Stevens *et al.* 2015).

Prevention

In contrast to LEDVT, pharmacologic prophylaxis has not clearly been demonstrated to reduce the risk for UEDVT. A Cochrane systematic review, which included 12 randomised clinical trials, found no significant decrease in UEDVT in cancer patients with a CVC/PICC treated with prophylactic heparin or vitamin K antagonists (RR 0.54, 95% CI 0.28–1.05 for symptomatic UEDVT) (Akl *et al.*, 2011). A recent case-control study which included patients without cancer did not reveal a statistically significant risk reduction with pharmacologic prophylaxis but, interestingly, revealed a lower risk of CVC/PICC-associated UEDVT in patients taking both aspirin and a statin (OR 0.31, 95%CI = 0.16–0.61) (Chopra *et al.*, 2015). This observation may merit additional research. Evidence-based clinical practice guidelines from the American College of Chest Physicians (ACCP) and the National Comprehensive Cancer Network (NCCN) recommend against anticoagulant prophylaxis solely on the basis of an indwelling CVC/PICC (Kahn *et al.*, 2012; Streiff *et al.*, 2010).

Table 22.1 Risk factors for venous access-associated upper extremity deep vein thrombosis (Joffe and Goldhaber, 2002; van Rooden *et al.*, 2005; Hull *et al.*, 1981).

Paget-Schroetter syndrome ('effort thrombosis')

Central venous catheterisation:
  PICC
  central venous catheters
  pacemakers
  diameter of intravascular device

Malignancy

Acquired thrombophilias
  antiphospholipid syndrome
  JAK-2 gene mutation

Heritable thrombophilias:
  Factor V Leiden
  Prothrombin GA20210
  antithrombin deficiency
  protein s deficiency
  protein c deficiency
  hyperhomocystinemia

Pregnancy

Oestrogen-based hormone therapy

Trauma

Surgery

Sepsis

Prior thrombosis

Immobilisation

Anesthesia

Chemotherapy

PICC diameter

Because the majority of UEDVTs are associated with CVC/PICCs, these should only be placed when definitively indicated, and only when the benefit of a CVC/PICC outweighs the risks. Clinicians should choose the smallest diameter catheter compatible with the indication, and ensure appropriate positioning of the catheter tip in the superior vena cava (SVC) or at the cavo-atrial junction (Evans *et al.*, 2010; Saber *et al.*, 2011). Since the duration of catheter use may also relate to thrombosis risk, they should be promptly removed when no longer needed (Chopra *et al.*, 2015).

Diagnosis

Studies of diagnostic methods may broadly be classified as 'accuracy' or 'management' trials. An accuracy study compares a diagnostic test against a reference standard, while a management study determines the clinical outcome of patients over a pre-defined period of follow-up after application of the diagnostic strategy. Management studies are preferred to inform clinical care (Bates *et al.*, 2012). Recent research has substantially advanced the level of evidence underlying the diagnostic approach to suspected UEDVT.

Signs, Symptoms, Clinical Pre-test Probability Assessment and D-dimer

The most common signs and symptoms of UEDVT are unilateral arm swelling, discomfort and erythema (Joffe *et al.*, 2004). History and physical examination are insufficiently accurate for treatment decisions, so diagnostic testing is required (Prandoni *et al.*, 1997; Constans *et al.*, 2008; Knudson *et al.*, 1990). A clinical pre-test probability score, used in combination with a sensitive D-dimer, was derived (Constans *et al.*, 2008) and recently validated in a prospective management study. There was a low rate of subsequent DVT or PE after a negative evaluation (0.4%; 95%CI, 0.0–2.2% for the full algorithm) – comparable to similar studies for suspected LEDVT (see Chapter 5) (Kleinjan *et al.*, 2014). A separate study showed that the sensitivity of D-dimer assays for UEDVT is similar to that for LEDVT (Sartori *et al.*, 2015a).

Diagnostic Imaging

Ultrasound

Until recently, only accuracy studies were available to support the use of ultrasound (US) to diagnose suspected UEDVT. A systematic review by di Nisio *et al.* (2010) revealed reassuring sensitivity and specificity of US versus contrast venography (CV); however, there were methodological limitations to the included studies. Nonetheless, the ACCP guidelines suggest US as the first imaging test for suspected UEDVT (Bates *et al.*, 2012).

Two management studies utilising US have now been published (Kleinjan *et al.*, 2014; Sartori *et al.*, 2015b). The first utilised US in cases in which the pre-test probability for UEDVT was high, and/or the D-dimer was abnormal. As noted above, the rate of subsequent VTE during follow-up was low with this strategy (Kleinjan *et al.*, 2014). In a separate study, duplex US was performed in all suspected cases of UEDVT, and anticoagulation was withheld if US showed no DVT (the US was repeated 5–7 days later if non-diagnostic). During a three-month follow-up, the rate of VTE after a negative US was 0.30% (95% CI, 0.05–1.68%) (Sartori *et al.*, 2015b). These findings validate US as the first-line imaging test for suspected UEDVT, and further support the ACCP statement (Bates *et al.*, 2012).

Contrast Venography

Contrast venography (CV) has been the accepted reference standard for suspected UEDVT, although the sensitivity of CV for suspected LEDVT is known to be imperfect. A management study of patients with suspected LEDVT, and a technically adequate, negative CV revealed a subsequent rate of DVT or PE of 1.2% (95% confidence interval, 0.2–4.4%) during three months of follow-up (Hull *et al.*, 1981). No such management study is available for CV use in suspected UEDVT. Furthermore, CV is invasive, requires patient exposure to radiation and intravenous contrast, and is technically demanding. CV is, therefore, broadly reserved for instances when the results of US are insufficient to reach a diagnostic conclusion, or when an US is negative but a high clinical suspicion for UEDVT persists.

Computed Tomography Venography

Computed tomography venography (CTV) is performed by imaging veins following contrast injection. A systematic review of accuracy studies of CTV in the diagnosis of LEDVT reported a pooled sensitivity of 95.9% (CI 93–97.8%) and specificity of 95.2% (CI 93.6–96.5%) (Thomas *et al.*, 2008). Limited data exist regarding its use for the upper extremities. A small study by Kim *et al.* (2003) reported 100% concordance between CTV and standard CV, in 27 patients with central venous obstruction. Drawbacks of CTV include exposure to ionising radiation and intravenous contrast.

Magnetic Resonance Venography

Magnetic resonance venography (MRV) may be performed using a variety of techniques and methods of image processing, some of which require gadolinium contrast. In a recent meta-analysis for MRV of the lower extremities, the pooled sensitivity and specificity versus CV were 91.5% and 94.8%, respectively (Sampson *et al.*, 2007). To date, however, no management studies have been performed. MRV does not expose patients to radiation or iodinated contrast, though gadolinium confers risk of nephrogenic systemic fibrosis in patients with renal insufficiency. MRV is able to produce images of the central veins of the thorax, a region where ultrasound has limitations.

Approach to the Diagnosis of Suspected UEDVT

Two possible approaches to the diagnosis of suspected UEDVT are presented in Figure 22.1. The first, in which US is employed as the initial diagnostic test in all suspected cases, is similar to the diagnostic algorithm in the ACCP guidelines (Bates *et al.*, 2012) (Figure 22.1a). The second utilises pre-test probability scoring and a D-dimer test, and reserves US for only a portion of the population (Figure 22.1b). It is presently unclear whether one approach is superior to the other. While not formally analysed, it is likely that the second strategy is less expensive.

(a)

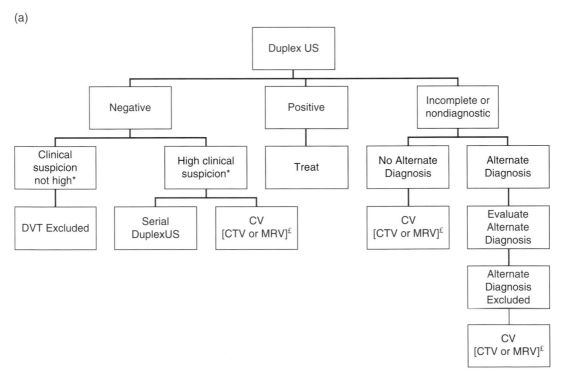

Figure 22.1 (a) Suggested diagnostic algorithm for suspected upper extremity DVT. Adapted from (Bates *et al.*, 2012).
US – ultrasound; CV – contrast venography; CTV – computed tomography venography; MRV – magnetic resonance venography.
* – Suspicion is based on clinician gestalt, as formal clinical prediction tools to quantify the pre-test probability of UEDVT are not well validated.
£ – CTV or MRV may be chosen in lieu of CV based on institutional experience, or patient-specific factors (such as contrast allergy, which would favour MRV).

(b)

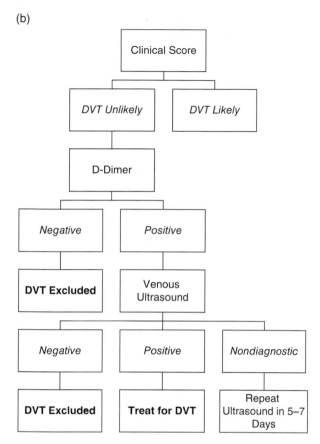

Figure 22.1 (b) Clinic Pre-test Probability and D-dimer based diagnostic algorithm for suspected upper extremity DVT. Adapted from Kleinjan, *et al.*, 2014.

Treatment

Goals of therapy of UEDVT include reduction or elimination of symptoms, prevention of DVT progression, or embolisation and reduction of the risk of post-thrombotic syndrome (PTS). In some cases, treatment is targeted to secondary prevention of new episodes of DVT. Due to limited data regarding treatment of UEDVT, many treatment recommendations are applied using indirect evidence from trials of LEDVT (Kearon *et al.*, 2008). In addition to anticoagulation, a number of interventional therapies for UEDVT have been described.

Anticoagulation

Anticoagulation, using the same approach as used for LEDVT, is the mainstay of therapy for UEDVT. Although no randomised-controlled trials exist for treatment of UEDVT, a retrospective analysis comparing conservative measures to anticoagulation reported a 48% and 70% rate of symptomatic resolution, respectively (Sajid *et al.*, 2007). Therapeutic anticoagulation decreases the risk of PE and recurrence by preventing thrombus extension. Complications from anticoagulation include a 2–4% rate of major bleeding (Kucher, 2011).

In contrast to LEDVT, indications for extended anticoagulation in UEDVT are uncertain. Unprovoked DVT has a lower rate of recurrence in the upper extremity than in the lower extremity (Laerum *et al.*, 1981;

Heijboer *et al.*, 1992; Cronan *et al.*, 1989; Linkins *et al.*, 2006) and is not, therefore, a compelling indication for long-term anticoagulation. ACCP guidelines recommend against extended anticoagulation (Kearon *et al.*, 2012). When the provocation for DVT is ongoing, such as active cancer, or when a CVC/PICC is not removed, extended duration anticoagulation is suggested (Kearon *et al.*, 2012). A guidance statement from the International Society of Thrombosis and Haemostasis (ISTH) also suggests extended anticoagulation for primary UEDVT with tight thoracic outlet which has not been surgically corrected (Baglin *et al.*, 2012).

The non-vitamin K antagonist anticoagulants (NOAC) have not been studied for the treatment of UE DVT. However, as mentioned above, randomised trials of conventional anticoagulants for treatment of UEDVT have not been performed, either; use of these agents is based on indirect evidence, clinical experience and retrospective data. In the opinion of the authors, NOACs are a reasonable therapeutic choice for treatment of UEDVT, and choice of agent should be based on the same principles used for LEDVT and PE (see Chapter 11).

Interventional and Endovascular Therapies

Anticoagulants do not result in fibrinolysis. Therefore, vein recanalisation depends on endogenous fibrinolytic processes. In a study of combined UEDVT and LEDVT, 82% of patients treated with anticoagulation had no detectable recanalisation (Goldhaber *et al.*, 1984). Residual clot has been associated with compromised valve function and a higher rate of PTS and possibly DVT recurrence (Vedantham, 2008). Various interventional therapies have been evaluated as a means of attempting to accelerate the process of recanalisation, with the goal of reducing the risk of PTS and, perhaps, the risk of DVT recurrence. In general, the level of evidence supporting these therapies is low, and evidence for use in UEDVT is often indirect.

Thrombolysis

Infusion of thrombolytic agents which activate fibrin-bound plasminogen has been studied as an additional therapy. As with LEDVT, systemic thrombolysis is rarely performed for UEDVT, as catheter-directed thrombolysis (CDT) is likely to result in fewer bleeding complications and better efficacy. Thrombolytic agents studied have included urokinase, alteplase and reteplase, but there is no data directly comparing their relative efficacy or safety (Vedantham *et al.*, 2006).

CDT utilises a multi-port catheter embedded directly into the thrombus under fluoroscopic guidance. For select cases of LEDVT, the Society of Interventional Radiology recommends a continuous high-volume drip regimen (25–100 ml/hour) with dilute thrombolytic and concomitant unfractionated heparin (Vedantham *et al.*, 2006). However, no published guideline specifies thrombolytic dosing for cases of upper extremity DVT. The patient is typically monitored in an intensive care or step-down unit during thrombolytic infusion. Laboratory monitoring for bleeding and fibrinogen are performed, so that the infusion may be stopped if bleeding is noted, or if fibrinogen becomes depleted (a possible predictor of increased bleeding risk). Repeat venography is periodically performed, to assess the degree of thrombolysis and to reposition the catheter.

The ideal duration of the procedure is unknown, as is the maximum dose of thrombolytic agent infused (Murphy *et al.*, 2010). Practitioners often terminate the procedure when complete thrombolysis is achieved, or after approximately 48 hours if residual thrombus remains. Therapeutically dosed anticoagulants are resumed following the procedure, and used for the same duration as would be the case without intervention (Sharafuddin *et al.*, 2002; Maleux *et al.*, 2010). Organised clots older than two weeks are generally less susceptible to thrombolysis, so interventional therapy is generally not entertained unless the thrombus is known to be acute (Vedantham, 2008).

They key patient-important outcomes from thrombolysis are reduction in the risk of PTS and the risk for recurrent DVT; however, no studies demonstrate clear improvement in these outcomes. A retrospective long-term analysis of 95 upper extremity DVT patients showed a 60% adjusted reduced risk for residual thrombosis after CDT, compared with anticoagulation alone (95% CI 0.2–0.9) (Enden *et al.*, 2009).

Rates of major bleeding for CDT for LEDVT range from 7–11% (Vedantham, 2008; Wicky, 2009; Engelberger *et al.*, 2014), and a registry of 3649 patients reported that patients undergoing CDT for LEDVT were twice as likely to be transfused, three times as likely to sustain intracranial haemorrhage, and 1.5 times as likely to sustain PE (Bashir *et al.*, 2014). The bleeding rate for CDT for UEDVT has not been well reported. Risk factors for bleeding include recent surgery, liver dysfunction, thrombocytopenia, advanced age, and prior stroke (Vedantham, 2008).

Given the lack of high-quality evidence, case selection for CDT is challenging. ACCP guidelines suggest thrombolysis be considered in cases meeting the following criteria: 'severe symptoms, thrombus involving most of the subclavian vein and the axillary vein, symptoms for 14 days or less, good functional status, life expectancy of 1 year, and low risk for bleeding' (Kearon *et al.*, 2012). NCCN guidelines recommend CDT in appropriate candidates based on institutional expertise (Lin *et al.*, 2006).

Percutaneous Mechanical Thrombectomy

Percutaneous mechanical thrombectomy (PMT) refers to a group of catheter-based devices that remove clot through aspiration, fragmentation, or maceration. PMT can be used in combination with pharmacologic thrombolysis (pharmaco-mechanical catheter-directed thrombolysis or PCDT), but may also be used as stand-alone treatment, such as in cases when thrombolytics are contraindicated. In a study of treatment of LEDVT, PCDT achieved a similar rate of recanalisation with lower thrombolytic dose, treatment time, and hospital stays than CDT (Lin *et al.*, 2006).

Efficacy and safety data for PMT and PCDT are very limited. Published rates of major bleeding from PCDT are 3-4% for DVT of both upper and lower extremities (Vedantham, 2008). Results of the National Heart, Lung, and Blood Institute randomized controlled trial for the treatment of proximal LEDVT with PCDT to assess PTS frequency at 24 months (ATTRACT Trial) demonstrated no difference in the development of post-thrombotic syndrome comparing the two groups (Vedantham, 2017).

Angioplasty and Endovascular Stenting

Balloon angioplasty of veins, along with endovascular stenting, has undergone limited evaluation for upper extremity DVT. A published series of 22 patients with PSS reported stent occlusion in all patients within six weeks (Urschel and Patel, 2003). Angioplasty use has been reported in conjunction with surgical decompression for PSS (see below) (Schneider *et al.*, 2004). Indications for these interventions are uncertain, and long-term outcome data is lacking.

Superior Vena Cava Filter

The goal of an SVC filter is to prevent PE from an UEDVT. Filters have been the subject of case reports, largely in patients with UEDVT and a contraindication to anticoagulation. A systematic review analysed 209 published SVC filter placements (Owens *et al.*, 2010). The rate of major complications was 3.8% – largely filter strut perforation through the SVC which led, in some cases, to cardiac tamponade, aortic perforation, and pneumothorax. Given the known risks and uncertain benefit of SVC filters, they have little, if any, role in the management of upper extremity DVT. No FDA-approved SVC filter exists. Evidence-based practice guidelines suggest that SVC filters should be reserved for 'exceptional circumstances in specialised centres' (Kearon *et al.*, 2012).

Surgical Treatment

Surgical correction with resection of the first rib aims to correct the extrinsic vein compression in PSS, with the goal of reducing the risk of recurrent thrombosis. The rationale for surgical correction arises from the observation that anticoagulation alone has been associated with persistent symptoms and recurrent thrombosis in more than 50% of PSS cases (Adams and DeWeese, 1971). No randomised trials of surgical intervention for PSS have been performed. A registry of 294 patients reported outcomes in three groups (initial anticoagulation alone, initial CDT, initial CDT plus prompt first rib resection). The latter groups required fewer subsequent thrombectomies, but there was no allocation concealment of patients, and assessments and interventions were not dictated by a study protocol (Urschel *et al.*, 2000). As noted above, angioplasty use has been described, in combination with surgical decompression (Schneider *et al.*, 2004). ACCP guidelines suggest that surgical correction should be reserved for highly select cases in specialised centres (Kearon *et al.*, 2012). High-quality studies assessing long-term outcomes are lacking. A review article has suggested a management algorithm (Naeem *et al.*, 2015).

Management of CVC/PICC Devices with UEDVT

Guidelines support leaving a functional CVC/PICC in place, if it has an ongoing indication for use (Kearon *et al.*, 2012) (Baglin *et al.*, 2012). Prospective studies have shown a low incidence of long-term complications in patients who continued catheter use during anticoagulation (Lee *et al.*, 2006). The ACCP recommends anticoagulation for three months when a CVC/PICC is removed shortly after diagnosis of upper extremity DVT in patients without cancer, and suggests the same duration in patients with cancer (Kearon *et al.*, 2012). The ISTH suggests a three-month course of anticoagulation (Baglin *et al.*, 2012). In patients with cancer and a CVC/PICC, the NCCN recommends anticoagulation during catheter use, and for a course of at least three months after the catheter is removed (Wagman *et al.*, 2008).

Prognosis and Complications

Reports cite a two-month death rate of 30%, and a 40% rate at 12 months following diagnosis of UEDVT; however, these studies included a large proportion of patients with significant comorbidities (Martinelli *et al.*, 2004; Hingorani *et al.*, 2005). There was an 11% mortality rate in the three months following UEDVT in the RIETE registry (Munoz *et al.*, 2008). Patients with PSS generally have good prognosis.

Symptomatic PE in the setting of upper extremity DVT ranges from 3–12% (Kuter, 2004; Prandoni *et al.*, 2004), with higher rates of asymptomatic PE. Prandoni *et al.* (2004) reported PE in 36% of patients UEDVT who underwent mandatory lung imaging. Nine percent of patients enrolled in the RIETE registry with UEDVT had symptomatic PE at presentation, versus 29% of patients with LEDVT (Munoz *et al.*, 2008).

UEDVT, even in unprovoked cases, is substantially less likely to recur than LEDVT. (Spencer *et al.*, 2007; Prandoni *et al.*, 1997, 2004; Lechner *et al.*, 2008). The annualised recurrence rate after a first UEDVT ranges from 2.3 to 4.7% (Spencer *et al.*, 2007; Isma *et al.*, 2010).

PTS following UEDVT occurs in 7–46%, the wide range reflecting the lack of a standardised definition in relevant studies (Elman and Kahn, 2006). Residual thrombosis has been associated with a four-fold increased risk of developing PTS following UEDVT (Joffe *et al.*, 2002). Compression garments were thought to decrease the risk of PTS following LEDVT, until a recent randomised controlled trial disproved this hypothesis (Kahn *et al.*, 2013). While no such studies have been performed for UEDVT, an evidence-based practice guideline suggests not using compression sleeves to prevent PTS, although it suggests a trial of compression therapy to treat symptoms of established PTS of the arm (Kearon *et al.*, 2012).

References

Adams JT, DeWeese JA (1971). Effort thrombosis of the axillary and subclavian veins. *Journal of Trauma* **11**(11): 923–30.

Akl EA, Vasireddi SR, Gunukula S, Yosuico VE, Barba M, Sperati F *et al.* (2011). Anticoagulation for patients with cancer and central venous catheters. *Cochrane Database of Systematic Reviews* (**4**): CD006468.

Anderson AJ, Krasnow SH, Boyer MW, Cutler DJ, Jones BD, Citron ML *et al.* (1989). Thrombosis: the major Hickman catheter complication in patients with solid tumor. *Chest* **95**(1): 71–5.

Baglin T, Bauer K, Douketis J, Buller H, Srivastava A, Johnson G. (2012). Duration of anticoagulant therapy after a first episode of unprovoked pulmonary embolus or deep vein thrombosis: guidance from the scientific and standardization committee of the international society on thrombosis and haemostasis. *Journal of Thrombosis and Haemostasis* **10**(4): 698–702.

Bashir R, Zack CJ, Zhao H, Comerota AJ, Bove AA. (2014) Comparative Outcomes of Catheter-Directed Thrombolysis Plus Anticoagulation vs Anticoagulation Alone to Treat Lower-Extremity Proximal Deep Vein Thrombosis. *JAMA Internal Medicine* **174**(9): 1494–501.

Bates SM, Jaeschke R, Stevens SM, Goodacre S, Wells PS, Stevenson MD *et al.* (2012). Diagnosis of DVT: Antithrombotic Therapy and Prevention of Thrombosis, 9th ed: American College of Chest Physicians Evidence-Based Clinical Practice Guidelines. *Chest* **141**(2 Suppl): e351S–418S.

Chan WS, Ginsberg JS (2006). A review of upper extremity deep vein thrombosis in pregnancy: unmasking the 'ART' behind the clot. *Journal of Thrombosis and Haemostasis* **4**(8): 1673–7.

Chopra V, Fallouh N, McGuirk H, Salata B, Healy C, Kabaeva Z *et al.* (2015). Patterns, risk factors and treatment associated with PICC-DVT in hospitalized adults: A nested case-control study. *Thrombosis Research* **135**(5): 829–34.

Chopra V, Flanders SA, Saint S, Woller SC, O'Grady NP, Safdar N *et al.* (2015). The Michigan Appropriateness Guide for Intravenous Catheters (MAGIC): results from a multispecialty panel using the RAND/UCLA appropriateness method. *Ann Intern Med.* **163**(6 suppl): S1–S40.

Constans J, Salmi LR, Sevestre-Pietri MA, Perusat S, Nguon M, Degeilh M *et al.* (2008). A clinical prediction score for upper extremity deep venous thrombosis. *Thrombosis and Haemostasis* **99**(1): 202–7.

Cronan JJ, Leen V (1989). Recurrent deep venous thrombosis: limitations of US. *Radiology* **170**(3 Pt 1): 739–42.

De Cicco M, Matovic M, Balestreri L, Panarello G, Fantin D, Morassut S *et al.* (1997). Central venous thrombosis: an early and frequent complication in cancer patients bearing long-term silastic catheter. A prospective study. *Thrombosis Research* **86**(2): 101–13.

Di Nisio M, Van Sluis GL, Bossuyt PM, Buller HR, Porreca E, Rutjes AW (2010). Accuracy of diagnostic tests for clinically suspected upper extremity deep vein thrombosis: a systematic review. *Journal of Thrombosis and Haemostasis* **8**(4): 684–92.

Ellis MH, Manor Y, Witz M (2000). Risk factors and management of patients with upper limb deep vein thrombosis. *Chest* **117**(1): 43–6.

Elman EE, Kahn SR (2006). The post-thrombotic syndrome after upper extremity deep venous thrombosis in adults: a systematic review. *Thrombosis Research* **117**(6): 609–14.

Enden T, Klow NE, Sandvik L, Slagsvold CE, Ghanima W, Hafsahl G *et al.* (2009). Catheter-directed thrombolysis vs. anticoagulant therapy alone in deep vein thrombosis: results of an open randomized, controlled trial reporting on short-term patency. *Journal of Thrombosis and Haemostasis* **7**(8): 1268–75.

Engelberger RP, Fahrni J, Willenberg T, Baumann F, Spirk D, Diehm N *et al.* (2014). Fixed low-dose ultrasound-assisted catheter-directed thrombolysis followed by routine stenting of residual stenosis for acute ilio-femoral deep-vein thrombosis. *Thrombosis and Haemostasis* **111**(6): 1153–60.

Evans RS, Sharp JH, Linford LH, Lloyd JF, Tripp JS, Jones JP *et al.* (2010). Risk of symptomatic DVT associated with peripherally inserted central catheters. *Chest* **138**(4): 803–10.

Evans RS, Sharp JH, Linford LH, Lloyd JF, Tripp JS, Woller SC *et al.* (2013). Reduction of Peripherally Inserted Central Catheter Associated Deep Venous Thrombosis. *Chest* **143**(3): 627–633.

Girolami A, Prandoni P, Zanon E, Bagatella P, Girolami B (1999). Venous thromboses of upper limbs are more frequently associated with occult cancer as compared with those of lower limbs. *Blood Coagulation & Fibrinolysis* **10**(8): 455–7.

Goldhaber SZ, Buring JE, Lipnick RJ, Hennekens CH (1984). Pooled analyses of randomized trials of streptokinase and heparin in phlebographically documented acute deep venous thrombosis. *American Journal of Medicine* **76**(3): 393–7.

Grant JD, Stevens SM, Woller SC, Lee EW, Kee ST, Liu DM *et al.* (2012). Diagnosis and management of upper extremity deep-vein thrombosis in adults. *Thrombosis and Haemostasis* **108**(6): 1097–108.

Heijboer H, Jongbloets LM, Buller HR, Lensing AW, ten Cate JW (1992). Clinical utility of real-time compression ultrasonography for diagnostic management of patients with recurrent venous thrombosis. *Acta Radiologica* **33**(4): 297–300.

Hingorani A, Ascher E, Lorenson E, DePippo P, Salles-Cunha S, Scheinman M *et al.* (1997). Upper extremity deep venous thrombosis and its impact on morbidity and mortality rates in a hospital-based population. *Journal of Vascular Surgery* **26**(5): 853–60.

Hingorani A, Ascher E, Markevich N, Yorkovich W, Schutzer R, Mutyala M *et al.* (2005). Risk factors for mortality in patients with upper extremity and internal jugular deep venous thrombosis. *Journal of Vascular Surgery* **41**(3): 476–8.

Hull R, Hirsh J, Sackett DL, Taylor DW, Carter C, Turpie AG *et al.* (1981). Clinical validity of a negative venogram in patients with clinically suspected venous thrombosis. *Circulation* **64**(3): 622–5.

Isma N, Svensson PJ, Gottsater A, Lindblad B (2010). Upper extremity deep venous thrombosis in the population-based Malmo thrombophilia study (MATS). Epidemiology, risk factors, recurrence risk, and mortality. *Thrombosis Research* **125**(6): e335–8.

Joffe HV, Goldhaber SZ (2002). Upper-extremity deep vein thrombosis. *Circulation* **106**(14): 1874–80.

Joffe HV, Kucher N, Tapson VF, Goldhaber SZ (2004). Upper-extremity deep vein thrombosis: a prospective registry of 592 patients. *Circulation* **110**(12): 1605–11.

Kahn SR, Lim W, Dunn AS *et al.* (2012). Prevention of VTE in nonsurgical patients: Antithrombotic Therapy and Prevention of Thrombosis, 9th ed: American College of Chest Physicians Evidence-Based Clinical Practice Guidelines. *Chest* **141**: e195S–226S.

Kahn SR, Shapiro S, Wells PS, Rodger MA, Kovacs MJ, Anderson DR *et al.* (2013). Compression stockings to prevent post-thrombotic syndrome: a randomised placebo-controlled trial. *Lancet* **383**(9920): 880–8.

Kearon C, Akl EA, Comerota AJ, Prandoni P, Bounameaux H, Goldhaber SZ *et al.* (2012). Antithrombotic Therapy for VTE Disease: Antithrombotic Therapy and Prevention of Thrombosis, 9th ed: American College of Chest Physicians Evidence-Based Clinical Practice Guidelines. *Chest* **141**(2 Suppl): e419S–94S.

Kearon C, Kahn SR, Agnelli G, Goldhaber S, Raskob GE, Comerota AJ (2008). Antithrombotic therapy for venous thromboembolic disease: American College of Chest Physicians Evidence-Based Clinical Practice Guidelines (8th Edition). *Chest* **133**(6 Suppl): 454S–545S.

Kim H, Chung JW, Park JH, Yin YH, Park SH, Yoon CJ *et al.* (2003). Role of CT venography in the diagnosis and treatment of benign thoracic central venous obstruction. *Korean Journal of Radiology* **4**(3): 146–52.

Kleinjan A, Di Nisio M, Beyer-Westendorf J, Camporese G, Cosmi B, Ghirarduzzi A *et al.* (2014). Safety and Feasibility of a Diagnostic Algorithm Combining Clinical Probability, d-Dimer Testing, and Ultrasonography for Suspected Upper Extremity Deep Venous ThrombosisA Prospective Management StudyDiagnostic Algorithm for Suspected Upper Extremity Deep Venous Thrombosis. *Annals of Internal Medicine* **160**(7): 451–7.

Knudson GJ, Wiedmeyer DA, Erickson SJ, Foley WD, Lawson TL, Mewissen MW *et al.* (1990). Color Doppler sonographic imaging in the assessment of upper-extremity deep venous thrombosis. *American Journal of Roentgenology* **154**(2): 399–403.

Korkeila P, Ylitalo A, Koistinen J, Airaksinen KE (2008). Progression of venous pathology after pacemaker and cardioverter-defibrillator implantation: A prospective serial venographic study. *Annals of Medicine* **41**(3): 216–23.

Kucher N (2011). Clinical practice. Deep-vein thrombosis of the upper extremities. *New England Journal of Medicine* **364**(9): 861–9.

Kuter DJ (2004). Thrombotic complications of central venous catheters in cancer patients. *Oncologist* **9**(2): 207–16.

Laerum F, Holm HA (1981). Postphlebographic thrombosis: a double-blind study with methylglucamine metrizoate and metrizamide. *Radiology* **140**(3): 651–4.

Lechner D, Wiener C, Weltermann A, Eischer L, Eichinger S, Kyrle PA (2008). Comparison between idiopathic deep vein thrombosis of the upper and lower extremity regarding risk factors and recurrence. *Journal of Thrombosis and Haemostasis* **6**(8): 1269–74.

Lee AY, Levine MN, Butler G, Webb C, Costantini L, Gu C *et al.* (2006). Incidence, risk factors, and outcomes of catheter-related thrombosis in adult patients with cancer. *Journal of Clinical Oncology* **24**(9): 1404–8.

Lin PH, Zhou W, Dardik A, Mussa F, Kougias P, Hedayati N *et al.* (2006). Catheter-direct thrombolysis versus pharmacomechanical thrombectomy for treatment of symptomatic lower extremity deep venous thrombosis. *American Journal of Surgery* **192**(6): 782–8.

Linkins LA, Stretton R, Probyn L, Kearon C (2006). Interobserver agreement on ultrasound measurements of residual vein diameter, thrombus echogenicity and Doppler venous flow in patients with previous venous thrombosis. *Thrombosis Research* **117**(3): 241–7.

Linnemann B, Meister F, Schwonberg J, Schindewolf M, Zgouras D, Lindhoff-Last E (2008). Hereditary and acquired thrombophilia in patients with upper extremity deep-vein thrombosis. Results from the MAISTHRO registry. *Thrombosis and Haemostasis* **100**(3): 440–6.

Luciani A, Clement O, Halimi P, Goudot D, Portier F, Bassot V *et al.* (2001). Catheter-related upper extremity deep venous thrombosis in cancer patients: a prospective study based on Doppler US. *Radiology* **220**(3): 655–60.

Maleux G, Marchal P, Palmers M, Heye S, Verhamme P, Vaninbroukx J *et al.* (2010). Catheter-directed thrombolytic therapy for thoracic deep vein thrombosis is safe and effective in selected patients with and without cancer. *European Radiology* **20**(9): 2293–300.

Martin C, Viviand X, Saux P, Gouin F (1999). Upper-extremity deep vein thrombosis after central venous catheterization via the axillary vein. *Critical Care Medicine* **27**(12): 2626–9.

Martinelli I, Battaglioli T, Bucciarelli P, Passamonti SM, Mannucci PM (2004). Risk factors and recurrence rate of primary deep vein thrombosis of the upper extremities. *Circulation* **110**(5): 566–70.

Munoz FJ, Mismetti P, Poggio R, Valle R, Barron M, Guil M *et al.* (2008). Clinical outcome of patients with upper-extremity deep vein thrombosis: results from the RIETE Registry. *Chest* **133**(1): 143–8.

Murphy EH, Fogarty TJ, Arko FR (2010). Endovascular intervention for lower extremity deep venous thrombosis. In: Fogarty TJ, White RA (eds). *Peripheral Endovascular Interventions*, 3rd edition, pp. 203–13. New York: Springer.

Naeem M, Soares G, Ahn S, Murphy T (2015). Paget-Schroetter syndrome: A review and Algorithm (WASPS-IR). *Phlebology* **30**(10): 675–86.

Owens CA, Bui JT, Knuttinen MG, Gaba RC, Carrillo TC (2010). Pulmonary embolism from upper extremity deep vein thrombosis and the role of superior vena cava filters: a review of the literature. *Journal of Vascular and Interventional Radiology* **21**(6): 779–87.

Prandoni P, Bernardi E, Marchiori A, Lensing AW, Prins MH, Villalta S *et al.* (2004). The long term clinical course of acute deep vein thrombosis of the arm: prospective cohort study. *BMJ* **329**(7464): 484–5.

Prandoni P, Polistena P, Bernardi E, Cogo A, Casara D, Verlato F *et al.* (1997). Upper-extremity deep vein thrombosis. Risk factors, diagnosis, and complications. *Archives of Internal Medicine* **157**(1): 57–62.

Saber W, Moua T, Williams EC, Verso M, Agnelli G, Couban S *et al.* (2011). Risk factors for catheter-related thrombosis (CRT) in cancer patients: a patient-level data (IPD) meta-analysis of clinical trials and prospective studies. *Journal of Thrombosis and Haemostasis* **9**(2): 312–9.

Sajid MS, Ahmed N, Desai M, Baker D, Hamilton G (2007). Upper limb deep vein thrombosis: a literature review to streamline the protocol for management. *Acta Haematologica* **118**(1): 10–8.

Sampson FC, Goodacre SW, Thomas SM, van Beek EJ (2007). The accuracy of MRI in diagnosis of suspected deep vein thrombosis: systematic review and meta-analysis. *European Radiology* **17**(1): 175–81.

Sartori M, Migliaccio L, Favaretto E, Cini M, Legnani C, Palareti G *et al.* (2015a). D-dimer for the diagnosis of upper extremity deep and superficial venous thrombosis. *Thrombosis Research* **135**(4): 673–8.

Sartori M, Migliaccio L, Favaretto E *et al.* (2015b). Whole-arm ultrasound to rule out suspected upper-extremity deep venous thrombosis in outpatients. *JAMA Internal Medicine* **175**(7): 1226–1227.

Schneider DB, Dimuzio PJ, Martin ND, Gordon RL, Wilson MW, Laberge JM *et al.* (2004). Combination treatment of venous thoracic outlet syndrome: open surgical decompression and intraoperative angioplasty. *Journal of Vascular Surgery* **40**(4): 599–603.

Sharafuddin MJ, Sun S, Hoballah JJ (2002). Endovascular management of venous thrombotic diseases of the upper torso and extremities. *Journal of Vascular and Interventional Radiology* **13**(10): 975–90.

Spencer FA, Emery C, Lessard D, Goldberg RJ (2007). Upper extremity deep vein thrombosis: a community-based perspective. *American Journal of Medicine* **120**(8): 678–84.

Stevens SM, Woller SC, Bauer KA, Kasthuri R, Chsuman M, Streiff M, Lim W, Douketis JD. J Thromb Thrombolysis. (2016) Jan; **41**(1): 154–64. doi: 10.1007/s11239-015-1316-1.

Streiff MB (2010). The National Comprehensive Cancer Center Network (NCCN) guidelines on the management of venous thromboembolism in cancer patients. *Thrombosis Research* **125**(Suppl 2): S128–33.

Thomas SM, Goodacre SW, Sampson FC, van Beek EJ (2008). Diagnostic value of CT for deep vein thrombosis: results of a systematic review and meta-analysis. *Clinical Radiology* **63**(3): 299–304.

Urschel HC, Jr., Razzuk MA (2000). Paget-Schroetter syndrome: what is the best management? *Annals of Thoracic Surgery* **69**(6): 1663–8; discussion 8–9.

Urschel HC, Jr., Patel AN (2003). Paget-Schroetter syndrome therapy: failure of intravenous stents. *Annals of Thoracic Surgery* **75**(6): 1693–6; discussion 6.

van Rooden CJ, Schippers EF, Barge RM, Rosendaal FR, Guiot HF, van der Meer FJ *et al.* (2005). Infectious complications of central venous catheters increase the risk of catheter-related thrombosis in hematology patients: a prospective study. *Journal of Clinical Oncology* **23**(12): 2655–60.

Vendantham S. Oral presentation at the Society of Interventional Radiology 2017 Washington, DC, USA. accessed on 2 September 2017: https://vascularnews.com/attract-fails-to-meet-primary-endpoint-but-experts-agree-results-are-hypothesis-generating/ 2017.

Vedantham S (2008). Interventions for Deep Vein Thrombosis: Reemergence of a Promising Therapy. *American Journal of Medicine* **121**(11): S28–S39.

Vedantham S, Millward SF, Cardella JF, Hofmann LV, Razavi MK, Grassi CJ *et al.* (2006). Society of Interventional Radiology position statement: treatment of acute iliofemoral deep vein thrombosis with use of adjunctive catheter-directed intrathrombus thrombolysis. *Journal of Vascular and Interventional Radiology* **17**(4): 613–6.

Wagman LD, Baird MF, Bennett CL, Bockenstedt PL, Cataland SR, Fanikos J *et al.* (2008). Venous thromboembolic disease. NCCN. Clinical practice guidelines in oncology. *Journal of the National Comprehensive Cancer Network* **6**(8): 716–53.

Wicky ST (2009). Acute deep vein thrombosis and thrombolysis. *Techniques in Vascular and Interventional Radiology* **12**(2): 148–53.

23

Management of Intra-abdominal Thrombosis

Serena M. Passamonti, Francesca Gianniello and Ida Martinelli

A. Bianchi Bonomi Hemophilia and Thrombosis Center, Fondazione IRCCS Ca' Granda - Ospedale Maggiore Policlinico, Milan, Italy

Thrombosis of abdominal veins other than the iliacs and the inferior vena cava are rare but clinically relevant, and have a wide spectrum of clinical presentations. Patients can be totally asymptomatic, or may present with acute abdominal pain. Abdominal veins collect blood from various organs, such as the liver, bowel, kidneys or ovaries, and their occlusion can cause an acute or chronic impairment of organ function, with long-term consequences that can affect the quality of life of the patients.

Portal vein thrombosis can lead to portal hypertension and oesophageal varices, with consequential risk of bleeding. Short-bowel syndrome can develop in patients who require extensive bowel resection for intestinal infarcts due to superior mesenteric vein thrombosis. Impairment of renal function due to thrombosis of the renal veins can damage the kidneys, leading to haemodialysis. In this chapter, we will describe various abdominal vein thromboses, their clinical implications, and strategies of treatment.

Splanchnic Vein Thrombosis

Epidemiology, Diagnosis and Risk Factors

Splanchnic vein thrombosis (SVT) is a heterogeneous group of diseases that includes hepatic vein thrombosis (Budd-Chiari syndrome, BCS), portal (PVT), splenic and mesenteric vein thrombosis (MVT). The concomitant involvement of more than one venous district is frequent. BCS is defined as the obstruction of the hepatic venous outflow, from the small hepatic veins to the junction of the inferior vena cava and the right atrium. This is considered the most frightening intra-abdominal vein thrombosis, because it may lead to liver transplantation, and has an overall mortality rate at six months of 10% (Janssen *et al.*, 2003; Darwish Murad *et al.*, 2009).

PVT is defined as the obstruction of the extra-hepatic portal vein, with or without the involvement of the intra-hepatic portal or other splanchnic veins (i.e. splenic and superior mesenteric veins). PVT can lead to the formation of portal cavernoma and the development of portal hypertension (Sarin *et al.*, 2006). BCS and PVT are rare, with an annual incidence of less than 1 case and 4 cases per million individuals, respectively (Valla, 2004; Almdal and Sorensen, 1991). MVT is more frequent, with an incidence of 2.7 cases per 100.000 individuals (Acosta *et al.*, 2008). Symptoms such as abdominal pain, nausea, vomiting, haematemesis and melena depend on the extension of thrombosis. and the number of involved veins.

Thrombosis can be fulminant, acute or chronic. In few cases, patients remain asymptomatic. Fulminant BCS occurs in 5% of cases and the acute form accounts for 20% of cases (Darwish Murad *et al.*, 2009). The overall survival of patients with PVT is 54% after ten years but, in the absence of cancer, cirrhosis and MVT, it increases up to 81%, with a mortality rate at one year of 5% (Janssen *et al.*, 2001). Acute MVT is associated with a risk of bowel infarction, and surgical resection is required in 22–33% of patients, with an early mortality rate of 20–30% (Acosta *et al.*, 2008; Morasch *et al.*, 2001). Prompt diagnosis of SVT is crucial. Doppler ultrasound has a sensitivity of 90% in PVT, and near 100% in BCS whereas, in MVT, it is lower because of the frequent presence of bowel gas (Kamath, 2006; Tessler *et al.*, 1991). Contrast-enhanced computed tomography and magnetic resonance imaging are techniques of first choice to diagnose MVT, while venography is reserved for selected cases.

SVT can be associated with a transient or persistent, local or systemic risk factor. In their absence, it is considered idiopathic. Risk factors associated with SVT are summarised in Table 23.1.

Risk factors differ according to age, site of thrombosis and geographical area of patients. For example, a local precipitating factor (i.e. abdominal surgery) is rare in BCS (Darwish Murad *et al.*, 2009), but not in PVT or MVT (Thatipelli *et al.*, 2010). Haematological disorders, autoimmune diseases and the use of hormonal therapies are the most common risk factors in BCS, whereas liver cirrhosis, abdominal cancer, inflammatory bowel diseases and abdominal surgery are the most common risk factors in PVT and MVT.

Table 23.1 Risk factors for splanchnic vein thrombosis.

Abdominal disorders and surgery

Acute

- Pancreatitis
- Peritonitis and sepsis
- Diverticulitis
- Splenectomy
- Hydatidosis
- Abdominal trauma

Chronic

- Cirrhosis
- Solid abdominal cancer
- Portal hypertension

Philadelphia chromosome negative chronic myelophrolipherative neoplasms

- Polycythaemia vera
- Essential thrombocytaemia
- Idiopathic myelofibrosis

Paroxysmal nocturnal haemoglobinuria

Thrombophilic states

- Antithrombin, protein C and protein S deficiency
- Factor V Leiden
- Prothrombin G20210A mutation
- Antiphospholipid antibodies

Gynaecological states

- Oral contraceptives/hormonal replacement therapy
- Pregnancy/puerperium

Miscellaneous

- Autoimmune disorders (Behçet disease)
- Hypereosinophilic syndrome

During the past years, myeloproliferative neoplasms, in particular those which are JAK2V617F mutation positive, have been recognised as an important systemic cause of SVT. SVT is the first clinical manifestation of myeloproliferative neoplasms in 25–65% of cases (Austin and Lambert, 2008). The prevalence of the JAK2V617F mutation in patients with SVT has been reported as high as 33%, ranging between 27% in non-malignant and non-cirrhotic patients with PVT, to 41% in patients with BCS (Smalberg *et al.*, 2012). Thus, routine screening for JAK2V617F mutation in patients with SVT is recommended (Smalberg *et al.*, 2012; Kiladjian *et al.*, 2008). Less common risk factors include autoimmune diseases, such as Behcet's disease and paroxysmal nocturnal haemoglobinuria.

Finally, the inherited thrombophilia abnormalities antithrombin, protein C or protein S deficiencies are infrequently diagnosed, and their inheritance is often complicated by liver impairment, resulting in reduced synthesis of procoagulant and anticoagulant factors. Factor V Leiden mutation is more strongly associated to BCS than PV, whereas the opposite is for the prothrombin G20210A mutation (Shetty and Ghosh, 2011; Dentali *et al.*, 2008).

Literature and Guidelines

Anticoagulant therapies include unfractionated heparin (UH), low molecular weight heparin (LMWH), vitamin K antagonists (VKA) and thrombolytic agents.

Guidelines on treatment of SVT are based on the result of observational studies and expert opinion, so the quality and the strength of the evidence are low. Concerning BCS, an increased long-term survival in anticoagulated, rather than in non-anticoagulated patients, was observed in a retrospective study investigating factors associated with survival in adult patients with BCS (Zeitoun *et al.*, 1999).

Two studies reported that anticoagulant therapy was prescribed in 72% of consecutive patients and in 86% of a case series with BCS (Darwish Murad *et al.*, 2009; Darwish *et al.*, 2004). Concerning non-cirrhotic patients with PVT, the rate of anticoagulant therapies varies from 55 to 90% (Spaander *et al.*, 2013). Thrombolytic treatment or invasive procedures are infrequently used both in patients with BCS (Sharma *et al.*, 2004) and in those with PVT (Rajani *et al.*, 2010; Condat *et al.*, 2001; Plessier *et al.*, 2010; Senzolo *et al.*, 2012), because of the high baseline risk of bleeding. The optimal management of PVT in cirrhotic patients is less well studied. The larger study included a cohort of 56 patients with non-malignant PVT, whose re-canalisation rate was higher in those treated with LMWH than in those not treated. In this study, LMWH therapy did not seem to worsen the risk of variceal bleeding (Senzolo *et al.*, 2012).

Anticoagulant therapy seems to be effective in reducing the risk of recurrent thrombosis independently of the site and the extension of SVT, although the evidence that VKA treatment favours re-canalisation, and reduces the recurrence rate without increasing the risk and severity of variceal bleeding, is limited (Condat *et al.*, 2001; Plessier *et al.*, 2010; Senzolo *et al.*, 2012). The risk of recurrence seems to be higher in patients with PVT (either isolated or extended to splenic or MVT) than in patients with isolated MVT (Amitrano *et al.*, 2007; Hedayati *et al.*, 2008).

A retrospective cohort study of patients with MVT treated with VKA reported an annual risk for recurrence of 4.6% person-years in 40% of patients who discontinue treatment (Dentali *et al.*, 2009). No data are available about the short or long-term risk of recurrence in patient with incidentally diagnosed SVT.

An international registry on 613 patients with SVT was recently completed (Ageno *et al.*, 2014). Onset of symptoms, risk factors, type and duration of anticoagulant therapies, bleeding events and recurrent thrombosis were collected. Eighty percent of patients received anticoagulant treatment, and the drug of choice was LMWH in the acute phase (66%), switched to VKA in 50% of cases. Patients who continued LMWH therapy instead of switching to VKA had mainly solid cancer, cirrhosis and low platelet count. Sixty-five percent of patients with incidentally diagnosed SVT received anticoagulant treatment – in particular, LMWH. Patients who received no treatment within the first month after diagnosis were the most fragile ones, with gastrointestinal bleeding at presentation, thrombocytopenia, end stage cirrhosis, or were asymptomatic.

In the lack of strong evidence, current guidelines on anticoagulant treatment are based mainly on expert opinion. The 9th edition of the American College of Chest Physicians' guidelines on Antithrombotic Therapy and Prevention of Thrombosis recommend anticoagulation over no anticoagulation in symptomatic patients with SVT, and no anticoagulation for incidentally detected thrombosis in asymptomatic patients (Kearon *et al.*, 2012). However, the authors suggest anticoagulant therapy in the presence of extensive thrombosis or active cancer (Kearon *et al.*, 2012).

The optimal duration of anticoagulant treatment is not well established, but recommendations are similar to those made for patients with deep vein thrombosis of the lower limbs or pulmonary embolism (Kearon *et al.*, 2012). Lifelong therapy is suggested for BCS, longer duration is recommended in case of unprovoked thrombosis if the risk of bleeding is low or moderate, and a minimum of 3–6 months therapy is suggested for PVT in the presence of removable risk factors (Janssen *et al.*, 2003; Sarin *et al.*, 2006; Condat *et al.*, 2006; Martinelli *et al.*, 2008).

Prolonged anticoagulation is recommended in the presence of active solid cancer, myeloproliferative neoplasm and severe thrombophilia (i.e. antithrombin, protein C and protein S deficiency, homozygosity for factor V Leiden or the prothrombin G20210A mutation, the presence of antiphospholipid antibodies, combined abnormalities) (Mannucci *et al.*, 2015; Kraaijenhagen *et al.*, 2000; Pengo *et al.*, 2009). Also, the American Association for the Study of Liver Disease recommends anticoagulation for patients with acute PVT and BCS (DeLeve *et al.*, 2009), considering long term duration of therapy in those with permanent risk factors or the involvement of the mesenteric veins, as well as for patients with BCS (DeLeve *et al.*, 2009).

Recommendation on Treatment

The optimal management of SVT requires a multidisciplinary approach that includes hepatologists, experts on thrombosis, radiologists and surgeons. Anticoagulant treatment should be considered for all patients with diagnosed SVT, because available data suggest an improved survival and re-canalisation rate, a reduction of the risk of portal hypertension, portal cavernoma and recurrent events. Hence, patients with SVT should be promptly evaluated for their risk of bleeding, principally due to the concomitant presence of cirrhosis, portal hypertension with gastric or esophageal varices, and low platelet count.

Considering the concomitant risk of bleeding, in the acute phase, patients should be treated with LMWH, followed by oral VKA. The decision to avoid anticoagulant treatment at the time of diagnosis is justified for patients with active variceal bleeding or very high risk of bleeding (e.g. low platelet count) or short life expectance (e.g. solid cancer or cirrhosis at terminal stage). Figure 23.1 summarises different therapeutic strategies according to different clinical presentation of SVT.

In case of rapid progression of thrombosis despite anticoagulation, patients should be considered for systemic or local thrombolysis and/or invasive procedures (i.e. angioplasty, trans-jugular intrahepatic portosystemic or surgical porto-systemic shunt) (Janssen *et al.*, 2003; Hollingshead *et al.*, 2005), that have a variable efficacy (Spaander *et al.*, 2013; Sharma *et al.*, 2004; Hollingshead *et al.*, 2005; Kim *et al.*, 2005). Thrombolysis should be limited to selected patients with onset of symptoms within 72 hours and low risk of bleeding – for example, those with extended MVT and intestinal ischemia (Hollingshead *et al.*, 2005). Failure of the aforementioned interventions occurs in 10–20% of patients with BCS, who are, therefore, candidates for liver transplantation (Darwish Murad *et al.*, 2009; Valla, 2008).

Renal Vein Thrombosis

Epidemiology, Diagnosis and Risk Factors

The annual incidence of renal vein thrombosis (RVT) in the general population is less than one per million (Zöller *et al.*, 2011). In the paediatric population, RVT is the most prevalent non catheter-related thrombosis during the neonatal period, and accounts for 16–20% of all thromboembolic events in the newborn (Bokenkamp *et al.*, 2000; Brandão *et al.*, 2011).

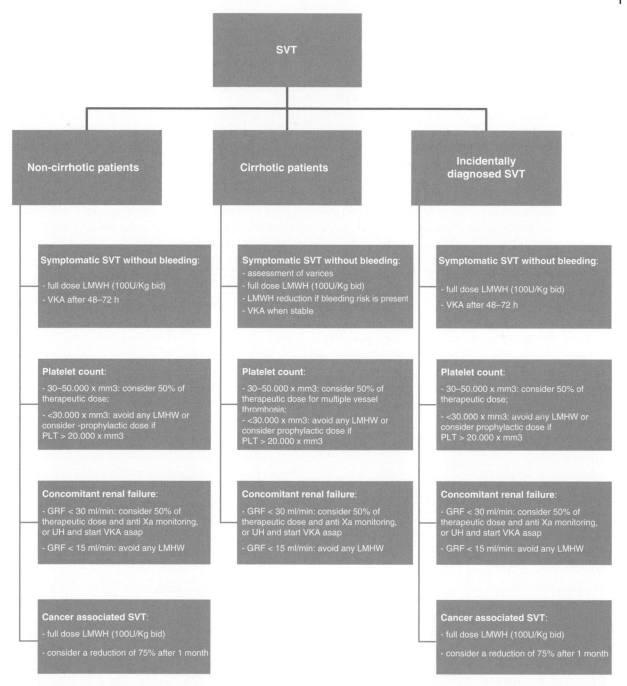

Figure 23.1 Suggested anticoagulant therapies for the acute-phase SVT in different situations.

Commonly, RVT has an insidious onset. The classic presentation includes microscopic or macroscopic haematuria, flank pain and worsen of renal function. Non-specific symptoms such as anorexia, nausea and vomiting are often present. The rapidity of venous occlusion and the development of venous collateral circulation are determinant of the clinical presentation and renal function impairment (Zöller *et al.*, 2011; Asghar *et al.*, 2007). In two-thirds of patients, RVT is asymptomatic and involves one or both renal veins (Zöller *et al.*, 2011).

Doppler ultrasound has a sensitivity of 85% and a specificity of 56% (Avashi *et al.*, 1983), but contrast computed tomography remains the imaging of choice for the diagnosis of RVT, with a sensitivity and specificity of almost 100% (Alvarez-Castells *et al.*, 2001). The disadvantages of computed tomography include radiation exposures and the use of nephrotoxic iodinated contrast media (Alvarez-Castells *et al.*, 2001). Magnetic resonance angiography is an alternative imaging, with a slightly lower sensitivity and specificity than computed tomography (Hodgson *et al.*, 2006).

Indirect radiographic signs of RVT include increased renal size, renal vein enlargement, prolonged cortico-medullary differentiation, thickening of renal fascia and stranding of perinephric fat. Inferior vena cava and renal venography are the gold standard test, although invasive and involving radiation exposure and injection of iodated contrast (Asghar *et al.*, 2007). Table 23.2 summarises common risk factors for RVT.

In adults, non-cancer-related RVT occurs mainly in patients with nephrotic syndrome that is, *per se*, associated with and increased risk of venous thromboembolism, because of the loss of the anticoagulant proteins antithrombin, protein C and protein S. The incidence of RVT in patients with nephrotic syndrome ranges from 5–62%, and is most common in membranous nephropathy (Singhal and Brimble, 2006). Concerning neoplasms, an intrinsic or extrinsic involvement of the renal vascular pedicle is common in renal cancer, as well as retroperitoneal tumours and lymphomas (Witz and Korzets, 2007). Other conditions related with RVT are blunt or surgical trauma, inferior vena cava filters and, in neonates, umbilical vein catheterisation (Witz and Korzets, 2007).

Table 23.2 Risk factors for renal and ovarian vein thrombosis.

Renal vein thrombosis	Ovarian vein thrombosis
Abdominal disorders and surgery	**Gynaecological states**
Cancer	Pregnancy/puerperium
Nephrotic syndrome	Cancer
Acute conditions	Pelvic infections
• urogenital infections	Gynaecological surgery
• other abdominal infection	
• sepsis	
Surgery	
• urologic, vascular, colorectal	
• renal transplantation	
Thrombophilic states	**Thrombophilic states**
• Antithrombin, protein C and protein S deficiency	• Antithrombin, protein C and protein S deficiency
• Factor V Leiden	• Factor V Leiden
• Prothrombin G20210A mutation	• Prothrombin G20210A mutation
• Antiphospholipid antibodies	• Antiphospholipid antibodies
Gynaecological states	
• Oral contraceptives/hormonal replacement therapy	
• Pregnancy/puerperium	
Miscellaneous	
• Vena cava filters	
• Umbilical vein catheterisation	

Finally, RVT can complicate 0.1–0.5% of renal transplantations (Salehipour *et al.*, 2009; Aktas *et al.*, 2011). Inherited thrombophilia abnormalities have been reported in approximately 50% of adult patients with RVT, similarly to what is observed in patients with deep vein thrombosis of the lower limbs (Wysokinski *et al.*, 2008). A case-control study carried out in newborns showed that factor V Leiden was associated with a nine-fold increased risk of RVT, whereas the presence of prothrombin G20210A mutation was not (Kosch *et al.*, 2004).

Recommendation on Treatment

For patients with RVT, a medical therapy, instead of a surgical approach (thrombectomy or nephrectomy), is recommended (Witz and Korzets, 2007). Regardless of aetiology, anticoagulant therapy with LMWH or UH, followed by VKA, is the treatment of choice for acute RVT. LMWH should be used with caution in patients with mild renal function impairment, and avoided in case of severe renal impairment, because of the drug accumulation in blood, with a potential increase of the risk of bleeding.

Patients with transient and no longer present risk factors should be treated with VKA for 3–6 months. Although the probability of recurrence is low (Wysokinski *et al.*, 2008), patients with idiopathic RVT, severe unremitting nephrosic syndrome or severe thrombophilia abnormalities should receive long-term anticoagulation (Zöller *et al.*, 2011; Witz and Korzets, 2007). In selected cases, thrombectomy and/or systemic or catheter-directed local thrombolysis is suitable (Kim *et al.*, 2009). These strategies should be performed within the first days after the onset of symptoms, to prevent irreversible damage to the kidneys. Such procedures are reserved for selected patients, such as those with bilateral RVT, RVT of a solitary native kidney or after renal transplantation, and those worsening despite medical treatment (Kim *et al.*, 2009; Janda, 2010).

Ovarian Vein Thrombosis

Epidemiology, Diagnosis and Risk Factors

Ovarian vein thrombosis (OVT) is a rare condition most commonly diagnosed in the post-partum period, complicating 1 : 500 to 1 : 2000 deliveries (Salomon *et al.*, 1999). A prospective observational study of more than 40 000 deliveries observed that the risk of OVT was higher for caesarean sections than vaginal deliveries, and for twin than single-child deliveries (Salomon *et al.*, 2010).

In 90% of cases, OVT occurs in the right ovarian vein, for anatomical reasons, due to the dextrotorsion of the puerperal enlarged uterus, which causes compression of the right ovarian vein. In addition, the right ovarian vein is longer than the left one, and has less competent valves, favouring local blood stasis. Finally, the diameter of the ovarian veins increases up to three times in pregnancy, and the flow rapidly declines after delivery. This may lead to partial collapse and blood stasis (Dessole *et al.*, 2003; Kominiarek and Hibbard *et al.*, 2006).

The incidence of recurrent OVT is 3% per patient-year, similar to that of recurrent deep vein thrombosis of the lower limbs (Wysokinska *et al.*, 2006). The clinical presentation of OVT is flank pain, fever in the first days after delivery and, occasionally, a tender abdominal mass can be appreciated. Additional symptoms are nausea, vomiting, malaise, ileus, dyspnoea and tachycardia. If OVT is not diagnosed and treated, it may extend to inferior vena cava or provoke pulmonary embolism (Kominiarek and Hibbard *et al.*, 2006). Objective diagnosis includes computed tomography, magnetic resonance or Doppler ultrasonography, with a sensitivity of 100%, 92% and 52%, respectively, and a specificity of 99%, 100% and 50%, respectively (Savader *et al.*, 1988; Twickler *et al.*, 1997).

Table 23.2 summarises the common risk factors for OVT. Uterine infection and sepsis are frequent determinants of OVT (Kominiarek and Hibbard *et al.*, 2006). Pregnancy-related hypercoagulability, which helps to maintain placental function during pregnancy and to minimise blood loss at delivery, may favour post-partum OVT (Greer, 1994). The haemostatic changes that characterise pregnancy include increased concentrations of most procoagulant factors (factors V, VII, VIII, IX, X, XII, fibrinogen and von Willebrand factor), the decrease of the natural anticoagulant protein S and reduced fibrinolytic activity (Greer, 1994). Other conditions associated to OVT are gynaecological cancers, pelvic infections, surgery and sepsis. Rarely, OVT has no recognised associated causes. Finally, thrombophilia abnormalities are present in 20–30% of patients with OVT (Salomon *et al.*, 1999, 2010).

Recommendation on Treatment

LMWH followed by VKA are generally recommended for 3–6 months in the presence of transient risk factors, whereas a prolonged duration is suggested for idiophatic OVT, cancer-related OVT, and in patients with severe thrombophilia abnormalities, in analogy to what is recommended for patients with the most common deep vein thrombosis of the limbs (Mannucci *et al.*, 2015; Salomon *et al.*, 2010).

Key Points

- Thrombosis of abdominal veins are rare but clinically relevant, with a wide spectrum of clinical presentations.
- Prompt diagnosis of splanchnic, renal and ovarian vein thrombosis is crucial, to limit organ damage and improve survival.
- Look for myeloproliferative neoplasms in patients with splanchnic vein thrombosis testing the JAK2V617F mutation.
- Look for the presence of gastric and esophageal varices in patients with splanchnic vein thrombosis.
- Full dose of LMWH followed by VKA is recommended, if not contraindicated.
- Sub-therapeutic doses of LMWH in the presence of thrombocytopenia, gastric and esophageal varices, or renal impairment.
- Consider thrombolysis or thrombectomy only in selected patients who worsen despite anticoagulant therapy.

Further Reading

De Stefano V, Martinelli I (2010). Splanchnic vein thrombosis: clinical presentation, risk factors and treatment. *Internal and Emergency Medicine* 5: 487–94.
Martinelli I, De Stefano V (2012). Extra-abdominal venous thromboses at unusual sites. *Best Practice & Research Clinical Haematology* 25: 265–74.
Ageno W, Dentali F, Squizzato A (2014). How I treat splanchnic vein thrombosis. *Blood* 124: 3685–91.
Kearon C, Akl EA, Comerota AJ *et al.* (2012). American College of Chest Physicians. Antithrombotic therapy for VTE disease: Antithrombotic Therapy and Prevention of Thrombosis, 9th ed: American College of Chest Physicians Evidence-Based Clinical Practice Guidelines. *Chest* 141(2 Suppl): e419S–94S.
Martinelli I, Bucciarelli P, Mannucci PM (2010). Thrombotic risk factors: basic pathophysiology. *Critical Care Medicine* 38(2 Suppl): S3–9.

References

Acosta S, Alhadad A, Svensson P *et al.* (2008). Epidemiology, risk and prognostic factors in mesenteric venous thrombosis. *British Journal of Surgery* 95: 1245–51.

Ageno W, Riva N, Schulman S *et al.* (2014). IRSVT study group. Antithrombotic treatment of splanchnic vein thrombosis: results of an international registry. *Seminars in Thrombosis and Hemostasis* **40**(1): 99–105.

Aktas S, Boyvat F, Sevmis S *et al.* (2011). Analysis of vascular complications after renal transplantation. *Transplantation Proceedings* **43**: 557–61.

Almdal TP, Sorensen TI (1991). Incidence of parenchymal liver diseases in Denmark, 1981 to 1985: analysis of hospitalization registry data. The Danish association for the study of the liver. *Hepatology* **13**: 650–5.

Alvarez-Castells A, Sebastia CC, Quiroga GS (2001). Computerized tomography angiography of renal vessels. *Archivos Españoles de Urología* **54**: 603–15.

Amitrano L, Guardascione MA, Scaglione M *et al.* (2007). Prognostic factors in noncirrhotic patients with splanchnic vein thromboses. *American Journal of Gastroenterology* **102**(11): 2464–2470.

Asghar M, Ahmed K, Shah SS *et al.* (2007). Renal vein thrombosis. *European Journal of Vascular and Endovascular Surgery* **34**: 217–23.

Austin SK, Lambert JR (2008). The JAK2 V617F mutation and thrombosis. *British Journal of Haematology* **143**: 307–20.

Avashi PS, Greene ER, Scholler C (1983). Noninvasive diagnosis of renal vein thrombosis by ultrasonic echo-doppler fluorimetry. *Kidney International* **23**: 882–7.

Bokenkamp A, von Kries R, Nowak-Gottl U *et al.* (2000). Neonatal renal vein thrombosis in Germany between 1992 and 1994: epidemiology, treatment and outcome. *European Journal of Pediatrics* **159**: 44–8.

Brandão LR, Simpson EA, Lau KK (2011). Neonatal renal vein thrombosis. *Seminars in Fetal and Neonatal Medicine* **16**: 323–8.

Condat B, Pessione F, Hillaire S *et al.* (2001). Current outcome of portal vein thrombosis in adults: risk and benefit of anticoagulant therapy. *Gastroenterology* **120**(2): 490–497.

Condat B, Valla D (2006). Nonmalignant portal vein thrombosis in adults. *Nature Clinical Practice Gastroenterology & Hepatology* **3**: 505–15.

Darwish Murad S, Valla DC, de Groen PC *et al.* (2004). Determinants of survival and the effect of portosystemic shunting in patients with Budd- Chiari syndrome. *Hepatology* **39**(2): 500–508.

Darwish Murad S, Plessier A, Hernandez-Guerra M *et al.* (2009). EN-Vie (European network for vascular disorders of the liver).Etiology, management, and outcome of the Budd–Chiari syndrome. *Annals of Internal Medicine* **151**: 167–75.

DeLeve LD, Valla DC, Garcia-Tsao G (2009). American association for the study liver diseases. Vascular disorders of the liver. *Hepatology* **49**: 1729–64.

Dentali F, Galli M, Gianni M, Ageno W (2008). Inherited thrombophilic abnormalities and risk of portal vein thrombosis. A meta-analysis. *Thrombosis and Haemostasis* **99**(4): 675–682.

Dentali F, Ageno W, Witt D *et al.* (2009). WARPED consortium. Natural history of mesenteric venous thrombosis in patients treated with vitamin K antagonists: a multi-centre, retrospective cohort study. *Thrombosis and Haemostasis* **102**(3): 501–504.

Dessole S, Capobianco G, Arru A *et al.* (2003). Postpartum ovarian vein thrombosis: an unpredictable event: two case reports and review of the literature. *Archives of Gynecology and Obstetrics* **267**: 242–6.

Greer I (1994). Haemostasis and thrombosis in pregnancy. In: Bloom Al, Forbes CD, Thomas DP, Tuddenham EGD (eds). *Haemostasis and Thrombosis*, pp 987–1016. Churchill Livingstone, Edinburgh.

Hedayati N, Riha GM, Kougias P *et al.* (2008). Prognostic factors and treatment outcome in mesenteric vein thrombosis. *Vascular and Endovascular Surgery* **42**(3): 217–224.

Hodgson D, Rankin S, Jan W et al. (2006). Magnetic Resonance imaging of living related kidney donor-an analysis of 111 consecutive cases. *BJU International* **97**: 584–6.

Hollingshead M, Burke CT, Mauro MA *et al.* (2005). Transcatheter thrombolytic therapy for acute mesenteric and portal vein thrombosis. *Journal of Vascular and Interventional Radiology* **16**: 651–61.

Janda SP (2010). Bilateral renal vein thrombosis and pulmonary embolism secondary to membranous glomerulonephritis treatedwith percutaneous catheter thrombectomy and localized thrombolytic therapy. *Indian Journal of Nephrology* **20**: 152–5.

Janssen HL, Wijnhound A, Haagsma EB *et al.* (2001). Extrahepatic portal vein thrombosis: aetiology and determinants of survival. *Gut* **49**: 720–4.

Janssen HL, Garcia-Pagan JC, Elias E *et al.* (2003). European group for the study of vascular disorders of the liver. Budd-Chiari syndrome: a review by an expert panel. *Journal of Hepatology* **38**: 364–71.

Kamath PS (2006). Budd-Chiari syndrome: Radiologic findings. *Liver Transplantation* **12**(11 Suppl 2): S21–S22.

Kearon C, Akl EA, Comerota AJ *et al.* (2012). American College of Chest Physicians. Antithrombotic therapy for VTE disease: Antithrombotic Therapy and Prevention of Thrombosis, 9th ed: American College of Chest Physicians Evidence-Based Clinical Practice Guidelines. *Chest* **141**(2 Suppl): e419S–94S.

Kiladjian JJ, Cervantes F, Leebeek FW, Marzac C, Cassinat B, Chevret S, Cazals-Hatem D, Plessier A, Garcia-Pagan JC, Darwish Murad S, Raffa S,Janssen HL, Gardin C, Cereja S, Tonetti C, Giraudier S, Condat B, Casadevall N, Fenaux P, Valla DC (2008). The impact of JAK2 and MPL mutations on diagnosis and prognosis of splanchnic vein thrombosis: a report on 241 cases. *Blood* **111**(10): 4922–9.

Kim HK, Choi HH, Lee JM *et al.* (2009). Acute renal vein thrombosis, oral contraceptives, and protein S deficiency: a successful catheter-directed thrombolysis. *Annals of Vascular Surgery* **23**: 687. e1–4.

Kim HS, Patra A, Khan J *et al.* (2005). Transhepatic catheter-directed thrombectomy and thrombolysis of acute superior mesenteric venous thrombosis. *Journal of Vascular and Interventional Radiology* **16**: 1685–91.

Kominiarek MA, Hibbard JU (2006). Postpartum ovarian vein thrombosis: an update. *Obstetrical & Gynecological Survey* **61**: 337–42.

Kosch A, Kuwertz-Broking E, Heller C *et al.* (2004). Renal venous thrombosis in neonates: prothrombotic risk factors and long term follow-up. *Blood* **104**: 1356–60.

Kraaijenhagen RA, in't Anker PS, Koopman MM, Reitsma PH, Prins MH, van den Ende A, Büller HR (2000). High plasma concentration of factor VIIIc is a major risk factor for venous thromboembolism. *Thrombosis and Haemostasis* **83**(1): 5–9.

Mannucci PM, Franchini M (2015). Classic thrombophilic gene variants. *Thrombosis and Haemostasis* **114**(5): 885–9.

Martinelli I, Franchini M, Mannucci PM (2008). How I treat rare venous thromboses. *Blood* **112**: 4818–23.

Morasch MD, Ebaugh JL, Chiou AC *et al.* (2001). Mesenteric venous thrombosis: a changing entity. *Journal of Vascular Surgery* **34**: 680–4.

Pengo V, Tripodi A, Reber G, Rand JH, Ortel TL, Galli M *et al.* (2009). Update of the guidelines for lupus anticoagulant detection. *Journal of Thrombosis and Haemostasis* **10**: 1737–40.

Plessier A, Darwish-Murad S, Hernandez-Guerra M *et al.* (2010). European Network for Vascular Disorders of the Liver (EN-Vie). Acute portal vein thrombosis unrelated to cirrhosis: a prospective multicenter follow-up study. *Hepatology* **51**(1): 210–218.

Rajani R, Björnsson E, Bergquist A *et al.* (2010). The epidemiology and clinical features of portal vein thrombosis: a multicentre study. *Alimentary Pharmacology & Therapeutics* **32**(9): 1154–1162.

Salehipour M, Salahi H, Jalaeian H *et al.* (2009). Vascular complications following 1500 consecutive living and cadaveric donor renal transplantations: a single center study. *Saudi Journal of Kidney Diseases and Transplantation* **20**: 570–2.

Salomon O, Apter S, Shaham D *et al.* (1999). Risk factors associated with postpartum ovarian vein thrombosis. *Thrombosis and Haemostasis* **82**: 1015–9.

Salomon O, Dulitzky M, Apter S (2010). New observations in postpartum ovarian vein thrombosis: experience of single center. *Blood Coagulation & Fibrinolysis* **21**: 16–9.

Sarin SK, Sollano JD, Chawla YK *et al.* (2006). Members of the APASL working party on portal hypertension. Consensus on extrahepatic portal vein obstruction. *Liver International* **26**: 512–9.

Savader SJ, Otero RR, Savader BL (1988). Puerperal ovarian vein thrombosis: evaluation with CT, US, and MR imaging. *Radiology* **167**: 637–9.

Senzolo M, M Sartori T, Rossetto V *et al.* (2012).Prospective evaluation of anticoagulation and transjugular intrahepatic portosystemic shunt for the management of portal vein thrombosis in cirrhosis. *Liver International* **32**(6): 919–927.

Sharma S, Texeira A, Texeira P *et al.* (2004). Pharmacological thrombolysis in Budd-Chiari syndrome: a single centre experience and review of the literature. *Journal of Hepatology* **40**: 172–80.

Shetty S, Ghosh K (2011). Thrombophilic dimension of Budd chiari syndrome and portal venous thrombosis – a concise review. *Thrombosis Research* **127**(6): 505–512.

Singhal R, Brimble KS (2006). Thromboembolic complications in the nephrotic syndrome: pathophysiology and clinical management. *Thrombosis Research* **118**: 397–407.

Smalberg JH, Arends LR, Valla DC, Kiladjian JJ, Janssen HLA, Leebeek FWG (2012). Myeloproliferative neoplasms in Budd-Chiari syndrome and portal vein thrombosis: a meta-analysis. *Blood* **120**(25): 4921–4928.

Spaander MCW, Hoekstra J, Hansen BE, Van Buuren HR, Leebeek FW, Janssen HLA (2013). Anticoagulant therapy in patients with noncirrhotic portal vein thrombosis: effect on new thrombotic events and gastrointestinal bleeding. *Journal of Thrombosis and Haemostasis* **11**(3): 452–459.

Tessler FN, Gehring BJ, Gomes AS *et al.* (1991). Diagnosis of portal vein thrombosis: value of color Doppler imaging. *American Journal of Roentgenology* **157**(2): 293–296.

Thatipelli MR, McBane RD, Hodge DO, Wysokinski WE (2010). Survival and recurrence in patients with splanchnic vein thromboses. *Clinical Gastroenterology and Hepatology* **8**(2): 200–205.

Twickler DW, Setiawan AT, Evans RS *et al.* (1997). Imaging of puerperal septic thrombophlebitis: prospective comparison of MR imaging, CT and sonography. *American Journal of Roentgenology* **169**: 1039–43.

Valla D (2004). Hepatic venous outflow tract obstruction etiopathogenesis: Asia versus the West. *Journal of Gastroenterology and Hepatology* **19**: S204–11.

Valla DC (2008). Budd-Chiari syndrome and veno-occlusive disease/sinusoidal obstruction syndrome. *Gut* **57**: 1469–78.

Witz M, Korzets Z (2007). Renal vein occlusion: diagnosis and treatment. *Israel Medical Association Journal* **9**: 402–5.

Wysokinska EM Hodge D, McBane 2nd RD (2006). Ovarian vein thrombosis: incidence of recurrent venous thromboembolism and survival. *Thrombosis and Haemostasis* **96**: 126–31.

Wysokinski WE, Gosk-Bierska I, Greene EL *et al.* (2008). Clinical characteristics and long-term follow-up of patients with renal vein thrombosis. *American Journal of Kidney Diseases* **51**: 224–32.

Zeitoun G, Escolano S, Hadengue A *et al.* (1999). Outcome of Budd-Chiari syndrome: a multivariate analysis of factors related to survival including surgical portosystemic shunting. *Hepatology* **30**(1): 84–89.

Zöller B, Li X, Sundquist J *et al.* (2011). Familial risks of unusual forms of venous thrombosis: a nationwide epidemiological study in Sweden. *Journal of Internal Medicine* **270**: 158–65.

24

Thrombosis in the Retinal Circulation

Wenlan Zhang and Paul Hahn

Department of Ophthalmology, Duke University Medical Center, Durham

Introduction

Retinal vein occlusion (RVO) and retinal artery occlusion (RAO) are retinal vascular disorders associated with significant vision impairment, which can affect the central or branch retinal vascular systems. While both RVO and RAO typically present as painless vision loss, with visual field loss depending on the area of retina affected, RVO and RAO are separate disease entities that have different clinical courses, work-ups, treatments and prognoses. This chapter focuses mainly on retinal vein occlusions, but will also briefly review retinal artery occlusions.

Basic Eye Anatomy

The eye is a complex light-sensing organ. The tear film, cornea and lens help to focus light on the neurosensory retina, which is comprised of multiple cell types that help convert light into electrical impulses that travel through the optic nerve to the brain. The macula measures about 5.5 mm in diameter, and is located between the optic disc and temporal vascular arcades. At the centre of the macula lies the fovea, which is responsible for high-resolution colour acuity.

The vascular supply to the retina comes from the ophthalmic artery, which arises from the internal carotid artery. The ophthalmic artery gives rise to the central retinal artery, which travels with the central retinal vein along the optic nerve within its dural sheath, branching into multiple branch retinal arteries and veins at the level of the scleral outlet and lamina cribosa (mesh-like perforations in the sclera) to nourish the inner retina. The ophthalmic artery also gives rise to multiple posterior ciliary arteries posterior to the level of the central retinal artery that nourishes the outer retina. Fifteen percent of people have a cilioretinal artery that supplies the inner retina at the macula derived from this ciliary circulation, and not from the central retinal artery (Schubert *et al.*, 2013). Oxygenated blood from the branched retinal arteries feed into an extensive capillary network that eventually collects in the venous system, and into the central retinal vein that exits the eye.

Retinal Vein Occlusion

Clinical Features

The immediate visual impact of an RVO depends on the location of the occluded vein. Patients who suffer from a central retinal vein occlusion (CRVO) usually present with sudden painless vision loss. Patients with a

Handbook of Venous Thromboembolism, First Edition. Edited by Jecko Thachil and Catherine Bagot.
© 2018 John Wiley & Sons Ltd. Published 2018 by John Wiley & Sons Ltd.

hemispheric retinal vein occlusion (HRVO) present with either a superior or inferior hemispheric visual field loss, corresponding to an inferior or superior occlusion of a large venous tributary, respectively. The level of visual impairment with branch retinal vein occlusion (BRVO) depends on the location and severity of occlusion, such that vision impairment is greater with any degree of macular involvement, while BRVOs away from the macula may be asymptomatic (Jaulim *et al.*, 2013).

RVO tends to be unilateral at presentation. However, it is estimated that 5–10% of BRVOs become bilateral, and that up to 7% of patients with one CRVO may develop a CRVO in the other eye within five years of the initial event (Central Vein Occlusion Study, 1993; Eye Disease Case-Control Study Group, 1993, 1996).

Presenting vision can range widely in RVO. In a study of 728 eyes with CRVO, 29% of affected eyes had visual acuity 20/40 or better, 43% had vision 20/50 to 20/200, and 28% had vision 20/250 or worse at the time of presentation. Median visual acuity was 20/80 (Central Vein Occlusion Study, 1993; Decroos and Fekrat, 2011). Visual acuity is typically better in BRVO eyes. In a study of 153 vision-impairing BRVO eyes, average visual acuity ranged from 20/50 to 20/60 (Thapa *et al.*, 2010). Notably, this did not include BRVOs occurring outside of the macula in peripheral retina, which can be entirely asymptomatic.

Clinical findings in RVO can be similar to diabetic retinopathy, hypertensive retinopathy, ocular ischemic syndrome, radiation retinopathy, leukemic retinopathy and trauma. Dilated ophthalmic evaluation, along with ophthalmic imaging such as fluorescein angiography, optical coherence tomography, electroretinography or visual field testing, may be necessary to make an appropriate diagnosis.

Complications of RVO include vision loss from macular oedema, retinal ischemia, epiretinal membrane formation, and ocular neovascularisation (of the iris, angle and retina). Uncontrolled neovascularisation can lead to vitreous haemorrhages, tractional retinal detachment, and neovascular glaucoma caused by neovascular membranes occluding the angle, the drainage system of the eye.

Perfusion status is an important classification for RVOs, especially for CRVO, where the entire retina is affected. Perfusion status is based clinically on the amount of retinal non-perfusion seen on fluorescein angiography – an imaging modality that examines retinal and choroidal circulation. Larger areas of non-perfusion are associated with higher risk of RVO complications and worse visual prognosis (Central Vein Occlusion Study Group, 1997; Hayreh *et al.*, 1990, 2011). Perfused (also known as non-ischemic, incomplete, partial) CRVOs can also convert to non-perfused CRVOs. The Central Vein Occlusion Study (CVOS), which studied the natural history of CRVO, found that 34% of initially perfused eyes converted to non-perfused status after three years (Central Vein Occlusion Study Group, 1997).

Epidemiology, Risk Factors, Associations

A pool of population-based studies, with 68751 participants from the United States, Europe, Asia and Australia, reported the prevalence of any RVO to be 0.52%, which estimates that nearly 16.4 million adults are affected by RVO (Rogers *et al.*, 2010). Another study, specific to the USA, reported a higher prevalence of RVO at 1.1% (Cheung *et al.*, 2008). Among the types of RVO, BRVOs are considered the most common, and the prevalence of BRVO has been estimated to range from 0.442–0.9% (Rogers *et al.*, 2010; Cheung *et al.*, 2008; Klein *et al.*, 2000), with a 5-year incidence of 0.6% (Klein *et al.*, 2000). The prevalence of CRVO has been reported to be < 0.1 to 0.4% (Rogers *et al.*, 2010; Klein *et al.*, 2000; Hayreh *et al.*, 1994; Mitchell *et al.*, 1996), with a five-year incidence of 0.2% (Klein *et al.*, 2000).

RVO creates significant morbidity that impacts healthcare. One study investigating Medicare reimbursements in elderly populations in the US found that BRVO and CRVO were associated with 16–22% higher one-year costs, and 12–15% higher three-year costs than hypertension and glaucoma controls (Fekrat *et al.*, 2010).

CRVO predominantly occurs in persons over the age of 65 years (Hayreh *et al.*, 1994), and it affects men and women equally (Hayreh *et al.*, 1994; Mitchell *et al.*, 1996). Similarly, BRVO typically affects individuals in their sixth or seventh decade of life (Eye Disease Case-Control Study Group, 1993). This older age group is reflective of the common risk factors for RVO development, which include systemic vascular diseases such as

Table 24.1 Retinal vein occlusion risk factors and associations.

Ocular Associations

- Glaucoma
- External compression of the eye and optic nerve: thyroid ophthalmopathy, intra-orbital masses, optic nerve head drusen, orbital trauma

Systemic vascular disease

- Hypertension, diabetes mellitus, hypercholesterolemia

Hypercoagulable states (Hayreh *et al.*, 2002)

- Protein C deficiency, protein S deficiency, activated protein C resistance, hyperhomocysteinemia, factor V Leiden, antiphospholipid antibody syndrome, antithrombin III deficiency, prothrombin gene mutations, abnormal fibrinogen levels

Hyperviscosity

- Blood dyscrasias, dysproteinemias, dehydration (Alghadyan, 1993)

Vasculitides

- Systemic lupus erythematous (Chang *et al.*, 2010), Sarcoidosis (Kimmel *et al.*, 1989)

Infections

- Syphilis (Primo, 1990), human immunodeficiency virus (Dunn, *et al.*, 2005), tuberculosis (O'Hearn *et al.*, 2007)

Medications

- Oral contraceptives (Matti *et al.*, 2010), anabolic steroids (Damasceno *et al.*, 2009), rofecoxib (Meyer *et al.*, 2005), hepatitis C treatment (Goncalves *et al.*, 2006)

---

hypertension, diabetes mellitus and hypercholesterolemia (Eye Disease Case-Control Study Group, 1993, 1996). Younger patients presenting with RVO may represent a different aetiology (Fong and Schatz, 1993; Gutman, 1983). Other disease associations and rare causes of RVO are summarised in Table 24.1.

Pathogenesis

The pathophysiology of RVO is not well understood, and proposed mechanisms differ for BRVOs and CRVOs. BRVOs are hypothesised to occur from thrombus formation at arteriovenous crossings as a result of arterial disease (Jaulim *et al.*, 2013). A mechanical compression theory postulates that systemic vascular disease and atherosclerosis leads to hypertrophy of the arterial wall, leading to arterial enlargement. Because arterio-venous crossings in the retina are comprised of an artery and vein that share a common adventitial sheath, this arterial enlargement causes compression and narrowing of the adjacent vein, leading to Virchow's triad of turbulent flow, increased viscosity and endothelial damage (Christoffersen and Larsen, 1999; Jefferies *et al.*, 1993; Staurenghi *et al.*, 1994; Weinberg, 1994; Zhao *et al.*, 1993).

Another theory that has been proposed involves venous constriction that is induced by vasoconstrictive molecules, such as endothelin-1, diffusing from adjacent hypoxic atherosclerotic arteries or tissues (Fraenkl *et al.*, 2010). This second theory bypasses the necessity for mechanical compression to be present to explain venous occlusion.

There are multiple theories for CRVO pathophysiology. Histopathology of eyes enucleated following CRVO demonstrate thrombus formation in the central retinal vein near the lamina cribosa, suggesting a role for particular anatomical variations of the lamina cribosa (Green *et al.*, 1981). It has been proposed that the location of the central retinal vein at the lamina cribosa may be more sensitive to mechanical compression, which could account for the associations reported between CRVO and atherosclerosis and glaucoma (Hahn *et al.*, 2011). However, another theory proposes that CRVO occurs posterior to the lamina cribosa from hemodynamic alterations, leading to Virchow's triad, rather than compression or strangulation in the lamina cribosa. This theory suggests a role implicating concurrent retinal artery insufficiency or occlusion, similar to the theory describing BRVO pathophysiology (Hayreh, 2005).

Work-up

It is important to involve an ophthalmologist in the care of patients with RVOs, as frequent eye exams are needed to monitor for vision-threatening complications, such as macular oedema and neovascularisation. Identifying these problems early allows for appropriate and timely initiation of treatment to optimise visual rehabilitation.

Careful assessment of medical history, ocular history, family history and current medications should be performed. Patients should be questioned about underlying hypertension, diabetes, heart disease, history of thrombosis or other hypercoagulable states, and also history of vasculitis or other inflammatory disorders. The Eye Disease Case-Control Study Group, which studied the natural history of RVOs, suggested surveying cardiovascular risk profile, and counselling on weight, diet, and exercise control in these patients (Eye Disease Case-Control Study Group, 1993, 1996).

Generally, a systemic work-up is not indicated in individuals older than 60 years of age who present with known systemic vascular risk factors (Hayreh *et al.*, 2002). However, it is important that, after the initial RVO assessment, patients are advised to continue monitoring and addressing risk factors for cardiovascular morbidity, as studies have shown greater risk of future cardiovascular disease (Martin *et al.*, 2002). Younger patients without vascular risk factors, and those presenting with bilateral simultaneous RVOs or other mixed retinal vascular occlusion, may warrant a limited systemic work-up that may include an erythrocyte sedimentation rate, C-reactive protein, antinuclear antibody, fasting plasma homocysteine level, and rapid plasma reagin (Central Vein Occlusion Study Group, 1997; Fong and Schatz, 1993; Lahey *et al.*, 2002). In situations where a hypercoagulable or inflammatory disorder is suspected, further work-up coordinated with haematology or rheumatology may be necessary.

Treatment

Systemic Treatment

Systemic prophylaxis with aspirin, heparin or warfarin for RVOs attributable to vascular risk factors is controversial. Unlike prophylaxis for deep vein thrombosis and pulmonary emboli, anticoagulation has not been shown to prevent or alter the natural history of RVOs (Hayreh, 2005; Browning and Fraser, 2004; Koizumi *et al.*, 2007). Moreover, RVOs can occur despite being on systemic anticoagulation, for non-ocular reasons (Hayreh *et al.*, 2002; Browning and Fraser, 2004).

Current ocular treatments are not aimed at the underlying thrombus or occlusion in RVOs but, rather, for the vision-threatening sequelae, especially macular oedema and ocular neovascularisation.

Intravitreal Anti-Vascular Endothelial Growth Factors

First-line therapy for macular oedema associated with RVO includes anti-vascular endothelial growth factors (anti-VEGF) agents or corticosteroids injected into the intravitreal space of the eye. Laser treatment, discussed below, is also a first-line treatment for macular oedema associated with BRVO, but not CRVO. Available intravitreal anti-VEGF agents include bevacizumab 1.25 mg, used off-label (Genentech, Inc., San Francisco, CA), ranibizumab 0.5 mg (Lucentis, Genentech, Inc.), and aflibercept 2 mg (Eylea, Regeneron, Inc., Tarrytown, NY).

While there are theoretical systemic risks to anti-VEGF use, such as stroke and myocardial infarction, reports suggest low risk of systemic adverse events to intravitreal anti-VEGF agents, although long-term effects are still unknown (Curtis *et al.*, 2010; Epstein *et al.*, 2012; Fintak *et al.*, 2008). The most significant ocular risk after injection is endophthalmitis, which has been reported to occur with an incidence of approximately one in 4500 injections (Fintak *et al.*, 2008).

Multiple studies have demonstrated resolution of macular oedema and vision improvement with bevacizumab use (Epstein *et al.*, 2012; Ehlers *et al.*, 2011; Ferrara *et al.*, 2007; Kriechbaum *et al.*, 2008; Priglinger *et al.*, 2007; Stahl *et al.*, 2007; Zhang *et al.*, 2011). However, due to its off-label use, and the lack of large randomised controlled trials with bevacizumab, its safety profile data in RVO treatment has not been rigorously studied.

Ranibizumab has been well studied with regards to RVO-related macular oedema treatment (Branch Retinal Vein Occlusion: Evaluation of Efficacy and Safety (BRAVO) study and Central Retinal Vein Occlusion Study: Evaluation of Efficacy and Safety (CRUISE) trial) The success of using aflibercept in CRVO treatment was demonstrated in the Controlled Phase 3 Evaluation of Repeated intravitreal administration of VEGF Trap-Eye In Central Retinal Vein Occlusion: Utility and Safety (COPERNICUS) trial, and the General Assessment Limiting Infiltration of Exudates in Central Retinal Vein Occlusion with VEGF Trap-Eye (GALILEO) study.

Following the initial six-month period of scheduled monthly injections, subjects often still require maintenance injections, but the optimal frequency of these ongoing injections remains unclear, and a large randomised head-to-head efficacy comparison between available anti-VEGF agents has not been performed (Mitry *et al.*, 2013; Braithwaite *et al.*, 2014).

Intravitreal Corticosteroids

Corticosteroids include intravitreal injection of triamcinolone acetonide 1–4 mg, used off-label for RVO in the United States, and sustained release dexamethasone implant 0.7 mg (Ozurdex, Allergan, Inc., Irvine, CA), which is FDA approved for treatment of macular oedema associated with RVO. The Standard Care Versus Corticosteroids for Retinal Vein Occlusion (SCORE) study and the Global Evaluation of Implantable Dexamethasone in Retinal Vein Occlusion with Macular Oedema (GENEVA) trial showed good outcomes with these treatments (Haller *et al.*, 2011). In these large-centre trials, primary ocular adverse events associated with corticosteroid use included cataract formation and elevated intraocular pressure requiring medical treatment (Ip *et al.*, 2009; Scott *et al.*, 2009; Haller *et al.*, 2011).

Laser Treatment

Argon laser photocoagulation is another readily available in-office procedure used in the treatment of RVO sequelae. Along with intravitreal injections, it is a first-line treatment option for BRVO-related macular oedema in perfused eyes with reduced vision of 20/40 to 20/200 (Branch Vein Occlusion Study Group, 1984). Focal treatment directed towards leaking microvascular abnormalities and oedematous retina in the area drained by the obstructed vein has demonstrated 2-line gain of visual acuity in 65% of treated eyes, compared with 37% of untreated eyes (Branch Vein Occlusion Study Group, 1984). In CRVO-related macular oedema, laser treatment was found to reduce the amount of macular oedema on angiographic studies, but was not found to improve visual acuity and, therefore, is not recommended (Central Vein Occlusion Study Group (1995).

Additionally, panretinal scatter laser photocoagulation directed to peripheral retinal areas affected by capillary nonperfusion is the gold standard treatment for the regression of ocular neovascularisation in RVO (Schubert *et al.*, 2013; Hahn and Fekrat, 2012). While larger areas of retinal nonperfusion confer a greater risk of ocular neovascularisation, studies have shown that prophylactic laser is not indicated for retinal ischemia alone in the absence of neovascularisation (Branch Vein Occlusion Study Group, 1984; Central Vein Occlusion Study Group (1995). Anti-VEGF agents can also temporise neovascularisation in RVOs, but laser photocoagulation is the definitive treatment for neovascularisation.

Surgical Treatment

When medical treatments are unsuccessful, vitrectomy surgery can address complications from CRVO, including non-clearing vitreous haemorrhage, ocular neovascularisation, epiretinal membranes and traction retinal detachments (Lam and Blumenkranz, 2002). Vitrectomy with membrane peeling may also be helpful for treatment of RVO-associated macular oedema but, in the era of anti-VEGF therapeutics for RVO, it is not commonly performed, and is generally reserved for refractory cases of macular oedema (DeCroos *et al.*, 2009; Liang *et al.*, 2007; Park and Kim, 2010).

Prognosis

Without treatment, approximately 50–60% of patients with BRVO maintain visual acuity of 20/40 or better, while about 20% are 20/200 or worse after one year (Branch Vein Occlusion Study Group, 1986). In CRVO, the natural history for visual outcome is largely predicted by vision at presentation. In the CVOS study, without treatment, those with presenting vision of 20/40 or better typically maintained that, while those with vision less than 20/200 only had a 20% chance for improvement (Central Vein Occlusion Study Group, 1997). Those presenting with intermediate vision of 20/50 to 20/200 had a 21% chance of improving, a 41% of remaining the same, and a 38% chance of worsening (Central Vein Occlusion Study Group, 1997). However, with the availability and promise of intravitreal pharmacotherapy, which has revolutionised RVO treatment, there is now greater potential for more favourable visual prognosis.

Retinal Artery Occlusion

Introduction

Retinal artery occlusion (RAO) is a vascular occlusive disorder that presents with sudden, unilateral, painless vision loss. Presenting visual acuity varies with the location of the arterial occlusion. Vision loss is more dramatic in central retinal artery occlusion (CRAO), compared with branch retinal artery occlusion (BRAO), which can be asymptomatic. CRAO is considered the ocular equivalent to a cerebral ischemic stroke (Varma *et al.*, 2013). Notably, in a prospective study of 244 patients with CRAO, 12–20% of patients had a history of amaurosis fugax before the acute event (Hayreh and Zimmerman, 2005).

Clinical Features

Ophthalmic examination shows evidence of acute retinal ischemia, usually manifesting as retinal whitening, corresponding to oedematous opacification in the distribution of the occluded artery. In cases of CRAO, a cherry-red spot in the area of the fovea may be appreciated.

These classic features are most apparent in the hours after the CRAO event, but fade over time (Hayreh and Weingeist, 1980). Moreover, examination may reveal the presence of 'box-carring' of the blood column within retinal vessels and, in CRAO, may also reveal a relative afferent pupillary defect (Varma *et al.*, 2013; Hayreh *et al.*, 2009a, 2009b). Fluorescein angiography, which images retinal vasculature, may demonstrate absence or marked stasis of circulation in affected arteries. In some cases of RAO, retinal emboli can be observed to be lodged at arteriolar bifurcations. Optical coherence tomography (OCT) reveals disruption of the inner retinal layers, classically demonstrating atrophy following the acute ischemic event. Visual field testing may demonstrate diffuse visual field loss in CRAO and altitudinal or sector defects in BRAO (Hayreh *et al.*, 2009a).

Epidemiology, Risk Factors and Associations, Pathogenesis

CRAO accounts for one in 10000 ophthalmological outpatient visits, and has an estimated incidence of 1–1.8 in 100000 (Rumelt *et al.*, 1999; Leavitt *et al.*, 2011; Park *et al.*, 2014). There are few large epidemiological studies of CRAO, but these studies report a 1.47–2.4 times higher incidence of CRAO in men over women, and increasing incidence with increasing age (Leavitt *et al.*, 2011; Park *et al.*, 2014). There are fewer reports of BRAO incidence, although a study of 212 BRAO eyes reported a mean age of 61 years (Hayreh *et al.*, 2009a).

Systemic vascular disease, such as hypertension, hyperlipidaemia, cardiovascular disease, diabetes and smoking, are risk factors for RAOs (Hayreh *et al.*, 2009a; Coisy *et al.*, 2013; Schmidt *et al.*, 2007). Embolisation and thrombosis can cause occlusion at any site. The three main types of emboli include cholesterol emboli (Hollenhorst plaques) arising in the carotid arteries, platelet-fibrin emboli associated with large vessel arteriosclerosis, and calcific emboli arising from diseased cardiac valves, which travel to the retinal vascular

Table 24.2 Retinal artery occlusion risk factors and associations.

Ocular associations

- Central retinal vein occlusion (Hayreh and Zimmerman, 2005), retinal surgery, peribulbar anesthesia, and forehead or periorbital corticosteroid injection

Systemic vascular disease (Hayreh and Zimmerman, 2005; Coisy *et al.*, 2013; Schmidt *et al.*, 2007)

- Carotid disease, Cardiovascular disease, Hypertension, Hyperlipidemia, Diabetes mellitus, Hypercholesterolemia

Emboli

- Carotid disease, Cardiac valvular disease (eg: mitral valve prolapse), Arrhythmias, Cardiac myxoma (Schmidt *et al.*, 2005), Fat emboli from trauma, infectious

Hypercoagulable states

- Hyperhomocysteinemia, high lupus anticoagulant

Hyperviscosity

- Blood dyscrasias, Dysproteinemias, Pregnancy (Greven *et al.*, 1995)

Inflammatory and vasculitides

- Susac's, Giant cell arteritis, Polyarteritis nodosa, Behcet's disease, Sarcoidosis, Crohn's disease

Infections

- Syphilis, Human immunodeficiency virus, Toxoplasmosis, Lyme disease, Whipple disease

Medications

- Oral contraceptives, Viagra

Other: Snake bites

---

system in the setting of a patent foramen ovale or other atrial septal defect (Schubert *et al.*, 2013). Rarely, CRAO is associated with Giant Cell Arteritis (GCA, also known as Temporal Arteritis) and other rare causes (Table 24.2).

Work-up

It is suggested that patients presenting with CRAO undergo work-up for common vascular risk factors, as well as investigation for embolic sources, such as carotid imaging and echocardiogram. In patients over 50 years old, Giant Cell Arteritis should be considered, unless a clear embolic source is identified. Further work-up for other rare causes of CRAO (Table 24.2), in younger patients or patients with an otherwise negative work-up, can also be considered (Varma *et al.*, 2013).

Treatment

There are no current treatments for RAO with proven beneficial effect (Rumelt *et al.*, 1999; Hayreh, 2011; Fraser and Adams, 2009). Attempts to dislodge emboli through ocular massage, inducing intraocular pressure reduction by medical and surgical means to increase retinal perfusion, inducing central retinal artery vasodilation through re-breathing expired CO_2, thrombolysis, systemic anticoagulation, high-dose steroids and hyperbaric oxygen, have not proved to be better than placebo (Fraser and Adams, 2009).

One common complication of CRAO is ocular ischemia leading to neovascular glaucoma, an event also seen in central retinal vein occlusion (CRVO) (Hayreh, 2011). Onset of neovascularisation in CRAO has been reported to occur from two weeks to four months post-occlusive event. The reported prevalence of neovascularisation ranges widely, from 2.5% to 18.2%, with one report as high as 31.6% (Hayreh and Zimmerman, 2005; Hayreh, 2011; Rudkin *et al.*, 2010). While there is debate regarding the aetiology of neovascularisation in CRAO (Hayreh *et al.*, 2009b; Duker and Brown, 1989), the treatment remains panretinal photocoagulation (PRP) of the peripheral retina, to reduce the incidence of neovascular glaucoma (Duker and Brown, 1989).

Prognosis

Vision recovery is minimal in most, but may occur within seven days of onset (Hayreh and Zimmerman, 2005; Hayreh *et al.*, 2009a, 2009b). The natural history of visual acuity in BRAO suggests final acuity of 20/40 or better in 89–100%, depending on the type of BRAO (Hayreh *et al.*, 2009a, 2009b). Prognosis after CRAO is poor, but vision may improve in 22% of eyes, show no change in 66%, and worsen in 12%, with the presence of a ciliary artery conferring improved visual prognosis (Hayreh and Zimmerman, 2005; Hayreh *et al.*, 2009b).

Conclusions

Retinal vein and artery occlusions are retinal vascular disorders that result in significant ocular morbidity. While they share similar risk factors, such as systemic vascular disease (cardiovascular disease, hypertension, diabetes), and similar complicating sequelae such as ocular neovascularisation, they are different disease entities, with different pathophysiology, work-ups and treatments.

Key Points

- Retinal vein occlusions and retinal artery occlusions are retinal vascular disorders that present with sudden painless unilateral vision loss.
- Retinal vein occlusions are a different disease entity than retinal artery occlusions.
- Acute central retinal artery occlusion is an ocular emergency and requires a systemic vascular evaluation.
- The vast majority of retinal vein occlusions occur as a result of underlying hypertension, hyperlipidaemia, diabetes and heart disease. Retinal artery occlusions commonly occur from systemic vascular disease, with emboli from carotid arteries, cardiac valvular disease and arrhythmias.
- Rare causes of retinal vein and artery occlusions include a history of thrombosis or other hypercoagulable states, vasculitis or other inflammatory disorders, infection and medications.
- Systemic anticoagulation, such as aspirin, warfarin and heparin, has not proved to be beneficial in either retinal vein occlusions or retinal artery occlusions, but may be helpful for associated systemic conditions.
- Development of intravitreal anti-VEGF agents has revolutionised treatment for the sequelae of retinal vein occlusions, especially macular oedema.
- Intravitreal injections with anti-VEGF agents and corticosteroids are first line treatment for macular oedema related to retinal vein occlusions, and are temporising agents in sequelae of ocular neovascularisation. Laser is also first-line treatment in macular oedema related to branch retinal vein occlusions, but not central retinal vein occlusions.
- There are no proven treatments available to improve vision in retinal artery occlusion.

Further Reading

Fraser SG, Adams W (2009). Interventions for acute non-arteritic central retinal artery occlusion. *The Cochrane Database of Systematic Reviews*. doi: 10.1002/14651858.CD001989.pub2: Cd001989.

Hahn P, Mruthyunjaya P, Fekrat S (2011). Central Retinal Vein Occlusion. In: Sadda S (ed). *Stephen J. Ryan Retina*, 5th edition. Elsevier.

Hayreh SS, Podhajsky PA, Zimmerman MB (2009). Retinal Artery Occlusion: Associated Systemic and Ophthalmic Abnormalities. *Ophthalmology* **116**(10): 1928–1936.

Jaulim A, Ahmed B, Khanam T, Chatziralli IP (2013). Branch retinal vein occlusion: epidemiology, pathogenesis, risk factors, clinical features, diagnosis, and complications. An update of the literature. *Retina* **33**(5): 901–910.

Rumelt S, Dorenboim Y, Rehany U (1999). Aggressive systematic treatment for central retinal artery occlusion. *American Journal of Ophthalmology* **128**(6): 733–738.

The Central Vein Occlusion Study (1993). Baseline and early natural history report. *Archives of Ophthalmology* **111**(8): 1087–1095.

The Central Vein Occlusion Study Group (1997). Natural history and clinical management of central retinal vein occlusion. *Archives of Ophthalmology* **115**(4): 486–491.

The Eye Disease Case-control Study Group (1993). Risk factors for branch retinal vein occlusion. *American Journal of Ophthalmology* **116**(3): 286–296.

The Eye Disease Case-Control Study Group (1996). Risk factors for central retinal vein occlusion. *Archives of Ophthalmology* **114**(5): 545–554.

Conflicts of Interest/disclosures

Paul Hahn reports consulting agreements unrelated to the submitted work with Second Sight Medical Products and Bausch & Lomb. Wenlan Zhang has no disclosures to report.

References

Alghadyan, AA (1993). Retinal vein occlusion in Saudi Arabia: possible role of dehydration. *Annals of Ophthalmology* **25**: 394–398.

Arevalo, JF, Garcia, RA, Wu, L *et al.* (2008). Radial optic neurotomy for central retinal vein occlusion: results of the Pan-American Collaborative Retina Study Group (PACORES). *Retina* **28**: 1044–1052.

Boyer, D, Heier, J, Brown, DM *et al.* (2012). Vascular Endothelial Growth Factor Trap-Eye for Macular Edema Secondary to Central Retinal Vein Occlusion: Six-Month Results of the Phase 3 COPERNICUS Study. *Ophthalmology* **119**: 1024–1032.

Braithwaite, T, Nanji, AA, Lindsley, K, Greenberg, PB (2014). Anti-vascular endothelial growth factor for macular oedema secondary to central retinal vein occlusion. *The Cochrane Database of Systematic Reviews* **5**: Cd007325.

Branch Vein Occlusion Study Group (1986). Argon laser scatter photocoagulation for prevention of neovascularization and vitreous hemorrhage in branch vein occlusion. A randomized clinical trial. *Archives of Ophthalmology* **104**: 34–41.

Brown, DM, Heier, J, Clark, WL *et al.* (2012). Intravitreal Aflibercept Injection for Macular Edema Secondary to Central Retinal Vein Occlusion: 1-year Results from the Phase 3 COPERNICUS Study. *American Journal of Ophthalmology* **155**(3): 429–437.

Browning, DJ, Fraser, CM (2004). Retinal vein occlusions in patients taking warfarin. *Ophthalmology* **111**: 1196–1200.

Campochiaro, PA, Heier, JS, Feiner, L *et al.* (2010). Ranibizumab for macular edema following branch retinal vein occlusion: six-month primary end point results of a phase III study. *Ophthalmology* **117**: 1102–1112 e1101.

Chang, PC, Chen, WS, Lin, HY, Lee, HM, Chen, SJ (2010). Combined central retinal artery and vein occlusion in a patient with systemic lupus erythematosus and anti-phospholipid syndrome. *Lupus* **19**: 206–209.

Cheung, N, Klein, R, Wang, JJ *et al.* (2008). Traditional and novel cardiovascular risk factors for retinal vein occlusion: the multiethnic study of atherosclerosis. *Investigative Ophthalmology & Visual Science* **49**: 4297–4302.

Christoffersen, NL, Larsen, M (1999). Pathophysiology and hemodynamics of branch retinal vein occlusion. *Ophthalmology* **106**: 2054–2062.

Coisy, S, Leruez, S, Ebran, JM, Pisella, PJ, Milea, D, Arsene, S (2013). Systemic conditions associated with central and branch retinal artery occlusions. *Journal Français d'Ophtalmologie* **36**: 748–757.

Curtis, LH, Hammill, BG, Schulman, KA, Cousins, SW (2010). Risks of mortality, myocardial infarction, bleeding, and stroke associated with therapies for age-related macular degeneration. *Archives of Ophthalmology* **128**: 1273–1279.

Damasceno, EF, Neto, AM, Damasceno, NA, Horowitz, SA, de Moraes Jr, HV (2009). Branch retinal vein occlusion and anabolic steroids abuse in young bodybuilders. *Acta Ophthalmologica* **87**: 580–581.

DeCroos, FC, Shuler, RK, Jr, Stinnett, S, Fekrat, S (2009). Pars plana vitrectomy, internal limiting membrane peeling, and panretinal endophotocoagulation for macular edema secondary to central retinal vein occlusion. *American Journal of Ophthalmology* **147**: 627–633 e621.

Decroos, FC, Fekrat, S (2011). The natural history of retinal vein occlusion: what do we really know? *American Journal of Ophthalmology* **151**: 739–741 e732.

Duker, JS, Brown, GC (1989). The efficacy of panretinal photocoagulation for neovascularization of the iris after central retinal artery obstruction. *Ophthalmology* **96**: 92–95.

Dunn, JP, Yamashita, A, Kempen, JH, Jabs, DA (2005). Retinal vascular occlusion in patients infected with human immunodeficiency virus. *Retina* **25**: 759–766.

Ehlers, JP, Decroos, FC, Fekrat, S (2011). Intravitreal bevacizumab for macular edema secondary to branch retinal vein occlusion. *Retina* **31**: 1856–1862.

Elman, MJ (1996). Thrombolytic therapy for central retinal vein occlusion: results of a pilot study. *Transactions of the American Ophthalmological Society* **94**: 471–504.

Epstein, DL, Algvere, PV, von Wendt, G, Seregard, S, Kvanta, A (2012). Benefit from Bevacizumab for Macular Edema in Central Retinal Vein Occlusion: Twelve-Month Results of a Prospective, Randomized Study. *Ophthalmology* **119**(12): 2587–91.

Fekrat, S, Goldberg, MF, Finkelstein, D (1998). Laser-induced chorioretinal venous anastomosis for nonischemic central or branch retinal vein occlusion. *Archives of Ophthalmology* **116**: 43–52.

Fekrat, S, de Juan, E, Jr (1999). Chorioretinal venous anastomosis for central retinal vein occlusion: transvitreal venipuncture. *Ophthalmic Surgery and Lasers* **30**: 52–55.

Fekrat, S, Shea, AM, Hammill, BG *et al.* (2010). Resource use and costs of branch and central retinal vein occlusion in the elderly. *Current Medical Research and Opinion* **26**: 223–230.

Feltgen, N, Junker, B, Agostini, H, Hansen, LL (2007). Retinal endovascular lysis in ischemic central retinal vein occlusion: one-year results of a pilot study. *Ophthalmology* **114**: 716–723.

Ferrara, DC, Koizumi, H, Spaide, RF (2007). Early bevacizumab treatment of central retinal vein occlusion. *American Journal of Ophthalmology* **144**: 864–871.

Fintak, DR, Shah, GK, Blinder, KJ *et al.* (2008). Incidence of endophthalmitis related to intravitreal injection of bevacizumab and ranibizumab. *Retina* **28**: 1395–1399.

Fong, AC, Schatz, H (1993). Central retinal vein occlusion in young adults. *Survey of Ophthalmology* **37**: 393–417.

Fraenkl, SA, Mozaffarieh, M, Flammer, J (2010). Retinal vein occlusions: The potential impact of a dysregulation of the retinal veins. *The EPMA Journal* **1**: 253–261.

Fraser, SG, Adams, W (2009). Interventions for acute non-arteritic central retinal artery occlusion. *The Cochrane Database of Systematic Reviews*. doi: 10.1002/14651858.CD001989.pub2: Cd001989.

Ghazi, NG, Noureddine, B, Haddad, RS, Jurdi, FA, Bashshur, ZF (2003). Intravitreal tissue plasminogen activator in the management of central retinal vein occlusion. *Retina* **23**: 780–784.

Goncalves, LL, Farias, AQ, Goncalves, PL, D'Amico, EA, Carrilho, FJ (2006). Branch retinal vein thrombosis and visual loss probably associated with pegylated interferon therapy of chronic hepatitis C. *World Journal of Gastroenterology* **12**: 4602–4603.

Green, WR, Chan, CC, Hutchins, GM, Terry, JM (1981). Central retinal vein occlusion: a prospective histopathologic study of 29 eyes in 28 cases. *Retina* **1**: 27–55.

Greven, CM, Slusher, MM, Weaver, RG (1995). Retinal arterial occlusions in young adults. *American Journal of Ophthalmology* **120**: 776–783.

Gutman, F. A (1983). Evaluation of a patient with central retinal vein occlusion. *Ophthalmology* **90**: 481–483.

Hahn, P, Mruthyunjaya, P, Fekrat, S (2011). Central Retinal Vein Occlusion. In: Sadda, S (ed). *Stephen J Ryan Retina*, 5th Edition. Elsevier.

Hahn, P, Fekrat, S (2012). Best practices for treatment of retinal vein occlusion. *Current Opinion in Ophthalmology* **23**: 175–181.

Haller, JA, Bandello, F, Belfort, R, Jr *et al.* (2011). Dexamethasone intravitreal implant in patients with macular edema related to branch or central retinal vein occlusion twelve-month study results. *Ophthalmology* **118**: 2453–2460.

Hattenbach, LO, Steinkamp, G, Scharrer, I, Ohrloff, C (1998). Fibrinolytic therapy with low-dose recombinant tissue plasminogen activator in retinal vein occlusion. *Ophthalmologica* **212**: 394–398.

Hattenbach, LO, Friedrich Arndt, C, Lerche, R *et al.* (2009). Retinal vein occlusion and low-dose fibrinolytic therapy (R.O.L.F.): a prospective, randomized, controlled multicenter study of low-dose recombinant tissue plasminogen activator versus hemodilution in retinal vein occlusion. *Retina* **29**: 932–940.

Hayreh, SS (2005). Prevalent misconceptions about acute retinal vascular occlusive disorders. *Progress in Retinal and Eye Research* **24**: 493–519.

Hayreh, SS (2011). Acute retinal arterial occlusive disorders. *Progress in Retinal and Eye Research* **30**: 359–394.

Hayreh, SS, Weingeist, TA (1980). Experimental occlusion of the central artery of the retina. *I. Ophthalmoscopic and fluorescein fundus angiographic studies. British Journal of Ophthalmology* **64**: 896–912.

Hayreh, SS, Zimmerman, MB (2005). Central Retinal Artery Occlusion: Visual Outcome. *American Journal of Ophthalmology* **140**: 376.e371–376.e.

Hayreh, SS, Klugman, MR, Beri, M, Kimura, AE, Podhajsky, P (1990). Differentiation of ischemic from non-ischemic central retinal vein occlusion during the early acute phase. *Graefe's Archive for Clinical and Experimental Ophthalmology* **228**: 201–217.

Hayreh, SS, Zimmerman, MB, Podhajsky, P (1994). Incidence of various types of retinal vein occlusion and their recurrence and demographic characteristics. *American Journal of Ophthalmology* **117**: 429–441.

Hayreh, SS, Zimmerman, MB, Podhajsky, P (2002). Hematologic abnormalities associated with various types of retinal vein occlusion. *Graefe's Archive for Clinical and Experimental Ophthalmology* **240**: 180–196.

Hayreh, SS, Podhajsky, PA, Zimmerman, MB (2009a). Branch Retinal Artery Occlusion: Natural History of Visual Outcome. *Ophthalmology* **116**: 1188–1194.e1184.

Hayreh, SS, Podhajsky, PA, Zimmerman, MB (2009b). Retinal Artery Occlusion: Associated Systemic and Ophthalmic Abnormalities. *Ophthalmology* **116**: 1928–1936.

Hayreh, SS, Podhajsky, PA, Zimmerman, MB (2011). Natural history of visual outcome in central retinal vein occlusion. *Ophthalmology* **118**: 119–133 e111–112.

Heier, JS, Campochiaro, PA, Yau, L *et al.* (2012). Ranibizumab for macular edema due to retinal vein occlusions: long-term follow-up in the HORIZON trial. *Ophthalmology* **119**: 802–809.

Ip, M. S, Scott, IU, VanVeldhuisen, PC *et al.* (2009). A randomized trial comparing the efficacy and safety of intravitreal triamcinolone with observation to treat vision loss associated with macular edema secondary to central retinal vein occlusion: the Standard Care vs Corticosteroid for Retinal Vein Occlusion (SCORE) study report 5. *Archives of Ophthalmology* **127**: 1101–1114.

Jaulim, A, Ahmed, B, Khanam, T, Chatziralli, IP (2013). Branch retinal vein occlusion: epidemiology, pathogenesis, risk factors, clinical features, diagnosis, and complications. An update of the literature. *Retina* **33**: 901–910.

Jefferies, P, Clemett, R, Day, T (1993). An anatomical study of retinal arteriovenous crossings and their role in the pathogenesis of retinal branch vein occlusions. *Australian and New Zealand Journal of Ophthalmology* **21**: 213–217.

Keane, PA, Sadda, SR (2011). Retinal vein occlusion and macular edema – critical evaluation of the clinical value of ranibizumab. *Clinical Ophthalmology* **5**: 771–781.

Kimmel, AS, McCarthy, MJ, Blodi, CF, Folk, JC (1989). Branch retinal vein occlusion in sarcoidosis. *American Journal of Ophthalmology* **107**: 561–562.

Klein, R, Klein, BE, Moss, SE, Meuer, SM (2000). The epidemiology of retinal vein occlusion: the Beaver Dam Eye Study. *Transactions of the American Ophthalmological Society* **98**: 133–141; discussion 141–133.

Koizumi, H, Ferrara, DC, Brue, C, Spaide, RF (2007). Central retinal vein occlusion case-control study. *American Journal of Ophthalmology* **144**: 858–863.

Korobelnik, JF, Holz, FG, Roider, J *et al.* (2014). Intravitreal Aflibercept Injection for Macular Edema Resulting from Central Retinal Vein Occlusion: One-Year Results of the Phase 3 GALILEO Study. *Ophthalmology* **121**: 202–208.

Kriechbaum, K, Michels, S, Prager, F *et al.* (2008). Intravitreal Avastin for macular oedema secondary to retinal vein occlusion: a prospective study. *British Journal of Ophthalmology* **92**: 518–522.

Lahey, JM, Tunc, M, Kearney, J *et al.* (2002). Laboratory evaluation of hypercoagulable states in patients with central retinal vein occlusion who are less than 56 years of age. *Ophthalmology* **109**: 126–131.

Lam, HD, Blumenkranz, M. S (2002). Treatment of central retinal vein occlusion by vitrectomy with lysis of vitreopapillary and epipapillary adhesions, subretinal peripapillary tissue plasminogen activator injection, and photocoagulation. *American Journal of Ophthalmology* **134**: 609–611.

Leavitt, JA, Larson, TA, Hodge, DO, Gullerud, RE (2011). The incidence of central retinal artery occlusion in Olmsted County, Minnesota. *American Journal of Ophthalmology* **152**: 820–823.e822.

Liang, XL, Chen, HY, Huang, YS *et al.* (2007). Pars plana vitrectomy and internal limiting membrane peeling for macular oedema secondary to retinal vein occlusion: a pilot study. *Annals of the Academy of Medicine, Singapore* **36**: 293–297.

Martin, S. C, Butcher, A, Martin, N *et al.* (2002). Cardiovascular risk assessment in patients with retinal vein occlusion. *British Journal of Ophthalmology* **86**: 774–776.

Martinez-Jardon, CS, Meza-de Regil, A, Dalma-Weiszhausz, J *et al.* (2005). Radial optic neurotomy for ischaemic central vein occlusion. *British Journal of Ophthalmology* **89**: 558–561.

Matti, AI, Lee, AW, Chen, CS (2010). Concurrent branch retinal vein occlusion and cerebral venous thrombosis from oral contraceptive pill use. *Canadian Journal of Ophthalmology* **45**: 541–542.

McAllister, IL, Constable, IJ (1995). Laser-induced chorioretinal venous anastomosis for treatment of nonischemic central retinal vein occlusion. *Archives of Ophthalmology* **113**: 456–462.

McAllister, IL, Douglas, JP, Constable, IJ, Yu, DY (1998). Laser-induced chorioretinal venous anastomosis for nonischemic central retinal vein occlusion: evaluation of the complications and their risk factors. *American Journal of Ophthalmology* **126**: 219–229.

McAllister, IL, Gillies, ME, Smithies, LA *et al.* (2010). The Central Retinal Vein Bypass Study: a trial of laser-induced chorioretinal venous anastomosis for central retinal vein occlusion. *Ophthalmology* **117**: 954–965.

Meyer, CH, Schmidt, JC, Rodrigues, EB, Mennel, S (2005). Risk of retinal vein occlusions in patients treated with rofecoxib (vioxx). *Ophthalmologica* **219**: 243–247.

Mitchell, P, Smith, W, Chang, A (1996). Prevalence and associations of retinal vein occlusion in Australia. The Blue Mountains Eye Study. *Archives of Ophthalmology* **114**: 1243–1247.

Mitry, D, Bunce, C, Charteris, D (2013). Anti-vascular endothelial growth factor for macular oedema secondary to branch retinal vein occlusion. *The Cochrane Database of Systematic Reviews* **1**: Cd009510.

O'Hearn, TM, Fawzi, A, Esmaili, D, Javaheri, M, Rao, NA, Lim, JI (2007). Presumed ocular tuberculosis presenting as a branch retinal vein occlusion in the absence of retinal vasculitis or uveitis. *British Journal of Ophthalmology* **91**: 981–982.

Opremcak, EM, Bruce, RA (1999). Surgical decompression of branch retinal vein occlusion via arteriovenous crossing sheathotomy: a prospective review of 15 cases. *Retina* **19**: 1–5.

Opremcak, EM, Bruce, RA, Lomeo, MD, Ridenour, CD, Letson, AD, Rehmar, AJ (2001). Radial optic neurotomy for central retinal vein occlusion: a retrospective pilot study of 11 consecutive cases. *Retina* **21**: 408–415.

Opremcak, EM, Rehmar, AJ, Ridenour, CD, Kurz, DE (2006). Radial optic neurotomy for central retinal vein occlusion: 117 consecutive cases. *Retina* **26**: 297–305.

Park, DH, Kim, IT (2010). Long-term effects of vitrectomy and internal limiting membrane peeling for macular edema secondary to central retinal vein occlusion and hemiretinal vein occlusion. *Retina* **30**: 117–124.

Park, SJ, Choi, N K, Seo, KH, Park, KH, Woo, SJ (2014). Nationwide incidence of clinically diagnosed central retinal artery occlusion in Korea, 2008 to 2011. *Ophthalmology* **121**: 1933–1938.

Peyman, GA, Kishore, K, Conway, MD (1999). Surgical chorioretinal venous anastomosis for ischemic central retinal vein occlusion. *Ophthalmic Surgery and Lasers* **30**: 605–614.

Priglinger, SG, Wolf, AH, Kreutzer, TC *et al.* (2007). Intravitreal bevacizumab injections for treatment of central retinal vein occlusion: six-month results of a prospective trial. *Retina* 27: 1004–1012.

Primo, S (1990). Central retinal vein occlusion in a young patient with seropositive syphilis. *Journal of the American Optometric Association* 61: 896–902.

Rogers, S, McIntosh, RL, Cheung, N *et al.* (2010). The prevalence of retinal vein occlusion: pooled data from population studies from the United States, Europe, Asia, and Australia. *Ophthalmology* 117: 313–319 e311.

Rudkin, AK, Lee, AW, Chen, CS (2010). Ocular neovascularization following central retinal artery occlusion: prevalence and timing of onset. *European Journal of Ophthalmology* 20: 1042–1046.

Rumelt, S, Dorenboim, Y, Rehany, U (1999). Aggressive systematic treatment for central retinal artery occlusion. *American Journal of Ophthalmology* 128: 733–738.

Schmidt, D, Hetzel, A, Geibel-Zehender, A (2005). Retinal arterial occlusion due to embolism of suspected cardiac tumors – report on two patients and review of the topic. *European Journal of Medical Research* 10: 296–304.

Schmidt, D, Hetzel, A, Geibel-Zehender, A, Schulte-Monting, J (2007). Systemic diseases in non-inflammatory branch and central retinal artery occlusion – an overview of 416 patients. *European Journal of Medical Research* 12: 595–603.

Schubert, H, Atebara, N, Kaiser, R *et al.* (2013). In: Skuta, G, Cantor, L. and Cioffi, G. (eds). *Retina and Vitreous*. San Francisco, CA: American Academy of Ophthalmology.

Scott, IU, Ip, MS, VanVeldhuisen, PC *et al.* (2009). A randomized trial comparing the efficacy and safety of intravitreal triamcinolone with standard care to treat vision loss associated with macular Edema secondary to branch retinal vein occlusion: the Standard Care vs Corticosteroid for Retinal Vein Occlusion (SCORE) study report 6. *Archives of Ophthalmology* 127: 1115–1128.

Stahl, A, Agostini, H, Hansen, LL, Feltgen, N (2007). Bevacizumab in retinal vein occlusion-results of a prospective case series. *Graefe's Archive for Clinical and Experimental Ophthalmology* 245: 1429–1436.

Staurenghi, G, Lonati, C, Aschero, M, Orzalesi, N (1994). Arteriovenous crossing as a risk factor in branch retinal vein occlusion. *American Journal of Ophthalmology* 117: 211–213.

Thapa, R, Paudyal, G, Bernstein, PS (2010). Demographic characteristics, patterns and risk factors for retinal vein occlusion in Nepal: a hospital-based case–control study. *Clinical & Experimental Ophthalmology* 38: 583–590.

The Branch Vein Occlusion Study Group (1984). Argon laser photocoagulation for macular edema in branch vein occlusion. *American Journal of Ophthalmology* 98: 271–282.

The Central Vein Occlusion Study (1993). Baseline and early natural history report. *Archives of Ophthalmology* 111: 1087–1095.

The Central Vein Occlusion Study Group N report (1995). A randomized clinical trial of early panretinal photocoagulation for ischemic central vein occlusion. *Ophthalmology* 102: 1434–1444.

The Central Vein Occlusion Study Group (1997). Natural history and clinical management of central retinal vein occlusion. *Archives of Ophthalmology* 115: 486–491.

The Eye Disease Case-control Study Group (1993). Risk factors for branch retinal vein occlusion. *American Journal of Ophthalmology* 116: 286–296.

The Eye Disease Case-Control Study Group (1996). Risk factors for central retinal vein occlusion. *Archives of Ophthalmology* 114: 545–554.

Varma, DD, Cugati, S, Lee, AW, Chen, CS (2013). A review of central retinal artery occlusion: clinical presentation and management. *Eye* 27: 688–697.

Weinberg, D (1994). Arteriovenous crossing as a risk factor in branch retinal vein occlusion. *American Journal of Ophthalmology* 118: 263–265.

Weizer, JS, Stinnett, SS, Fekrat, S (2003). Radial optic neurotomy as treatment for central retinal vein occlusion. *American Journal of Ophthalmology* 136: 814–819.

Zhang, H, Liu, ZL, Sun, P, Gu, F (2011). Intravitreal Bevacizumab for Treatment of Macular Edema Secondary to Central Retinal Vein Occlusion: Eighteen-Month Results of a Prospective Trial. *Journal of Ocular Pharmacology and Therapeutics* 26(3): 279–84.

Zhao, J, Sastry, SM, Sperduto, RD, Chew, EY, Remaley, NA (1993). Arteriovenous crossing patterns in branch retinal vein occlusion. The Eye Disease Case-Control Study Group. *Ophthalmology* 100: 423–428.

Section VI

Long-term Sequelae of VTE

25

Post-thrombotic Syndrome

Andrew Busuttil and Alun H. Davies

Academic Section of Vascular Surgery, Charing Cross Hospital, Imperial College London, UK

Introduction

As survival rates from deep venous thrombosis (DVT) have improved dramatically with the introduction of anticoagulant medication, interest has developed in the long-term sequelae of DVT, namely the post-thrombotic syndrome (PTS). Pulmonary embolism is less frequent, due to wider use of early anti-coagulation, better recognition of DVT risk factors, and the availability of multiple imaging modalities for suspected DVT cases. Post-thrombotic syndrome is a collection of signs and symptoms of chronic venous insufficiency following an episode of DVT. These can range from mild symptoms, with some lower limb swelling and a minimal impact on quality of life, to severe ulceration with debilitating effects on quality of life.

Pathophysiology

There are two main mechanisms in the pathophysiology of PTS – namely, venous outflow obstruction and valvular incompetence or reflux. Both are a consequence of a previous episode of DVT. Outflow obstruction results from incomplete clot resorption, and/or scarring of the vein wall secondary to the inflammatory processes occurring during thrombosis. The same inflammatory process may also lead to valvular damage and eventual venous reflux, despite complete resorption of the thrombus.

Reflux and outflow obstruction lead to chronic venous hypertension, due to the presence of higher ambulant venous pressure during normal exercise, as opposed to a drop in ambulant venous pressure seen in healthy patients. Chronic venous hypertension is thought to give rise to an inflammatory cascade in capillary beds, resulting in the appearance of fibrin cuffs around capillaries and a leukocyte response. This leads to increased vascular permeability and the typical lipodermatosclerosis seen in venous insufficiency.

Signs and Symptoms

Patients often present with lower limb swelling, aching and even venous claudication, six months to two years after having an episode of DVT. Signs on examination include oedema, venous ectasia (venous flaring), skin changes ranging from venous eczema to lipodermatosclerosis (most often seen in the gaiter area), venous ulcers and evidence of past ulceration. Patients may also have pain on compression of their calf muscles, and symptoms have a tendency to be worse towards the end of the day.

Handbook of Venous Thromboembolism, First Edition. Edited by Jecko Thachil and Catherine Bagot.
© 2018 John Wiley & Sons Ltd. Published 2018 by John Wiley & Sons Ltd.

Risk Factors for Developing PTS

Risk factors for developing PTS include location of the thrombus, with ilio-femoral DVTs more likely to result in PTS. The incidence of PTS following DVT varies according to the location and extent of the clot and, to a lesser degree, the diagnostic criteria applied, as there are various scoring systems being used in clinical practice. In a 2006 article by Kahn *et al.*, (2006), which used data from the VETO trial, the diagnosis of PTS is made according to a minimum score obtained on disease specific scores, such as the Villalta scale or Ginsberg criteria, and this varies the incidence considerably.

Overall, the incidence of PTS after an ilio-femoral DVT is 50–60% at two years (Baldwin *et al.*, 2013). This is considerably lower when below-knee or femoropopliteal DVTs are concerned, and one must interpret the incidence with some caution, as the majority of patients will only have minor PTS symptoms. The reason for the difference in incidence is that the saphenous venous system acts as a collateral in femoropopliteal deep venous occlusion, while the iliac veins do not have such collaterals.

Recurrent DVT at the same location is also more likely to lead to PTS; however, the evidence for this is not robust. When it comes to other variables, such as age and gender, there is no consensus on whether these have a significant impact on rates of PTS, although several reports in published literature do exist. However, no large, adequately powered trials to address the risk factors for PTS development have been published to date (Kahn, 2009).

Quality of Life

The impact of PTS on patients' quality of life correlates with the severity of PTS, and this has been demonstrated in a number of studies. Patients with moderate PTS have quality of life scores which are worse than those for patients suffering from chronic lung disease or arthritis, and patients with severe PTS patients have scores similar to patients suffering from congestive heart failure or cancer (Baldwin *et al.*, 2013). Patients with moderate or severe PTS often have to forgo employment, especially if it involves prolonged periods of standing. The cost of chronic venous disease to the economy is estimated to be about 2% of the total healthcare expenditure, in both direct and indirect costs.

Scoring Systems

A number of scoring systems have been developed to help clinicians and researchers stratify patients' symptoms and monitor responses to interventions, although some controversy exists as to which is most suitable for routine use. A recently published study (Soosainathan *et al.*, 2013) identified the Villalta score (Villalta *et al.*, 1994; Table 25.1) to be the most consistent and easy-to-reproduce score, which takes both clinical signs and patient symptoms into account. It does not, however, take into account any anatomical considerations which are found in the CEAP (Eklof *et al.*, 2004) classification (Table 25.2).

The Villalta score allows patients and physicians to assign a score of 0, 1, 2 or 3 to each symptom or sign, depending on severity (0 not present, 1 mild, 2 moderate and 3 severe), and allows a stratification of severity for PTS with a diagnosis of mild PTS made with a score of 5–9, moderate PTS with a score of 10–14 and severe PTS with a score of 15. The presence of ulceration automatically classifies the disease as severe. The Villalta score is recommended for use by the International Society on Thrombosis and Haemostasis.

The CEAP classification (Clinical, Aetiology, Anatomy and Pathophysiology) is useful as a research tool to grade the pattern of disease in chronic venous disease patients. It is difficult to monitor response to treatment using this classification, but it provides an accurate description of the pathophysiology, anatomy and clinical symptoms.

Table 25.1 Villalta score.

Symptom/sign	None (0)	Mild (1)	Moderate (2)	Severe (3)
Heaviness				
Pain				
Cramps				
Pruritus				
Parasthaesia				
Pretibial oedema				
Induration of the skin				
Hyperpigmentation				
Venous ectasia				
Redness				
Pain on calf compression				
Ulcer				
Total				

Table 25.2 CEAP classification – patients are assigned a value for each category C, E, A and P. For example, a typical PTS patient would score $C_{4B}E_SA_DP_O$.

C – Clinical Class	Characteristics	E – Aetiology
0	No clinical findings	C – Congenital
1	Telangiectasia	S – Secondary
2	Varicose veins	P – Primary
3	Oedema (only venous in origin)	A – Anatomy
4	a) Pigmentation and/or eczema	Superficial
	b) Lipodermatosclerosis	Deep
5	Prior ulceration (healed)	Perforator
6	Active ulcer	P – Pathophysiology
Symptomatic	Asymptomatic	Reflux
	Symptomatic	Obstruction

The Ginsberg criteria (Kahn *et al.*, 2006) for the diagnosis of PTS is useful in helping make the diagnosis of PTS, but is not able to provide a clinician or researcher with a severity score. The Ginsberg criteria are pain and swelling in a limb on a daily basis, typical of venous incompetence (worse at the end of the day and better with elevation), and present six months after an episode of DVT. This must be accompanied by evidence of venous insufficiency, for a positive diagnosis. The criteria also include a global rating questionnaire, which allows monitoring for improving or worsening of symptoms with time.

The venous clinical severity scoring (VCSS) is a broader scoring system developed by the American Venous Forum (AVF), and takes into account the size of ulcer and the number of ulcers, amongst other factors (Table 25.3).

Table 25.3 Venous clinical severity score.

	None: 0	Mild: 1	Moderate: 2	Severe: 3
Pain or other discomfort (i.e. aching, heaviness, fatigue, soreness or burning). Presumes venous origin.		Occasional pain or other discomfort (i.e. not restricting regular daily activities).	Daily pain or other discomfort (i.e. interfering with but not preventing daily activities).	Daily pain or discomfort (i.e. limits most regular daily activities).
Varicose veins				
Varicose veins > 3 mm in diameter to qualify in the standing position.		Few: scattered (i.e. isolated branch varicosities or clusters). Also includes corona phlebetcatica (ankle flare).	Confined to calf or thigh.	Involves calf and thigh.
Venous oedema				
Presumes venous origin.		Limited to foot and ankle area.	Extends above ankle gut below knee.	Extends to knee and above.
Skin pigmentation				
Presumes venous origin. Does not include focal pigmentation over varicose veins or pigmentation due to other chronic diseases.	None or focal.	Limited to perimalleolar area.	Diffuse over lower third of calf.	Wider distribution above lower third of calf.
Inflammation				
More than just recent pigmentation (i.e. erythema; cellulitis; venous eczema; dermatitis).		Limited to perimalleolar area.	Diffuse over lower third of calf.	Wider distribution above lower third of calf.
Induration				
Presumes venous origin of secondary skin and subcutaneous changes (i.e. chronic oedema with fibrosis; hypodermitis). Includes white atrophy and lipodermatosclerosis.		Limited to perimalleolar area.	Diffuse over lower third of calf.	Wider distribution above lower third of calf.
Active ulcer number	0	1	2	>3
Active ulcer duration (longest active).	N/A	<3 months	>3 months but < 1 year	Not healed for > 1 year
Active ulcer size (largest active)		Diameter < 2 cm	Diameter 2–6 cm	Diameter > 6 cm
Use of compression therapy	0: not used	1: intermittent use of stockings	2: wears stockings most days	3: full compliance; stockings

Investigations

The diagnosis of PTS is a clinical one, with investigation used for characterisation of the lesion and detection of reflux, and also to aide with planning treatment.

Duplex ultrasound is a non-invasive technique that is able to provide clinicians with information on the location of the lesion and reflux within the imaged segment, with limitations in visualisation of the iliac veins and inferior vena cava in certain patients. In most patients, particularly when good images have been obtained, it is all that is needed to monitor and plan treatment.

When considering venous stenting, venography is an invaluable tool, and is either performed separately, as a pre-operative planning procedure, or performed during the same procedure for stenting. Venography is an invasive procedure, and requires significant expertise both to perform and interpret the images. Digital sub-traction techniques are used, and contrast is injected via a sheath placed into the popliteal vein. This allows for ascending and descending venography, which is brought about by tilting the patient cranially and caudally, and observing the flow of contrast.

Computerised tomography (CT) venography is also used to help delineate the proximal extent of a stenotic lesion and to help identify any extrinsic compressive lesions and any anatomical abnormalities, such as congenital absence of the inferior vena cava (IVC) or a bifid IVC system. Unfortunately, CT venography is not a dynamic study, and is not able to demonstrate reflux or dynamic venous compression.

Magnetic resonance venography is another imaging modality which allows for dynamic sequencing to show reflux. It is a useful modality when patients are not able to have intravenous iodinated contrast, but it requires specialist radiologists for interpretation.

The latest technique in evaluating venous stenotic lesions is intravascular ultrasound (IVUS). This is used with increasing frequency for stent deployment, as two-dimensional digital subtraction venography is likely to miss a stenotic lesion if only one plane of imaging is used. The use of IVUS is more likely to identify stenotic lesions, such as in the May-Thurner syndrome, which is important in acute venous stenting to prevent re-thrombosis (and lower the incidence of PTS).

Treatment

Lifestyle Changes and Conservative Management

Patients should be encouraged to avoid prolonged periods of standing, and to elevate legs whenever possible. Weight loss may aid with venous drainage, and patients should be encouraged to exercise as much as they feel is possible. Recent studies looking into exercise for patients with PTS has shown it to be safe, and it may reduce the severity of the symptoms. However, this is often limited by pain from venous claudication, and the data is not robust, with randomised controlled trials lacking in this area.

Compression

The use of compression therapy in chronic venous insufficiency has long been the mainstay of treatment – particularly so when skin ulceration develops. Compression therapy works by reducing the venous pressure, with decreasing grades of compression from the ankle proximally.

Compression stockings improve tissue perfusion with oxygenated blood, and reduce venous pooling (Agu *et al.*, 2004). There is no robust evidence for the use of stockings in PTS patients, and some recent studies demonstrate that they do not provide any improvement in symptoms, or reduce PTS rates following DVT events. Nonetheless, the American College of Chest Physicians and the American Heart Association both recommend the use of compression stockings in PTS patients.

Provided there are no contra-indications to using compression stockings, their use is believed to help with symptomatology, particularly lower limb swelling, which is often seen in PTS patients.

The latest addition to compression therapy are pneumatic compression devices, which have been shown to improve quality of life scores, as well as Villalta scores for patients. However, further adequately powered trials are needed.

Pharmacological Agents

There is great debate on the use of pharmacological agents for the treatment of PTS, such as micronised purified flavonoid fractions (MPFF) (Daflon) and pentoxyfiline. The theory behind their efficacy is their ability to reduce the circulating inflammatory markers, and they may help reduce the inflammatory process associated with chronic venous insufficiency. Two studies have shown that the use of MPFF leads to improved ulcer healing rates when combined with compression. In a large study, the consistent use of MPFF has been shown to improve the CEAP score of patients. There is a lack of robust evidence from randomised controlled placebo trials, and this is most likely the reason why their use is not widespread. They are extensively used in mainland Europe, but not in the UK or USA.

Venous Stenting

Venous stenting is rapidly becoming the treatment of choice for patients with deep venous obstruction, particularly at the level of the iliac veins. In recent years, we have seen the introduction of a number of venous specific stents, such as the VICI stent (Veniti) and Zilver Vena Stent (Cook), among others, and an ever growing number of centres who perform these procedures.

Venous stents differ from arterial stents in many ways, as these stents need not cope with high pressures and flows, but need to have a high radial force to maintain patency of the vessel. They are often oversized, as the diameter of larger veins fluctuates considerably during respiration. These first-generation venous specific stents are bare metal stents, and require anti-coagulation and anti-platelet therapy to maintain patency. Recent studies have shown that primary, assisted primary and secondary patency rates are very promising, and that they have a significant impact on the disease trajectory and ulcer healing. Further study into their use is needed to determine their long-term benefit and cost-effectiveness, as there have been no randomised controlled trials to date.

Venous stenting may be performed for chronic iliac vein occlusions, non-thrombotic iliac vein lesions (such as May-Thurner syndrome, where the right common iliac artery compresses the left common iliac vein), and also as an adjunct in catheter-directed thrombolysis for ilio-femoral DVT.

Anticoagulation regimens following the placement of venous stents are still a matter of debate, but work is being undertaken to establish the most appropriate agent and duration of treatment.

Venous stenting is fast replacing the need for deep venous bypass, as it has a much more acceptable morbidity profile.

Deep Venous Reconstruction

Surgical bypass of occluded venous segments has been performed for over 50 years now, with overall 50–80% patency rates, depending on a number of factors. These procedures are invasive, carry a significant morbidity and, due to their specialised nature, are only performed in a handful of centres. Deep venous reconstruction brings about an improvement in both symptoms and ulcer healing rates, but it is only suitable for a small number of individuals, based on the anatomy of the obstruction and patency of suitable conduits for bypass/reconstruction.

Valve Repair

Open valvuloplasty involves a venotomy and plication of the loose valve leaflets, but this is invasive and carries significant morbidity, and there are no robust studies from which to draw conclusions. As with deep venous bypass, these procedures are carried out in a handful of centres, and require careful patient selection.

Deep Venous Valve Prosthesis

The idea of a biomedical device that could be implanted into patients' veins to treat deep venous reflux is not new. However, no such device currently exists, and there are a number of groups developing prosthetic valves from a wide range of materials. The pioneer of such techniques, Pavnick, conducted a small trial involving four patients with deep venous reflux. He used a prototype valve he developed, and he was able to demonstrate an improvement in symptoms and improved ulcer healing. Unfortunately, due to the nature of blood flow in the venous system and the propensity for thrombosis, no large-scale trials of any device have yet been undertaken. There are a number of groups attempting to produce prosthetic venous valves from a variety of materials – both biological as well as prosthetic – and it is hoped that such a device would bring yet another treatment option for patients with deep venous reflux.

Prevention Strategies

It is clear that, whereas venous stenting offers a treatment option for patients, the focus should be in reducing the incidence of PTS. The first step would be accurate risk assessment of hospital patients and appropriate DVT prophylaxis, in order to reduce DVT rates. Prompt anticoagulation has been proved to reduce the incidence of PTS. In fact, anticoagulation is, so far, the best-proven method for reducing PTS in proximal DVT patients. For this reason, further efforts must be made to deliver timely anticoagulation.

Prompt Anticoagulation

To date, the best evidence for reducing PTS in DVT patients is anticoagulation. Several studies have shown that effective bridging and tight control of anticoagulation leads to lower PTS rates. The time spent below the therapeutic range when using vitamin K antagonists (VKA) has shown to strongly correlate with an increased risk of PTS.

Trials comparing low molecular weight heparin (LMWH) versus VKA have shown the former to be more effective in reducing PTS in DVT patients. This is thought to be due to the constant therapeutic effect of LMWH, and the sometimes haphazard international normalised ratio control with the use of VKA. It is not yet clear what effect the direct oral anticoagulants, such as rivaroxaban or apixaban, will have on PTS rates, and further study into the effect of these drugs is required.

Elastic Compression Stockings (ECS)

The use of ECS following a diagnosis of a DVT and for a duration of up to two years has been proved to reduce the incidence of PTS in a number of studies. This firmly held belief has, however, come into question with the publication of the SOX (Kahn *et al.*, 2014) trial results. This randomised controlled trial compared the use of appropriately fitted ECS with a placebo (ECS two sizes too large) in DVT patients, and followed up patients for two years. Both patients and researchers were blind to the treatment, and this was effectively demonstrated in the manuscript. The authors demonstrated no difference in the PTS rates in patients using ECS, compared with placebo stockings and, while this was the first trial of its kind, further evidence is needed before one may be able to draw meaningful long-term conclusions on the topic.

Several other studies, with different designs, have produced a mixed body of evidence. Currently, most guidelines recommend the use of ECS for a period of two years following the diagnosis of a DVT to reduce the incidence of PTS. However, the revised 2014 National Institute of Healthcare and Clinical Excellence (NICE) guidelines cast some doubt as to the efficacy of ECS and whether or not they should be used.

Early Thrombus Removal

Over the past 50 years, early thrombus removal has seen a considerable shift in techniques. Open surgical thrombectomy was effective in removal of ilio-femoral venous thrombus, but carried with it significant morbidity. With the discovery of streptokinase, and later recombinant tissue plasminogen activator (TPA), thrombolysis became an option. Systemic administration of these medications was able to bring about satisfactory thrombus dissolution rates, but at a cost of significant bleeding complications, as well as intra-cranial haemorrhages. Catheter-directed thrombolysis (CDT) and, later, mechanically assisted thrombolysis, have led to lower doses of thrombolytic agent needed for thrombus resolution, significantly reducing the incidence of bleeding complications.

There are many devices on the market for pharmaco-mechanical thrombolysis (PMT), and these are all undergoing further study. To date, the only randomised controlled study published on CDT and its long-term benefits was the CAVENT (Enden *et al.*, 2012) study, which was a randomised controlled multi-centred trial, comparing CDT and anticoagulation to anticoagulation alone, in patients with ilio-femoral DVT. The authors found an absolute risk reduction of 14.4% in PTS rates in the CDT arm. One must note that, although the PTS rates were lower, there was no significant improvement in the quality of life scores at two years between the two groups.

Since the publication of this trial, there have been significant additions to the armamentarium for treating proximal DVT, such as the EKOS device, which is an ultrasound-accelerated CDT catheter, using even smaller amounts of thrombolytic agent, with good thrombus dissolution rates.

The ATTRACT (Vedantham *et al.*, 2013) trial is another RCT looking at both PMT and CDT and the effects they have on PTS reduction, and results were expected to be published in 2016. This will continue to add to the body of evidence supporting the use of early thrombus removal.

Current guidance from NICE and the AVF/Society for Vascular Surgery recommend that patients with ilio-femoral DVT should be considered for CDT, providing they are within two weeks of presentation, are expected to live longer than one year, have no contra-indication to thrombolytic therapy and have good pre-morbid levels of functionality.

Key Points

- Post-thrombotic syndrome is a common, under-recognised disease with significant effects on patients' quality of life.
- Diagnosis is a clinical one.
- Reducing the incidence of DVT through effective thromboprophylaxis plays a vital role in preventing the development of PTS.
- A number of PTS prevention strategies exist, and results from further trials are expected in the coming years.
- Effective anticoagulation is crucial to help reduce the incidence of PTS.
- Eligibility criteria for catheter directed thrombolysis:
  - thrombosis less than two weeks old;
  - good pre-morbid mobility;
  - life expectancy greater than one year;
  - no contraindication to thrombolysis;
  - ilio-femoral DVT.

Further Reading

Agu O, Baker D, Seifalian AM (2004). Effect of graduated compression stockings on limb oxygenation and venous function during exercise in patients with venous insufficiency. *Vascular* **12**(1): 69–76.

Baldwin MJ, Moore HM, Rudarakanchana N, Gohel M, Davies AH (2013). Post-thrombotic syndrome: a clinical review. *Journal of Thrombosis and Haemostasis* **11**(5): 795–805.

Eklof B, Rutherford RB, Bergan JJ, Carpentier PH, Gloviczki P, Kistner RL, et al. (2004). Revision of the CEAP classification for chronic venous disorders: consensus statement. *Journal of Vascular Surgery* **40**(6): 1248–52.

Enden T, Haig Y, Klow NE, Slagsvold CE, Sandvik L, Ghanima W, et al. (2012). Long-term outcome after additional catheter-directed thrombolysis versus standard treatment for acute -emoral deep vein thrombosis (the CaVenT study): A randomised controlled trial. *The Lancet* **379**(9810): 31–8.

Kahn SR, Desmarais S, Ducruet T, Arsenault L, Ginsberg JS (2006). Comparison of the Villalta and Ginsberg clinical scales to diagnose the post-thrombotic syndrome: correlation with patient-reported disease burden and venous valvular reflux. *Journal of Thrombosis and Haemostasis* **4**(4): 907–8.

Kahn SR, Shapiro S, Wells PS, Rodger MA, Kovacs MJ, Anderson DR, et al. (2014). Compression stockings to prevent post-thrombotic syndrome: a randomised placebo-controlled trial. *The Lancet* **383**(9920): 880–8.

Kahn SR (2009). Post-thrombotic syndrome after deep venous thrombosis: Risk factors, prevention, and therapeutic options. *Clinical Advances in Hematology and Oncology* **7**(7): 433–5.

Soosainathan A, Moore HM, Gohel MS, Davies AH (2013). Scoring systems for the post-thrombotic syndrome. *Journal of Vascular Surgery* **57**(1): 254–61.

Vedantham S, Goldhaber SZ, Kahn SR, Julian J, Magnuson E, Jaff MR, et al. (2013). Rationale and design of the ATTRACT Study: A multicenter randomized trial to evaluate pharmacomechanical catheter-directed thrombolysis for the prevention of postthrombotic syndrome in patients with proximal deep vein thrombosis. *American Heart Journal* **165**(4): 523–30.e3.

Villalta S, Bagatella, P., Piccioli, A., Lensing, A.W., Prins, M.H., Prandoni, P (1994). Assessment of validity and reproducibility of a clinical scale for the post thrombotic syndrome. *Haemostasis* **24**(suppl. 1): 158A.

26

Chronic Thromboembolic Pulmonary Hypertension

Demosthenes G. Papamatheakis and William R. Auger

University of California, San Diego, USA

Introduction

In the last 25 years, there have been significant changes in our understanding of pulmonary hypertension, which have led to disease stratification revisions, as well as paradigm shifts in management. One of the most intriguing categories of pulmonary hypertension is the one due to chronic thromboembolic disease, defined as an elevated pulmonary artery (PA) pressure (mean > 25 mm Hg) in the presence of organised pulmonary emboli, suggested by persistent perfusion defects on lung perfusion scintigraphy, and confirmed radiographically with catheter-based, computed tomographic (CT) or magnetic resonance (MR) angiography.

In addition to having a different pathophysiological basis relative to pulmonary arterial hypertension (PAH), chronic thromboembolic pulmonary hypertension (CTEPH) is the only potentially curable form of pulmonary hypertension with a pulmonary endarterectomy (Mayer *et al.*, 2011). However, despite the considerable progress achieved over the past decades in the detection, evaluation, and management of this unique group of patients, there remain multiple unanswered questions about CTEPH, ranging from the epidemiology of this disease, its pathobiology and the optimal diagnostic pathway to select patients appropriate for endarterectomy. The recent availability of an FDA-approved PAH directed medical therapy for subgroups of CTEPH patients, and the evolving role of balloon pulmonary angioplasty in the treatment of some selected patients, will be additional topics reviewed in this chapter.

Epidemiology

CTEPH has been viewed as a rare outcome in those patients having survived one or more acute pulmonary embolic events, though experience suggests that this disease is under-recognised (Lang, 2004). The incidence and prevalence of CTEPH have not been clearly defined. Several studies have attempted to define incidence rates of CTEPH after acute pulmonary embolism (PE), ranging between 0.57% and 8.8% (Pengo *et al.*, 2004; Miniati *et al.*, 2006; Becattini *et al.*, 2006; Dentali *et al.*, 2009; Klok *et al.*, 2010; Korkmaz *et al.*, 2012; Guerin *et al.*, 2014).

In 2004, Pengo and colleagues reported on the incidence of CTEPH in 223 patients (initial cohort of 314 patients), followed prospectively after an acute episode of pulmonary embolism. These patients did not have a prior history of venous thromboembolism, and were evaluated for CTEPH if they manifested symptoms of persistent unexplained dyspnoea leading confirmatory testing. The cumulative incidence was noted to be 3.8% at two years (Pengo *et al.*, 2004).

Handbook of Venous Thromboembolism, First Edition. Edited by Jecko Thachil and Catherine Bagot.

In an attempt to identify patients with asymptomatic CTEPH, Dentali and colleagues looked at consecutive patients within 6–12 months after their first episode of PE. They reported an incidence rate of 8.8% in their 91-patient cohort, half of these patients without cardiopulmonary symptoms (Dentali *et al.*, 2009). In order to replicate these results in a more robust fashion, Klok and colleagues investigated the incidence of CTEPH in a cohort of 866 consecutive patients diagnosed with an acute PE. They reported a CTEPH incidence of only 0.57%. For those patients with a history of unprovoked pulmonary embolism, a CTEPH incidence of 1.5% was observed. Although this study was designed to look at all patients, regardless of symptoms, a large number of patients did not undergo study screening, and the final number of confirmed CTEPH patients was primarily established through record review (Klok *et al.*, 2010).

The most recent study addressing the development of CTEPH in the post-PE population was published in 2014 by Guerin and colleagues. Patients were evaluated yearly for a median of 26 months, with dyspnoea questionnaires and echocardiography using a pre-defined algorithm. Of the 146 patients that were followed for approximately two years after their acute PE, the confirmed prevalence of CTEPH was 4.8%. CTEPH patients were older (>70 years), exhibited higher PA pressures on initial presentation, more frequently had prior thromboembolic events, and demonstrated more proximal thromboembolic disease. Unique was the observation that, in review of CT angiographic studies at the time of presentation, all of the patients eventually diagnosed with CTEPH showed radiographical signs of chronic thrombus. This suggested that the initial presentation for these patients might have been CTEPH, and not acute pulmonary embolism (Guerin *et al.*, 2014).

The variability of reported CTEPH incidence likely resulted from differences in study design, with non-uniformity in PH evaluation (i.e. echocardiographical screening vs. right heart catheterisation), inconsistent exclusion of other causes of PH in enrolled patients, and selection bias. The limited 2–3 year follow-up after the thromboembolic event may have also rendered an inaccurate incidence assessment.

Leading to further uncertainty as to overall prevalence of CTEPH is evidence that a substantive number of patients with CTEPH do not have a reported history of venous thromboembolism. Results from the International CTEPH Registry published in 2011 revealed that 25.2% of enrolled patients were without a confirmed diagnosis of a previous pulmonary embolism; 43.9% had not experienced a previous deep vein thrombosis (Pepke-Zaba *et al.*, 2011). In this patient group, the incident pulmonary embolic event was evidently asymptomatic, and the initial clinical presentation of these patients a manifestation of established CTEPH, as in the report of Guerin and colleagues (2014).

Pathophysiology

Most cases of CTEPH are thought to have evolved from a prior episode of acute pulmonary embolism (PE), although the latter may have been asymptomatic and never diagnosed (Pepke-Zaba *et al.*, 2011). Although efforts at identifying the pathophysiological mechanisms of CTEPH have been focused on the transition from an acute thromboembolism to a chronic, endothelialised, endovascular 'scar', the process is not completely understood. In addition to a genetic pre-disposition for inadequate thrombus dissolution, for which there is limited published data, hypotheses include the concepts of local inflammation, ineffective angiogenesis, and endothelial dysfunction (Lang *et al.*, 2013; Quarck *et al.*, 2015).

White blood cell-derived inflammatory infiltrates within the thrombus/vessel wall complex may result in a chemokine cascade that promotes smooth muscle cell proliferation, fibroblast migration and proliferation, apoptosis inhibition and endothelin-1 production. Although the specifics are not clear, it appears that the inflammatory milieu results in maladaptive vessel-wall remodelling, with poor thrombus dissolution and lumen recanalisation. This theory is supported by published data on inflammatory markers and endarterectomised material analysed from CTEPH patients (Lang *et al.*, 2013; Quarck *et al.*, 2015; Bernard and Yi, 2007; Wynants *et al.*, 2012).

Endothelial activation is an important component in the process of thrombus dissolution, mostly through vessel recanalisation. A dysfunctional endothelium does not allow for effective angiogenesis, including fibrinolysis and thrombus contraction and absorption, resulting instead in fibroblast proliferation and deregulation of myofibroblast differentiation. This hypothesis, taken together with a 'localised inflammation' theory, as well as reports of abnormal fragmentation of fibrinogen variants (Morris *et al.*, 2009), provide a plausible mechanism for abnormal thrombus dissolution and maladaptive vessel wall remodelling, bridging the gap between acute pulmonary embolus and chronic thromboembolic disease (Lang *et al.*, 2013; Zabini *et al.*, 2012; Sakao *et al.*, 2011; Firth *et al.*, 2010).

In addition, published data provide a better characterisation of patients at risk for CTEPH, these risk factors mostly identified through international registries (Pepke-Zaba *et al.*, 2011) and large case series (Firth *et al.*, 2010). Some of these risk factors are thrombophilic states: antiphospholipid antibody syndromes or lupus anticoagulant (Pepke-Zaba *et al.*, 2011; Bonderman *et al.*, 2009; Wolf *et al.*, 2000), elevated levels of factor VIII (Bonderman *et al.*, 2003), factor V Leiden (Wong *et al.*, 2010), and von Willebrand factor (Bonderman *et al.*, 2003; Wong *et al.*, 2010), which have been found at a higher incidence in CTEPH patients, compared with non-thrombotic pulmonary hypertension and/or control subjects.

Other risk factors associated with higher CTEPH incidence include larger perfusion defects or higher levels of pulmonary hypertension at the time of initial PE diagnosis, recurrent PE, splenectomy, ventriculo-atrial shunts, infected pacemakers, non-O blood group, thyroid replacement therapy, and history of malignancy (Pengo *et al.*, 2004; Guerin *et al.*, 2014; Wolf *et al.*, 2000).

An essential aspect of the pathophysiological pathway leading to CTEPH is the development of a distal pulmonary vasculopathy, which occurs in varying degrees in addition to the upstream large vessel occlusion or narrowing with chronic thrombus. Early observations revealed small vessel disease with pathologic changes similar to PAH, including vessel wall muscularisation, intimal fibrosis, medial hypertrophy and even plexiform lesions (Moser and Bloor, 1993).

However, a recent study reports post-capillary remodelling in CTEPH patients, associated with bronchial-to-pulmonary venous shunting and collateral blood flow, suggesting a much more complex distal vasculopathy than previously appreciated (Dorfmüller *et al.*, 2014). Moreover, it remains unclear whether this downstream vascular pathology evolves as a function of the duration of established chronic thromboembolic disease, is provoked by a relative high flow state in the vascular bed uninvolved with obstructing thrombus, is associated with a particular genetic predisposition, or is related to the presence of an infectious process or other medical condition(s) (Lang *et al.*, 2013).

Clinical Presentation and Patient Evaluation

The most common presenting symptom of CTEPH is exertional dyspnoea, and patients may only initially perceive unexpected exercise intolerance. Moreover, once the patient does seek medical attention, there needs to be a certain level of suspicion by the treating physician in order to initiate the proper evaluation. It is not uncommon for patient's chronic thromboembolic disease to go undiagnosed or misdiagnosed for prolonged periods of time. Other symptoms related to CTEPH can include cough, haemoptysis, palpitations or atypical chest pain, but these tend to be relatively uncommon. In cases of advanced disease, however, symptoms or right heart failure may predominate, such as peripheral oedema, abdominal distention due to ascites, and chest pain, light-headedness or syncope with exertion.

To facilitate a prompt and appropriate diagnosis of CTEPH, several clinical observations should be considered. As a prior history of thromboembolic disease may be remote or, as indicated above, lacking altogether, patients presenting with cardiopulmonary symptoms without an evident cause should prompt an assessment for pulmonary vascular disease – notably, pulmonary hypertension and chronic thromboembolic disease. The clinician should also be aware that, even in the absence of resting pulmonary hypertension, the presence of chronic thromboemboli may be associated with exertional dyspnoea and an unacceptable decline in exercise capabilities. Symptoms in these cases are thought to be due to either poor augmentation of right ventricular function during exercise (despite relatively normal function at rest), the development of pulmonary hypertension during exertion, or symptomatic dead space ventilation during exercise (van der Plas *et al.*, 2010).

Klok and colleagues have described the pulmonary and cardiac compromise experienced by these patients as a sequela of the post-PE syndrome, and possibly an earlier stage of the more 'extreme' manifestation of this syndrome, CTEPH (Klok *et al.*, 2014). Nevertheless, despite the lack of hemodynamic derangement at rest, these patients should be considered potential candidates for PTE surgery.

On physical examination, abnormal findings can be very subtle, or not present at all. With more advanced disease, classic signs of pulmonary hypertension, such as a split second heart sound (S2) and accentuated pulmonic component (P2), a palpated right ventricular impulse, a murmur due to tricuspid regurgitation and an S4 gallop, can be noted. In addition, in advanced cases with right ventricular dysfunction or failure, signs of pulmonary venous congestion can be seen, such as an S3 gallop, elevated jugular venous pressure, lower extremity oedema, ascites and hepatomegaly.

Additional physical findings may be related to prior DVT and venous stasis changes of the extremities, such as varicose veins or skin discoloration. Hypoxia may be present from right to left shunt through a patent foramen ovale, significant right heart compromise, or severe VQ mismatch, causing cyanosis (Kapitan *et al.*, 1989). Clubbing is not observed when CTEPH is the principal diagnosis. Finally, pulmonary flow murmurs or bruits may be heard when auscultating the lungs, due to turbulent blood flow through partially obstructed or narrowed vessels. Although this finding is not exclusive to CTEPH, it is not found in pulmonary hypertension arising from more distal pulmonary artery disease.

The initial work-up is similar to that with any patient evaluation for dyspnoea, including basic laboratory tests, pulmonary function testing and a chest X-ray. Though these tests have value in the evaluation of the patient with CTEPH, they are particularly useful for the detection of comorbidities. The essential role of 'routine' laboratory testing is in the evaluation for anaemia, thrombocytopenia and a coagulopathy (PT, aPTT) which affect operability risks. The presence of liver and renal function abnormalities, which can be compromised as a result of right ventricular dysfunction, also impact the risks surrounding surgery.

Screening for hypercoagulable states is recommended, as the presence of inherited thrombophilia or antiphospholipid antibodies (lupus anticoagulant, anticardiolipin antibodies) will impact the approach to anticoagulation pre- and post-operatively. Basic pulmonary function tests are primarily useful, to rule out coexisting restrictive or obstructive lung disease. DLCO may also be reduced in CTEPH patients, even in the absence of any spirometric obstruction or restriction (Steenhuis *et al.*, 2000).

A chest radiograph has value in identifying any other evident thoracic pathology that might explain abnormal VQ scan findings, including hemi-diaphragm position. Radiographic findings that can be observed in CTEPH include enlarged pulmonary arteries, cardiomegaly with enlarged right sided heart chambers (Satoh *et al.*, 2005) and, on occasion, 'avascular' parenchyma, representing lung regions supplied by pulmonary vessels occluded with chronic thromboemboli.

Without an evident cause for a patient's dyspnoea and progressing exercise intolerance, pulmonary vascular disease should be considered (Figure 26.1).

To screen for pulmonary hypertension and right heart dysfunction, transthoracic echocardiography should be obtained (Kim *et al.*, 2013). Doppler estimate of right ventricular systolic pressure, an assessment of right ventricular and atrial chamber size and function, along with interventricular septal motion, are features discernible with this non-invasive imaging modality. An echocardiogram possesses an additional value in assessing

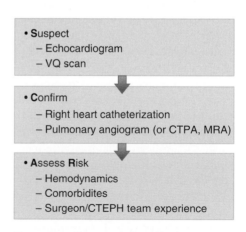

Figure 26.1 Suggested algorithm for stepwise approach in evaluation, diagnosis and management of CTEPH. Reprinted with permission from the *Journal of the American College of Cardiology* (Kim *et al.*, 2013).

whether there is valvular or left heart disease, either as a comorbid condition, or as the possible alternative aetiology of pulmonary hypertension (Lang *et al.*, 2015; Marston *et al.*, 2015; Raisinghani and Ben-Yehuda, 2006).

With echocardiogram results suggesting pulmonary hypertension, the next step in the evaluation algorithm should be a VQ scan, as a screen for mismatched perfusion defects and chronic thromboembolic disease.

As some cases of CTEPH may have normal resting hemodynamics, if the level of suspicion for pulmonary vascular disease is high in the appropriate clinical setting, a VQ scan should be obtained, even with a normal echocardiogram. Despite recent advances in CT imaging of the pulmonary vascular bed, the VQ scan remains the recommended standard in screening for CTEPH (Kim *et al.*, 2013), with several studies showing a greater sensitivity in disease detection compared to CT angiography (Tunariu *et al.*, 2007; Soler *et al.*, 2012).

The pattern of perfusion abnormality has additional value, in that VQ scan with a more peripheral pattern of perfusion abnormality ('mottled') suggests small vessel pulmonary vascular disease, while segmental and larger perfusion abnormalities with defined margins are indicative of more proximal vessel involvement (Lisbona *et al.*, 1985). The greatest value of this study centres on the observation that a normal perfusion scan excludes the diagnosis of operable CTEPH. However, an abnormal perfusion scan is not pathognomonic for CTEPH, as other disease may present with similar findings (Kerr *et al.*, 1995; Rossi *et al.*, 2001; Kerr, 2005; Wijesuriya *et al.*, 2013). As a result, additional confirmatory diagnostic studies are required.

Catheter-based digital subtraction pulmonary angiography (DSA), which can safely be performed even in severe pulmonary hypertension (Nicod *et al.*, 1987; Pitton *et al.*, 1996), has been considered the gold standard test for confirming the presence of chronic thromboembolic disease, and providing the diagnostician with an anatomic blueprint of chronic thromboembolic lesion location and extent (Figure 26.2).

The availability of biplane image acquisition further allows for greater detail in evaluating certain areas (e.g. right middle lobe and lingula) that may not be well visualised on anterior-posterior imaging only. Angiographic findings of chronic thromboembolic disease are diverse and, in most patients, are found in combination. These include 'pouch' defects, complete obstruction of major vessels, pulmonary artery 'webs' or 'bands', pulmonary artery wall irregularities and distinct vessel narrowing, occasionally accompanied by post-stenotic dilatation (Auger *et al.*, 1992).

Other imaging modalities which are utilised in the evaluation of CTEPH patients include CT pulmonary angiography (CTPA) and MR pulmonary angiography (MRA). These modalities can play a pivotal role in the work-up of the CTEPH patient, especially when competing diagnoses are under consideration (Wijesuriya *et al.*, 2013). Evaluation of the lung parenchyma, mediastinum and cross-sectional definition of the pulmonary vasculature provide supplemental information to DSA, to confirm the diagnosis of CTEPH (or verify the presence of an alternative diagnosis) and assess for coexistent lung disease.

Although CTPA has been increasingly substituted for DSPA (Reichelt *et al.*, 2009; Ley *et al.*, 2012; Sugiura *et al.*, 2013) in the CTEPH patient evaluation, persistent shortcomings with defining distal vessel disease, along with interpretive inconsistencies, are ongoing challenges in using this modality for operative assessment. Similarly, MRA has replaced DSA in some experienced CTEPH centres (Coulden, 2006), providing the required detail for the evaluation of the pulmonary vascular bed and in determining operability (Kreitner *et al.*, 2007; Nikolaou *et al.*, 2005; Rajaram *et al.*, 2012). Moreover, cardiac MR allows for evaluation of the cardiac chambers, collateral pulmonary circulation, the presence of congenital cardiac or pulmonary venous abnormalities, RV- LV interaction, and provides data on RV function and muscle mass (Kreitner *et al.*, 2004; Alfakih *et al.*, 2004).

The next step in the work up is defining disease severity from a hemodynamic perspective with right heart catheterisation (RHC). The information provides for pre-operative risk stratification, given evidence that a high pulmonary vascular resistance (greater than 1000 to 1200 dyn*s*cm^{-5}) and severe right heart dysfunction increase perioperative mortality risk (Darteville *et al.*, 2004; Madani *et al.*, 2012; de Perrot *et al.*, 2015). It can also evaluate the pulmonary hemodynamic response to exercise in those uncommon cases with mild derangement or normal pulmonary artery pressures at rest, despite persistent perfusion defects on V/Q scan. This provides objective documentation of abnormal pulmonary vascular physiology that may explain exertional cardiopulmonary symptoms.

(a)

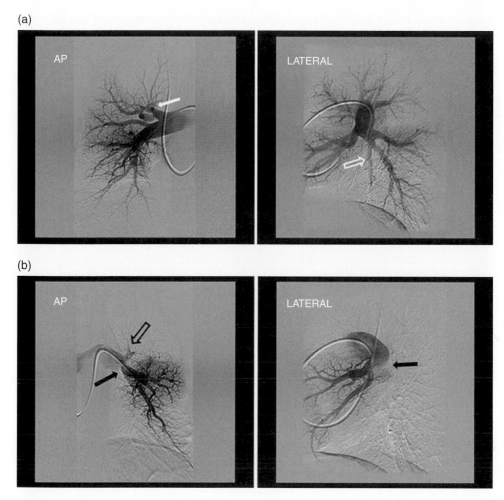

(b)

Figure 26.2 (a) Proximal vessel narrowing in right upper lobe (solid white arrow) and on lateral view, intimal irregularities anterior right lower lobe vessel (open white arrow). (b) Segmental level narrowing left upper lobe arteries (open black arrow), with what appears to be 'web' narrowing of proximal left descending PA. That on lateral view was the lingula artery (solid black arrow); the left descending PA was completely occluded beyond the lingula. These angiographic findings are consistent with organized thromboembolic disease.

The final step in the evaluation of the CTEPH patient is an assessment of surgical candidacy. This process necessitates a thorough evaluation, at an experienced CTEPH centre, of the operability of the chronic thromboembolic lesions. Such a determination is not only based on a careful review of the diagnostic studies above, but also depends on the capabilities of the surgical team responsible for performing the endarterectomy. Surgical candidacy is further impacted by patient comorbidities, overall preoperative conditioning, and the anticipation that the potential benefits of symptom relief and pulmonary hemodynamic improvement will outweigh the attendant risks of this surgical procedure.

Treatment

The treatment option providing the greatest opportunity for cure for patients with CTEPH is surgical removal of the thromboembolic material via pulmonary thromboendarterectomy (PTE) surgery (also known as pulmonary endarterectomy, PEA), followed by life-long anticoagulation. Centres with more experienced diagnosticians and surgeons, and with an understanding of the perioperative management necessary to support these patients, are now resecting chronic thromboembolic disease at the distal segmental and sub-segmental level, previously thought to be inoperable.

Since its inception, pulmonary thromboendarterectomy surgery has evolved significantly (Daily and Auger, 1999), and various studies have looked into modifying specific aspects of the technique (Hagl *et al.*, 2003; Mikus *et al.*, 2008; Thompson *et al.*, 2008; Morsolini *et al.*, 2012). However, the fundamental elements of the procedure have remained relatively unchanged over the past two decades. In its current iteration, a thrombo-endarterectomy necessitates a median sternotomy, cardiopulmonary bypass, and deep hypothermia (for tissue protection), with circulatory arrest periods in order to provide a bloodless surgical field. This allows for an optimal visual field for as complete a dissection as possible.

The favourable short- and long-term outcomes of the surgery with reduction of PA pressures, and improvement in RV function and functional status, have been consistently reported by multiple centres worldwide (Madani *et al.*, 2012; Mayer *et al.*, 2011; de Perrot *et al.*, 2011; Ogino *et al.*, 2006; Maliyasena *et al.*, 2012). Moreover, as longer-term data have become available, the haemodynamic and resultant functional status improvements are sustained in most patients, along with a favourable impact on long-term survivorship (Condliffe *et al.*, 2008; Saouti *et al.*, 2009; Freed *et al.*, 2011; Corsico *et al.*, 2008; Ishida *et al.*, 2012).

Although there are data indicating a higher mortality rate with exceptionally high pre-operative PVR ($>1000\,\mathrm{dyn^*s^*cm^{-5}}$), the growing experience at CTEPH centres worldwide has resulted in a marked decline in in-hospital mortality over the past decade. Initial reports noted a five- to seven-fold increase in postoperative PTE deaths (Darteville *et al.*, 2004; Hartz *et al.*, 1996) in high-PVR ($>1,100\,\mathrm{dyn^*s^*cm^{-5}}$) patients. More recent data indicate an increased risk, though with baseline mortality rates much lower than previously recorded.

Madani and colleagues reported a declining overall operative mortality risk of 2.2% following PTE surgery in 500 patients operated on between 2006 and 2010. In this cohort, those patients with a preoperative $\mathrm{PVR}>1000\,\mathrm{dyn^*s^*cm^{-5}}$ experienced a mortality rate of 4.1%, compared with 1.6% in those patients with a PVR less than $1000\,\mathrm{dyn^*s^*cm^{-5}}$ (Madani *et al.*, 2012). Similarly, de Perrot and colleagues reported an overall mortality of 4% in a cohort of 120 CTEPH patients undergoing endarterectomy surgery between 2005 and 2013, with all deaths occurring in patients presenting with $\mathrm{TPR}>1,200\,\mathrm{dyn^*s^*cm^{-5}}$ and clinical evidence for decompensated right heart failure (de Perrot *et al.*, 2015).

Though the definition of residual pulmonary hypertension varies between reporting centres, there are patients who do not achieve normal pulmonary pressures and right heart function following PTE surgery. Occurrence estimates vary between 5% and 35% of operated patients, though long-term information as to what level of residual pulmonary hypertension negatively impacts functional status and survivorship is lacking (Condliffe *et al.*, 2008; Freed *et al.*, 2011; Corsico *et al.*, 2008; Bonderman *et al.*, 2007; Thistlethwaite *et al.*, 2006). Possible explanations for this postoperative outcome include residual chronic thromboembolic disease that could not be surgically resected, or a significant amount of coexisting distal vessel arteriopathy. Catheter-based procedures to 'partition' the vascular resistance between proximal and distal components, in an effort to provide objective criteria to predict poor outcomes following endarterectomy surgery, are difficult to perform, and have not been consistently reliable (Kim *et al.*, 2004; Toshner *et al.*, 2012).

Treatment options for CTEPH patients appropriately deemed not to be surgical candidates include PAH-directed medical therapy and, recently, in some centres, balloon pulmonary angioplasty. In patients with inoperable CTEPH, and in those with residual pulmonary hypertension following PTE surgery, only a few randomised controlled studies examining the efficacy of PAH directed medical therapy have been conducted. In a small cohort of patients receiving sildenafil (9 of 19 patients, 12 week trial) (Suntharalingam *et al.*, 2008), and in a larger study examining the efficacy of bosentan (77 of 157 patients receiving drug, 16 week trial) (Jais *et al.*, 2008), a pulmonary haemodynamic benefit for those patients receiving drug was achieved, though a significant improvement in the primary endpoint, six-minute walk distance, was not realised in either study.

However, a recent randomised, controlled 16-week trial (CHEST-1) examined the efficacy of a soluble guanylate cyclase stimulator, riociguat, in patients with inoperable CTEPH, or in those with persistent pulmonary hypertension following pulmonary endarterectomy. This study demonstrated a significant improvement in six-minute walk distance (39 m increase in the riociguat group vs. a 6 m decrease in the placebo group), a pulmonary hemodynamic benefit (PVR decrease of 226 dyn*s*cm^{-5} in the riociguat group vs. increase of 23 dyn*s*cm^{-5} in the placebo group), a better World Health Organisation functional class, and a reduction of pro-b natriuretic peptide levels in patients on this medication, compared with placebo (Ghofrani *et al.*, 2013). A subsequent open-label, long-term extension study (CHEST-2), providing riociguat to those patients previously receiving placebo, confirmed the exercise and functional status benefit of this medication for up to a year, with a similar safety profile achieved in CHEST-1 (Simonneau *et al.*, 2015).

Another treatment option that has emerged in the last few years is percutaneous trans-catheter balloon pulmonary angioplasty (BPA). Though early reports (Voorburg *et al.*, 1988; Feinstein *et al.*, 2001; Pitton *et al.*, 2003) suggested that some pulmonary hemodynamic benefit could be achieved in selected patients ('inoperable' CTEPH, poor surgical candidates), a resurgence of this procedure, primarily from centres in Japan and Norway, has documented significant hemodynamic improvements as long as one year after BPA in selected CTEPH patients (Sugimura *et al.*, 2012; Katoaka *et al.*, 2012; Mizoguchi *et al.*, 2012; Andreassen *et al.*, 2013; Fukui *et al.*, 2014; Taniguchi *et al.*, 2014).

The ultimate utility of this procedure in the treatment of CTEPH patients requires further study, as questions remain regarding appropriate patient selection, the optimal procedural approach and timing of repeat procedures, as well as technical adjustments to avoid reperfusion lung injury or pulmonary vascular injury. Also, as thromboendarterectomy surgery has been consistently demonstrated to be a potentially curative therapy for CTEPH patients, the burden of proof as to short- and long-term effectiveness of BPA is essential. Figure 26.3 depicts an expert suggested management algorithm.

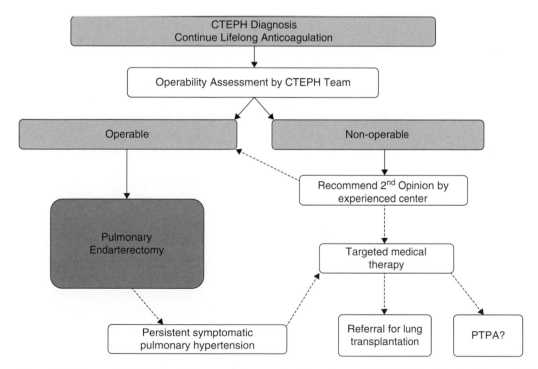

Figure 26.3 Suggested algorithm for treatment approaches for patients with CTEPH. Reprinted with permission from the *Journal of the American College of Cardiology* (Kim *et al.*, 2013).

Summary

Chronic thromboembolic pulmonary hypertension is the only form of pulmonary hypertension that is potentially curable. CTEPH incidence is ill-defined, estimated between 0.57% and 8.8% after an acute PE, though approximately 25% of patients with CTEPH do not report such an event. The disease pathophysiology is also poorly defined, and is theorised to be based on a combination of endothelial dysfunction, local inflammation and ineffective angiogenesis. Most patients present with dyspnoea on exertion, or exaggerated exercise intolerance, and a high level of suspicion is required in order to initiate the appropriate evaluation and avoid delays in diagnosis.

Echocardiography provides valuable information regarding pulmonary artery pressures and right ventricular characteristics, whereas routine laboratory tests, a hypercoagulable work-up, chest radiography, and pulmonary function testing help in the evaluation for comorbidities and for patient risk stratification. The screening test for chronic thromboembolic disease is the VQ scan, and confirmatory testing includes digital subtraction pulmonary angiography and right heart catheterisation, although CT angiography and magnetic resonance imaging provide valuable diagnostic information. Pulmonary thromboendarterectomy surgery, followed by life-long anticoagulation, remains the cornerstone of CTEPH treatment, with success rates related to the experience of the treatment centre. PH targeted medical therapy is now available and FDA-approved for inoperable cases or patients with residual pulmonary hypertension post-operatively, and balloon pulmonary angioplasty is a newly emerging treatment modality.

Key Points

- CTEPH is a potentially surgically curable form of pulmonary hypertension.
- The incidence of CTEPH is estimated between 0.57% and 8.8% after an acute PE but may be higher, based on approximately 25% of patients presenting without a prior episode of PE.
- CTEPH pathophysiology is poorly defined, but is theorised to be based on a combination of endothelial dysfunction, local inflammation and ineffective angiogenesis.
- A high level of suspicion and prompt evaluation of the patient complaining of dyspnoea on exertion is important to avoid delays in diagnosis.
- VQ scanning is the recommended screening study for chronic thromboembolic disease screening.
- The diagnosis of CTEPH is confirmed with digital subtraction pulmonary angiography and right heart catheterisation; thoracic CT angiography and magnetic resonance imaging provide important diagnostic information.
- Pulmonary thromboendarterectomy surgery remains the treatment of choice for CTEPH patie

Further Reading

Kim NH, Delcroix M, Jenkins DP *et al.* (2013) Chronic thromboembolic pulmonary hypertension. *Journal of the American College of Cardiology* **62**: D92–D99.

Klok FA, van der Hulle T, den Exter PL, Lankeit M, Huisman MV, Konstantinides S (2014). The post-PE syndrome: a new concept for chronic complications of pulmonary embolism. *Blood Reviews* **28**: 221–226.

Lang IM, Pesavento R, Bonderman D, Yuan JX-J (2013). Risk factors and basic mechanisms of chronic thromboembolic pulmonary hypertension: a current understanding. *European Respiratory Journal* **41**: 462–468.

Madani MM, Auger WR, Pretorius V, Sakakibara N, Kerr KM, Kim NK, Fedullo PF, Jamieson SW (2012). Pulmonary endarterectomy: recent changes in a single institution's experience of more than 2,700 patients. *Annals of Thoracic Surgery* **94**: 97–103.

Mayer E, Jenkins D, Lindner J, D'Armini A, Kloek J, Meyns B, Ilkjaer LB, Klepetko W, Delcroix M, Lang I, Pepke-Zaba J, Simonneau G, Darteville P (2011). Surgical management and outcome of patients with chronic thromboembolic pulmonary hypertension: results from an international prospective registry. *Journal of Thoracic and Cardiovascular Surgery* **141**: 702–710.

Ogo T (2015). Balloon pulmonary angioplasty for inoperable chronic thromboembolic pulmonary hypertension. *Current Opinion in Pulmonary Medicine* **21**: 425–431.

Papamatheakis DG, Kim NH (2015). Advances in the management of chronic thromboembolic pulmonary hypertension. *Current Hypertension Reports* **17**: 75.

Pengo V, Lansing AWA, Prins MH *et al.* (2004). Incidence of chronic thromboembolic pulmonary hypertension after pulmonary embolism. *New England Journal of Medicine* **350**: 2257–2264.

Pepke-Zaba J, Delcroix M, Lang I *et al.* (2011). Chronic thromboembolic pulmonary hypertension (CTEPH): Results from an international prospective registry. *Circulation* **124**: 1973–1981.

Bibliography

Alfakih K, Reid S, Jones T, Sivananthan M (2004). Assessment of ventricular function and mass by cardiac magnetic resonance imaging. *European Radiology* **14**: 1813–1822.

Andreassen AK, Ragnarsson A, Gude E, Geiran O, Andersen R (2013). Balloon pulmonary angioplasty in patients with inoperable chronic thromboembolic pulmonary hypertension. *Heart* **99**: 1415–1420.

Auger WR, Fedullo PF, Moser KM, Buchbinder M, Peterson KL (1992). Chronic major- vessel chronic thromboembolic pulmonary artery obstruction: Appearance at angiography. *Radiology* **183**: 393–398.

Becattini C, Agnelli G, Pesavento R, Silingardi M, Poggio R, Taliani MR, Ageno W (2006). Incidence of chronic thromboembolic pulmonary hypertension after a first episode of pulmonary embolism. *Chest* **130**: 172–175.

Bernard J, Yi FS (2007). Pulmonary thromboendarterectomy: a clinicopathologic study of 200 consecutive pulmonary thromboendarterectomy cases in one institution. *Human Pathology* **38**: 871–877.

Bonderman D, Turecek PL, Jakowitsch J, Weltermann A, Adlbrecht C, Schneider B, Kneussl M, Rubun LJ, Kyrle PA, Klepetko W, Maurer G, Lang IM (2003). High prevalence of elevated clotting factor VIII in chronic thromboembolic pulmonary hypertension. *Thrombosis and Haemostasis* **90**: 372–376.

Bonderman D, Skoro-Sajer N, Jakowitsch J, Adlbrecht C, Dunkler D, Taghavi S, Klepetko W, Kneussl M, Lang IM (2007). Predictors of outcome in chronic thromboembolic pulmonary hypertension. *Circulation* **115**: 2153–2158.

Bonderman D, Wilkens H, Wakounig S, Schafers H-J, Jansa P, Linder J, Simkova I, Martischnig AM, Dudczak J, Sadushi R, Skoro-Sajer N, Klepetko W, Lang IM (2009). Risk factors for chronic thromboembolic pulmonary hypertension. *European Respiratory Journal* **33**: 325–331.

Condliffe R, Kiely DG, Gibbs JS, Corris PA, Peacock AJ, Jenkins DP, Hodgkins D, Goldsmith K, Hughes RJ, Sheares K, Tsui SSL, Armstrong IJ, Torpy C, Crackett R, Carlin CM, Das C, Coghlan JG, Pepke-Zaba J (2008). Improved outcomes in medically and surgically treated chronic thromboembolic pulmonary hypertension. *American Journal of Respiratory and Critical Care Medicine* **177**: 1122–1127.

Corsico AG, D'Armini AM, Cerveri I, Klersy C, Ansaldo E, Niniano R, Gatto E, Monterosso C, Morsolini M, Nicolardi S, Tramontin C, Pozzi E, Vigano M (2008). Long term outcome after pulmonary thromboendarterectomy. *American Journal of Respiratory and Critical Care Medicine* **178**: 419–424.

Coulden R (2006). State-of-the-art imaging techniques in chronic thromboembolic pulmonary hypertension. *Proceedings of the American Thoracic Society* **3**: 577–583.

Daily PO, Auger WR (1999). Historical perspective: surgery for chronic thromboembolic disease. *Seminars in Thoracic and Cardiovascular Surgery* **11**: 143–151.

Darteville P, Fadel E, Mussot S, Chapelier A, Herve P, de Perrot M, Cerrina J, Ladurie FL, Lehouerou D, Humbert M, Sitbon O, Simmoneau G (2004). Chronic thromboembolic pulmonary hypertension. *European Respiratory Journal* **23**: 637–48.

de Perrot M, McRae K, Shargall Y, Pletsch L, Tan K, Slinger P, Ma M, Paul N, Moric J, Thenganatt J, Mak S, Granton JT (2011). Pulmonary thromboendarterectomy for chronic thromboembolic pulmonary hypertension: the Toronto experience. *Canadian Journal of Cardiology* **27**: 692–697.

de Perrot M, Thenganatt J, McRae K, Moric J, Mercier O, Pierre A, Mak S, Granton J (2015). Pulmonary endarterectomy in severe chronic thromboembolic pulmonary hypertension. *Journal of Heart and Lung Transplantation* **34**: 369–375.

Dentali F, Donadini M, Gianni M, Bertolini A, Squizzato A, Venco A, Ageno W (2009). Incidence of chronic pulmonary hypertension in patients with previous pulmonary embolism. *Thrombosis Research* **124**: 256–258.

Dorfmüller P, Günther S, Ghigna M-R, de Montpréville, Boulate D, Paul J-F, Jaïs X, Decante B, Simonneau G, Darteville P, Humbert M, Fadel E, Mercier O (2014). Microvascular disease in chronic thromboembolic pulmonary hypertension: a role for pulmonary veins and systemic vasculature. *European Respiratory Journal* **44**: 1275–1288.

Feinstein JA, Goldhaber SZ, Lock JE, Ferndandes SM, Landzberg MJ (2001). Balloon angioplasty for treatment of chronic thromboembolic pulmonary hypertension. *Circulation* **103**: 10–13.

Firth AL, Yao W, Ogawa A, Madani MM, Lin GY, Yuan JX (2010). Multipotent mesenchymal progenitor cells are present in endarterectomized tissues from patients with chronic thromboembolic pulmonary hypertension. *American Journal of Physiology. Cell Physiology* **298**: C1217–C1225.

Freed DH, Thomson BM, Berman M, Tsui SSL, Dunning J, Sheares KK, Pepke-Zaba J, Jenkins DP (2011). Survival after pulmonary thromboendarterectomy: effect of residual pulmonary hypertension. *Journal of Thoracic and Cardiovascular Surgery* **141**: 383–387.

Fukui S, Ogo T, Morita Y, Tsuji A, Tateishi E, Ozaki K, Sanda Y, Fukuda T, Yasuda S, Ogawa H, Nakanishi N (2014). Right ventricular reverse remodeling after balloon pulmonary angioplasty. *European Respiratory Journal* **43**: 1394–1402.

Ghofrani HA, D'Armini AM, Grimminger F, Hoeper MM, Kim NH, Mayer E, Simonneau G, Wilkins MR, Fritsch A, Neuser D, Weimann G, Wang C (2013). Riociguat for the treatment of chronic thromboembolic pulmonary hypertension. *New England Journal of Medicine* **369**: 319–29.

Guerin L, Couturaud F, Parent F, Revel MP, Gillaizeau F, Planquette B, Pontal D, Guégan M, Simonneau G, Meyer G, Sanchez O (2014). Prevalence of chronic thromboembolic pulmonary hypertension after acute pulmonary embolism. *Thrombosis and Haemostasis* **112**: 598–605.

Hagl C, Khaladj N, Peters T, Hoeper MM, Logemann F, Haverich A, Macchiarini P (2003). Technical advances of pulmonary thromboendarterectomy for chronic thromboembolic pulmonary hypertension. *European Journal of Cardio-Thoracic Surgery* **23**: 776–781.

Hartz RS, Byme JG, Levitsky S, Park J, Rich S (1996). Predictors of mortality in pulmonary thromboendarterectomy. *Annals of Thoracic Surgery* **62**: 1255–1260.

Ishida K, Masuda M, Tanabe N, Matsumiya G, Tatsumi K, Nakajima N (2012). Long-term outcome after pulmonary endarterectomy for chronic thromboembolic pulmonary hypertension. *Journal of Thoracic and Cardiovascular Surgery* **144**: 321–326.

Jais X, D'Armini A, Jansa P, Torbicki A, Delcroix M, Ghofrani HA, Hoeper MM, Lang IM, Mayer E, Pepke-Zapa J, Perchenet L, Morganti A, Simonneau G, Rubin LJ (2008). Bosentan for treatment of inoperable chronic thromboembolic pulmonary hypertension: BENEFiT (Bosentan effects in iNopErable Forms of chronIc Thromboembolic pulmonary hypertension), a randomized, placebo-controlled trial. *Journal of the American College of Cardiology* **52**: 2127–2134.

Kapitan KS, Buchbinder M, Wagner PD, Moser KM (1989). Mechanisms of hypoxemia in chronic thromboembolic pulmonary hypertension. *American Review of Respiratory Disease* **139**: 1149–1154.

Katoaka M, Inami T, Hayashida K, Shimura N, Ishiguro H, Abe T, Tamura Y, Ando M, Fukuda K, Yoshino H, Satoh T (2012). Percutaneous transluminal pulmonary angioplasty for the treatment of chronic thromboembolic pulmonary hypertension. *Circulation: Cardiovascular Interventions* **5**: 756–762.

Kerr KM, Auger WR, Fedullo PF, Channick RN, Yi ES, Moser KM (1995). Large vessel pulmonary arteritis mimicking chronic thromboembolic disease. *American Journal of Respiratory and Critical Care Medicine* **152**: 367–373.

Kerr KM (2005). Pulmonary artery sarcoma masquerading as chronic thromboembolic pulmonary hypertension. *Nature Clinical Practice Cardiovascular Medicine* **2**: 108–112.

Kim HS, Fesler P, Channick RN, Knowlton KU, Ben-Yehuda O, Lee SH, Naeije R, Rubin LJ (2004). Preoperative partitioning of pulmonary vascular resistance correlates with early outcome after thromboendarterectomy for chronic thromboembolic pulmonary hypertension. *Circulation* **109**: 18–22.

Kim NH, Delcroix M, Jenkins DP, Channick R, Darteville P, Jansa P, Lang I, Madani MM, Ogino H, Pengo V, Mayer E (2013). Chronic thromboembolic pulmonary hypertension. *Journal of the American College of Cardiology* **62**: D92–D99.

Klok FA, van Kralingen KW, van Dijk APJ, Heyning FH, Vliegen HW (2010). Prospective cardiopulmonary screening program to detect chronic thromboembolic pulmonary hypertension in patients after acute pulmonary embolism. *Haematologica* **95**: 970–975.

Klok FA, van der Hulle T, den Exter PL, Lankeit M, Huisman MV, Konstantinides S (2014). The post-PE syndrome: a new concept for chronic complications of pulmonary embolism. *Blood Reviews* **28**: 221–226.

Korkmaz A, Ozlu T, Ozsu S, Kazaz Z, Bulbul Y (2012). Long-term outcomes in acute pulmonary thromboembolism: the incidence of chronic thromboembolic pulmonary hypertension and associated risk factors. *Clinical and Applied Thrombosis/Hemostasis* **18**: 281–288.

Kreitner K-F, Ley S, Kauczor H-U, Mayer E, Kramm T, Pitton MB, Krummenauer F, Thelen M (2004). Chronic thromboembolic pulmonary hypertension: pre- and postoperative assessment with breath-hold magnetic resonance techniques. *Radiology* **32**: 535–543.

Kreitner K-F, Kunz RP, Ley S, Oberholzer K, Neeb D, Gast KK, Heussel C-P, Eberle B, Mayer E, Kauczor H-U, Duber C (2007). Chronic thromboembolic pulmonary hypertension - assessment by magnetic resonance imaging. *European Radiology* **17**: 11–21.

Lang IM (2004). Chronic thromboembolic pulmonary hypertension – not so rare after all. *New England Journal of Medicine* **350**: 2236–2238.

Lang IM, Pesavento R, Bonderman D, Yuan JX-J (2013). Risk factors and basic mechanisms of chronic thromboembolic pulmonary hypertension: a current understanding. *European Respiratory Journal* **41**: 462–468.

Lang RM, Badano LP, Mor-Avi V, Afilalo J, Armstrong A, Ernande L, Flachskampf FA, Foster E, Goldstein SA, Kuznetsova T, Lancellotti P, Muraru D, Picard MH, Rietzschel ER, Rudski L, Spencer KT, Tsang W, Voigt JU (2015). Recommendations for cardiac chamber quantification by echocardiography in adults: An update from the American Society of Echocardiography and the European Association of Cardiovascular Imaging. *Journal of the American Society of Echocardiography* **28**: 1–39.

Ley S, Ley-Zaporozhan J, Pitton MB, Schneider J, Wirth GM, Mayer E, Duber C, Kreitner K-F (2012). Diagnostic performance of state-of-the-art imaging techniques for morphological assessment of vascular abnormalities in patients with chronic thromboembolic pulmonary hypertension (CTEPH). *European Radiology* **22**: 607–616.

Lisbona R, Kreisman H, Novales-Diaz J, Derbekyan V (1985). Perfusion lung scanning: differentiation of primary from thromboembolic pulmonary hypertension. *American Journal of Roentgenology* **144**: 27–30.

Madani MM, Auger WR, Pretorius V, Sakakibara N, Kerr KM, Kim NK, Fedullo PF, Jamieson SW (2012). Pulmonary endarterectomy: recent changes in a single institution's experience of more than 2,700 patients. *Annals of Thoracic Surgery* **94**: 97–103.

Maliyasena VA, Hopkins PMA, Thomson BM, Dunning J, Wall DA, Nq BJ, McNeil KD, Mullany D, Kermeen FD (2012). An Australian tertiary referral center experience of the management of chronic thromboembolic pulmonary hypertension. *Pulmonary Circulation* **2**: 359–364.

Marston NA, Brown j, Olson N, Auger WR, Madani M, Wong D, Raisinghani AB, DeMaria AN, Blanchard DG (2015). Right ventricular strain before and after pulmonary thromboendarterectomy in patients with chronic thromboembolic pulmonary hypertension. *Echocardiography* **32**: 1115–1121.

Mayer E, Jenkins D, Lindner J, D'Armini A, Kloek J, Meyns B, Ilkjaer LB, Klepetko W, Delcroix M, Lang I, Pepke-Zaba K, Simonneau G, Dartevelle P (2011). Surgical management and outcome of patients with chronic thromboembolic pulmonary hypertension: results from an international prospective registry. *Journal of Thoracic and Cardiovascular Surgery* **141**: 702–710.

Mikus PM, Mikus E, Martin-Suarez S, Galie N, Manes A, Pastore S, Arpesella G (2008). Pulmonary endarterectomy: an alternative to circulatory arrest and deep hypothermia: mid-term results. *European Journal of Cardio-Thoracic Surgery* **34**: 159–163.

Miniati M, Monti S, Bottai M, Scoscia E, Bauleo C, Tonelli L, Dainelli A, Giuntini C (2006). *Survival and restoration of pulmonary perfusion in a long-term follow-up of patients after acute pulmonary embolism.* **85**: 253–262.

Mizoguchi H, Ogawa A, Munemasa M, Mikouchi H, Ito H, Matsubara H (2012). Refined balloon pulmonary angioplasty for inoperable patients with chronic thromboembolic pulmonary hypertension. *Circulation: Cardiovascular Interventions* **5**: 748–755.

Morris TA, Marsh JJ, Chiles PG, Magana MM, Liang NC, Soler X, Desantis DJ, Ngo D, Woods VL Jr. (2009). High prevalence of dysfibrinogenemia among patients with chronic thromboembolic pulmonary hypertension. *Blood* **114**: 1929–1936.

Morsolini M, Nicolardi S, Milanesi E, Sarchi E, Mattiucci G, Klersy C, D'Armini AM (2012). Evolving surgical techniques for pulmonary endarterectomy according to the changing features of chronic thromboembolic pulmonary hypertension patients during 17-year single-center experience. *Journal of Thoracic and Cardiovascular Surgery* **144**: 100–107.

Moser KM, Bloor CM (1993). Pulmonary vascular lesions occurring in patients with chronic major vessel thromboembolic pulmonary hypertension. *Chest* **103**: 685–692.

Nicod P, Peterson K, Levine M, Dittrich H, Buchbinder M, Chappuis F, Moser K (1987). Pulmonary angiography in severe chronic pulmonary hypertension. *Annals of Internal Medicine* **107**: 565–568.

Nikolaou K, Schoenberg SO, Attenberger U, Scheidler J, Dietrich O, Kuehn B, Rosa F, Huber A, Leuchte H, Baumgartner R, Behr J, Reiser MF (2005). Pulmonary arterial hypertension: diagnosis with fast perfusion imaging and high-spatial- resolution MR angiography – preliminary experience. *Radiology* **236**: 694–703.

Ogino H, Ando M, Matsuda H, Minatoya K, Sasaki H, Nakanishi N, Kyotani S, Imanaka H, Kitamura S (2006). Japanese single-center experience of surgery for chronic thromboembolic pulmonary hypertension. *Annals of Thoracic Surgery* **82**: 630–636.

Pengo V, Lansing AWA, Prins MH, Marchiori A, Davidson BL, Tiozzo F, Albanese P, Biasiolo A, Pegoraro C, Iliceto S, Prandoni P; Thromboembolic Pulmonary Hypertension Study Group (2004). Incidence of chronic thromboembolic pulmonary hypertension after pulmonary embolism. *New England Journal of Medicine* **350**: 2257–2264.

Pepke-Zaba J, Delcroix M, Lang I, Mayer E, Jansa P, Ambroz D, Traecy C, D'Armini AM, Morsolini M, Snijder R, Bresser P, Torbicki A, Kristensen B, Lewczuk J, Simkova I, Barbera JA, de Perrot M, Hoeper MM, Gaine S, Speich R, Gomez-Sanchez MA, Kovacs G, Hamid AM, Jais X, Simonneau G (2011). Chronic thromboembolic pulmonary hypertension (CTEPH): Results from an international prospective registry. *Circulation* **124**: 1973–1981.

Pitton MB, Düber C, Mayer E, Thelen M (1996). Hemodynamic effects of nonionic contrast bolus injection and oxygen inhalation during pulmonary angiography in patients with chronic major-vessel thromboembolic pulmonary hypertension. *Circulation* **94**: 2485–2491.

Pitton MB, Herber S, Mayer E, Thelen M (2003). Pulmonary balloon angioplasty of chronic thromboembolic pulmonary hypertension (CTEPH) in surgically inaccessible cases. *RöFo* **175**: 631–4.

Quarck R, Wynants M, Verbeken E, Meyns B, Delcroix M (2015). Contribution of inflammation and impaired angiogenesis to the pathobiology of chronic thromboembolic pulmonary hypertension. *European Respiratory Journal* **46**: 431–443.

Raisinghani A, Ben-Yehuda O (2006). Echocardiography in chronic thromboembolic pulmonary hypertension. *Seminars in Thoracic and Cardiovascular Surgery* **18**: 230–235.

Rajaram S, Swift AJ, Capener D, Telfer A, Davies C, Hill C, Condliffe R, Elliot C, Hurdman J, Kiely DG, Wild JM (2012). Diagnostic accuracy of contrast-enhanced MR angiography and unenhanced proton MR imaging compared with CT angiography in chronic thromboembolic pulmonary hypertension. *European Radiology* **22**: 310–317.

Reichelt A, Hoeper MM, Galamski M, Keberle M (2009). Chronic thromboembolic pulmonary hypertension: Evaluation with 64-detector row CT versus digital subtraction angiography. *European Journal of Radiology* **71**: 49–54.

Rossi SE, McAdams HP, Rosado-de-Christenson ML, Franks TJ, Galvin JR (2001). Fibrosing mediastinitis. *Radiographics* **21**: 737–757.

Sakao S, Hao H, Tanabe N, Kasahara Y, Kurosu K, Tatsumi K (2011). Endothelial-like cells in chronic thromboembolic pulmonary hypertension: crosstalk with myofibroblast-like cells. *Respiratory Research* **12**: 109.

Saouti N, Morshuis WJ, Heijmen RH, Snijder RJ (2009). Long-term outcome after pulmonary endarterectomy for chronic thromboembolic pulmonary hypertension: a single institution experience. *European Journal of Cardio-Thoracic Surgery* **35**: 947–952.

Satoh T, Kyotani S, Okano Y, Nakanishi N, Kunieda T (2005). Descriptive patterns of severe chronic pulmonary hypertension by chest radiography. *Respiratory Medicine* **99**: 329–336.

Simonneau G, D'Armini AM, Ghofrani H-A, Grimminger F, Hoeper MM, Jansa P, Kim NH, Wang C, Wilkins M, Fritsch A, Davie N, Colorado P, Mayer E (2015). Riociguat for the treatment of chronic thromboembolic pulmonary hypertension: along-term extension study (CHEST-2). *European Respiratory Journal* **45**: 1293–1302.

Soler X, Kerr KM, Marsh JJ, Renner JW, Hoh CK, Test VJ, Morris TA (2012). Pilot study comparing SPECT perfusion scintigraphy with CT pulmonary angiography in chronic thromboembolic pulmonary hypertension. *Respirology* **17**: 180–184.

Steenhuis LH, Groen HJM, Koeter GH, van der Mark TW (2000). Diffusion capacity and haemodynamics in primary and chronic thromboembolic pulmonary hypertension. *European Respiratory Journal* **16**: 276–281.

Sugimura K, Fukumoto Y, Satoh K, Nochioka K, Miura Y, Aoki T, Tatebe S, Miyamichi-Yamamoto S, Shimokawa H (2012). Percutaneous transluminal pulmonary angioplasty markedly improves pulmonary hemodynamics and long-term prognosis in patients with chronic thromboembolic pulmonary hypertension. *Circulation Journal* **76**: 485–488.

Sugiura T, Tanabe N, Matsuura Y, Shigeta A, Kawata N, Jujo T, Yanagawa N, Sakao S, Kasahara Y, Tatsumi K (2013). Role of 320-slice computed tomography in the diagnostic workup of patients with chronic thromboembolic pulmonary hypertension. *Chest* **143**: 1070–1077.

Suntharalingam J, Treacy CM, Doughty NJ, Goldsmith K, Soon E, Toshner MR, Sheares KK, Hughes R, Morrell NW, Pepke-Zaba J (2008). Long-term use of sildenafil in inoperable chronic thromboembolic pulmonary hypertension. *Chest* **134**: 229–236.

Taniguchi Y, Miyagawa K, Nakayama K, Kinutani H, Shinke T, Okada K, Okita Y, Hirata KI, Emoto N (2014). Balloon pulmonary angioplasty: an additional treatment to improve the prognosis of patients with chronic thromboembolic pulmonary hypertension. *EuroIntervention* **10**: 518–525.

Thistlethwaite PA, Kemp A, Du L, Madani MM, Jamieson SW (2006). Outcomes of pulmonary thromboendarterectomy for treatment of extreme thromboembolic pulmonary hypertension. *Journal of Thoracic and Cardiovascular Surgery* **131**: 307–313.

Thompson B, Tsui SSL, Dunning J, Goodwin A, Vuylsteke A, Latimer R, Pepke-Zaba J, Jenkins DP (2008). Pulmonary endarterectomy is possible and effective without the use of complete circulatory arrest – the UK experience in over 150 patients. *European Journal of Cardio-Thoracic Surgery* **33**: 157–163.

Toshner M, Suntharalingam J, Fesler P, Soon E, Sheares KK, Jenkins D, White P, Morrell NW, Naeije R, Pepke-Zaba J (2012). Occlusion pressure analysis role in partitioning of pulmonary vascular resistance in CTEPH. *European Respiratory Journal* **40**: 612–617.

Tunariu N, Gibbs SJ, Win Z, Gin-Sing W, Graham A, Gishen P, Al-Nahhas A (2007). Ventilation-perfusion scintigraphy is more sensitive than multidetector CTPA in detecting chronic thromboembolic disease as a treatable cause of pulmonary hypertension. *Journal of Nuclear Medicine* **48**: 680–684.

van der Plas MN, Reesink HJ, Roos CM (2010). Pulmonary endarterectomy improves dyspnea by the relief of dead space ventilation. *Annals of Thoracic Surgery* **89**: 347–352.

Voorburg JAI, Cats VM, Buis B, Bruschke AVG (1988). Balloon angioplasty in the treatment of pulmonary hypertension caused by pulmonary embolism. *Chest* **94**: 1249–1253.

Wijesuriya S, Chandratreya L, Medford AR (2013). Chronic pulmonary emboli and radiologic mimics on CT pulmonary angiography. A diagnostic challenge. *Chest* **143**: 1460–1471.

Wolf M, Boyer-Neumann C, Parent F, Eschwege V, Jaillet H, Meyer D, Simonneau G (2000). Thrombotic risk factors in pulmonary hypertension. *European Respiratory Journal* **15**: 395–399.

Wong CL Szydio R, Gibbs S, Laffan M (2010). Hereditary and acquired thrombotic risk factors for chronic thromboembolic pulmonary hypertension. *Blood Coagulation & Fibrinolysis* **21**: 201–206.

Wynants M, Quarck R, Ronisz A, Alfaro-Moreno E, Van Raemdonck D, Meyns B, Delcroix M (2012). Effects of C-reactive protein on human pulmonary vascular cells in chronic thromboembolic pulmonary hypertension. *European Respiratory Journal* **40**: 886–894.

Zabini D, Nagaraj C, Stacher E, Lang IM, Nierlich P, Klepetko W, Heinemann A, Olschewski H, Balint Z, Olschewski A (2012). Angiostatic factors in the pulmonary endarterectomy material from chronic thromboembolic pulmonary hypertension patients cause endothelial dysfunction. *PLoS One* **7**(8): e43793.

27

Predicting Recurrent VTE

R. Campbell Tait

Honorary Professor of Haemostasis and Thrombosis, Department of Haematology, Glasgow Royal Infirmary, Glasgow, UK

Following a first episode of venous thrombosis, treated with a finite period of anticoagulation, the risks of recurrent VTE (rVTE) are approximately 10%, 20%, 30% and 40% at one, three, five and ten years, respectively. Such recurrence rates are not insignificant, as are the potential consequences: post-thrombotic syndrome, chronic thromboembolic pulmonary hypertension (both discussed in previous chapters), and death. However, over a ten-year period, it is clear that the majority of patients will remain recurrence-free. Therefore, any decision to recommend indefinite anticoagulation must balance its benefits against the associated risks of major and fatal bleeding.

Long-term therapeutic anticoagulation has been shown to reduce the risk of recurrent VTE by 80–90%. However, the benefit to an individual patient will greatly depend on their own absolute risk of recurrence, so understanding the risk factors which influence recurrence rates is essential. The absolute rVTE rate which merits long-term anticoagulation (i.e. when the benefits clearly outweigh the risk) will vary from patient to patient, depending on the patient's bleeding risk and on the likely severity of any consequence of a rVTE event. The annual risk of major bleeding during anticoagulation with a vitamin K antagonist is 1–3%, with a case fatality rate of 9–13%, while the estimated fatality rate of a rVTE is 3.6–5%.

Based on these estimates, and consistent with current clinical practice, it is generally accepted that finite-term (e.g. three months) anticoagulation is indicated for patients with a perceived rVTE rate of ≤ 5% at one year or ≤ 15–20% at five years. Patients with higher predicted rVTE rates need individual risk assessments and consideration for indefinite anticoagulation. Established and putative risk factors which may influence the risk of rVTE are described below, and summarised in Table 27.1.

Factors Influencing Risk of Recurrent VTE

Provoked and Unprovoked VTE

Approximately one half of all VTE events occur without any obvious trigger, while the other half has an identifiable precipitating or provoking factor, which may be a transient or permanent risk factor. When there is a major persisting (e.g. cancer) or permanent risk factor (e.g. major immobility such as lower limb paresis), the risk of rVTE is high, so continuing anticoagulation as long as the risk factor persists is indicated. In contrast, following a first VTE associated with a transient risk factor, rates of rVTE are low, and indefinite anticoagulation is rarely indicated, especially when VTE has occurred after major surgery, following which rVTE rates are < 1% per year.

Meanwhile, rVTE following a non-surgical provoking event (e.g. trauma, temporary immobilisation, pregnancy or oestrogen use) has been recorded at 4.2%/year over the initial two years, but not as high as

Handbook of Venous Thromboembolism, First Edition. Edited by Jecko Thachil and Catherine Bagot.
© 2018 John Wiley & Sons Ltd. Published 2018 by John Wiley & Sons Ltd.

Table 27.1 Risk factors for recurrent VTE following a first unprovoked VTE.

Established risk factors *(hazard ratio >2.0 for recurrent VTE)*	Comment
PE or proximal DVT (*vs.* distal DVT)	
Elevated fibrin D-dimer four weeks after anticoagulant cessation	
Fibrin D-dimer prior to anticoagulant cessation	Non-low levels may only be discriminatory in females
Male sex	
Major Thrombophilia (antiphospholipid syndrome, antithrombin, protein C and protein S deficiency)	Evidence for inherited thrombophilias is relatively weak and based on studies of thrombophilia families
High Factor VIII or von Willebrand factor	Very high levels – above 75th or 90th percentiles
Post-thrombotic syndrome	May only be discriminatory in females
Weak or possible risk factor *(hazard ratio < 2.0 for recurrent VTE)*	
Residual vein occlusion	Meta-analysis suggests not a significant risk factor following unprovoked VTE
Age	Younger age may be more of a risk in males, while older age is a risk in females
Factor V Leiden or prothrombin *G20201A* variant	Meta-analyses report hazard ratios of 1.4–1.7 for recurrent VTE

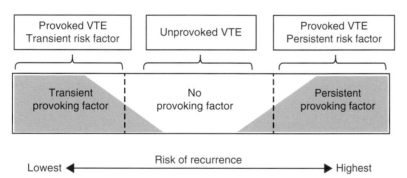

Figure 27.1 Conceptual framework for risk of recurrent VTE following provoked and unprovoked first VTE. *Source:* Kearon *et al.* (2016b). Reproduced with permission of International Society on Thrombosis and Haemostasis.

following an unprovoked VTE, when recorded recurrence rates are in the order of 7.4%/y over the initial two years. Indeed, a large observational cohort study reported rVTE rates, at one, three, five and ten years after anticoagulant cessation, respectively, of 6.6%, 12.3%, 16.1% and 22.5% following a VTE provoked by a transient risk factor, compared with 15%, 26.3%, 40.8% and 52.6% following unprovoked VTE.

This inverse association between the degree of provocation for an initial VTE and the risk of rVTE has been represented schematically (Figure 27.1) by the International Society on Thrombosis and Haemostasis, who have also suggested helpful definitions for major and minor provoking factors. Indeed, whether a VTE has been unprovoked is the single most important factor in deciding if a patient needs further assessment of their risk for rVTE and consideration for indefinite anticoagulation.

Site of VTE

The location of the initial VTE not only influences the risk of rVTE, but also the likely site for a recurrent event. The rVTE rate following a distal leg deep vein thrombosis (DVT) is approximately half of that following a proximal DVT or pulmonary embolism. Following a pulmonary embolism, the rVTE rates are similar to those following a proximal leg DVT, although the rVTE event is three times more likely to be a pulmonary embolism, which is then more likely to be fatal. The site of recurrence will also influence morbidity, with recurrent DVT being associated with a 2–3 fold higher risk of developing post-thrombotic syndrome and recurrent pulmonary embolism, associated with a 19 fold higher risk of developing chronic thromboembolic pulmonary hypertension.

Evidence for rVTE rates following VTE at unusual sites is limited. However, rVTE at any site following arm DVT, cerebral venous sinus thrombosis or abdominal vein thrombosis all appear to be lower than following proximal leg DVT or pulmonary embolism. Therefore, short-term anticoagulation is usually sufficient, following VTE with a transient risk factor or unprovoked VTE occurring at these unusual sites.

Duration of Initial Anticoagulant Therapy

Current evidence supports the need for at least three months anticoagulation following an initial VTE, and historical data demonstrate that an initial period of anticoagulation of ≤ 6 weeks is associated with a higher rVTE rate following anticoagulant cessation. In contrast, longer finite periods of anticoagulation, greater than 3–6 months, do not benefit patients with unprovoked VTE at potentially high risk of rVTE as, once anticoagulation is discontinued, rVTE rates are similar. Therefore, a patient with an unprovoked VTE should either receive 3–6 months or indefinite duration anticoagulation, the latter being reserved for those assessed as having a sufficiently high risk of rVTE.

Age, Sex and Obesity

While increasing age is associated with increased risk of first VTE, a similar risk associated with rVTE is less clear. Some studies show a small incremental risk with each ten-year age band for rVTE, while others do not. However, it appears that there may be an interaction with gender, in that higher rates of rVTE are seen in older women but in younger men.

Several observational studies have demonstrated higher rVTE rates in males, compared with females. The association is strongest following unprovoked VTE, when hazard ratios (HR) of around 2.2 for rVTE have been reported. Age at first VTE is generally lower in females compared with males and, in young women, it can often be associated with use of estrogenic hormonal preparations. However, even after adjusting for these confounders, rVTE appears more common in men.

The evidence for rVTE being more common in obese patients is mixed, with some studies suggesting a slight increased rVTE rate when BMI is ≥ 30, but this may be an association restricted to women.

Thrombophilia

High levels of procoagulant proteins and deficiencies of anticoagulant proteins, as well as the presence of the common Factor V Leiden and prothrombin G20210A thrombophilia variants, are recognised risk factors for first VTE. However, their influence on rVTE is thought to be minimal. Meta-analyses have generally shown statistically significant but small hazard ratios of 1.4–1.7 for rVTE in association with Factor V Leiden and prothrombin G20210A thrombophilia variants. Furthermore, in one study, homozygosity for either of these variants inferred no greater risk for rVTE than heterozygosity. Evidence regarding rVTE rates in the presence of a major thrombophilia, such as deficiency of antithrombin, protein C or protein S, is limited because of the relative rarity of these conditions. However, in studies of thrombophilic families with these conditions, there does appear to be a small increase in risk of rVTE (HR 2.8).

High levels of procoagulant proteins may also be associated with rVTE. Strongest associations have been demonstrated with very high levels of Factor VIII and von Willebrand factor, usually above the 75th or 90th percentile, when HR of 3–4 have been reported when measured at least three months after anticoagulant cessation.

Although generally accepted that individuals with antiphospholipid syndrome are at high risk of rVTE, the evidence supporting this is limited. In a moderately sized observational study, a single elevated anticardiolipin antibody measurement was associated with a two-fold higher risk of rVTE, while several small poorly controlled studies have suggest up to six-fold higher rVTE rates in lupus anticoagulant-positive patients.

Fibrin D-dimer

Markers of coagulation activation, or its potential, might reasonably be predictive for rVTE. Indeed, elevated levels of the fibrin degradation product D-dimer have consistently been associated with 2–2.5 fold higher rVTE rates. This is especially so following unprovoked VTE, but is also seen in some studies following VTE provoked by a transient risk factor. In most studies following unprovoked VTE, D-dimer has been assessed 3–4 weeks following anticoagulant cessation, when levels above the normal range are associated with higher risk of rVTE. However this association remains true at later time points. Also, at least in women, D-dimer levels within the lower half of the normal range (Vidas D-dimer, < 250 µg/l) prior to anticoagulant cessation are associated with a lower rVTE rate.

Thrombin generation has been assessed as a risk factor for rVTE. Initial reports suggested high peak thrombin levels may be associated with rVTE. However, subsequent studies show no association between any of the thrombin generation parameters and the risk of rVTE following unprovoked VTE.

Residual Vein Occlusion and Post-thrombotic Syndrome

Following DVT of the leg, there is gradual recanalisation of the thrombosed vessel. Serial ultrasound examinations demonstrate that at six months, approximately 40% of patients will have completely recanalised, with no evidence of residual venous occlusion (RVO) while, after three years, this figure will be nearer 75%. Initial reports have suggested that the absence of any residual vein occlusion is associated with a significantly lower rVTE rate. However, results from subsequent studies have been less promising, and a meta-analysis concluded that, following unprovoked DVT, residual vein occlusion at the time of anticoagulant cessation was not predictive of rVTE. Some guidelines recommend continuing anticoagulation following cerebral venous sinus thrombosis and abdominal vein thrombosis, until there is full recanalisation of the thrombosed vessel. However, this is expert opinion, rather than evidence-based.

Post-thrombotic syndrome of varying degrees develops in around 25% of patients with leg DVT, and has been associated with rVTE. In particular, the presence of any one of the three common signs (HER: hyperpigmentation, oedema and redness) at six months following an unprovoked proximal DVT of the leg has been associated with a 2.5–3 fold increase in rVTE in both men and women.

Other Factors

Pregnancy and the puerperium, and the use of oral oestrogen-containing hormonal preparations, are established transient risk factors for first VTE. Following a pregnancy-associated VTE, despite a 5–10% risk of rVTE during a subsequent pregnancy, the risk of unprovoked rVTE is very low. Use of oral oestrogen-containing hormonal preparations poses a lower risk of first VTE than does pregnancy. Therefore, some investigators have regarded such oral oestrogen associated VTE as unprovoked. However, in these studies, it is clear that their patients have a much lower risk of rVTE than other female patients with unprovoked VTE (HR typically around 0.5).

The above data on risk of rVTE is largely based on patients who have only had a single prior VTE. For those who have already had two VTE events, there is a temptation to automatically recommend indefinite anticoagulation after the second event. This is difficult to argue against when both events have been unprovoked. However, data from DURAC 1 and 2 studies would suggest that the cumulative rVTE rates following a second

VTE are very similar to those following a first event. Therefore, when only one of the two events has been unprovoked, there is probably merit in undertaking a standard risk assessment for rVTE, as would be done following a first unprovoked event.

Long term use of anticoagulant medication significantly reduces the risk of rVTE following unprovoked VTE. However long term use of other medications with potential antithrombotic properties have also been shown to have a modest effect on rVTE. Both the use of aspirin (HR 0.68, 95% CI, 0.51–0.90) and statins (HR 0.62, 95% CI, 0.45–0.85), particularly in patients without clinical arteriovascular disease, have been associated with small but significant reductions in rVTE rates.

Clinical Prediction Rules for Recurrent VTE

The majority of the above established and putative risk factors for rVTE, with hazard ratios in the range 1.5–2.5, have relatively small effects on the absolute rate of rVTE and are, therefore, insufficiently powerful predictors of rVTE to individually drive decision-making on long-term anticoagulation. However, several management studies in patients with unprovoked VTE have demonstrated the utility of D-dimer assessment, following cessation of anticoagulant therapy, in identifying a subgroup of patients who clearly benefit from continuing or re-starting long-term anticoagulant therapy.

A more individualised rVTE risk assessment may be gained by combining those risk factors which appear to be independent predictors of rVTE. This strategy has been tested in several large observational studies, including an individual patient data (IPD) meta-analysis, which have generated a variety of clinical prediction rules (CPR) or nomograms for rVTE following unprovoked DVT or pulmonary embolism (Table 27.2).

Table 27.2 Clinical prediction rules for recurrent VTE following unprovoked first VTE.

	Vienna prediction nomogram	HERDOO score (females only)	DASH score
Risk factors included:			
Fibrin D-dimer	Continuous variable	≥250 µg/l prior to stopping anticoagulant (1 point)	above reference range four weeks after stopping anticoagulant (2 points)
Male sex	Yes	–	Yes (1 point)
Age	–	≥65 years (1 point)	≤50 years (1 point)
BMI ≥ 30	–	Yes (1 point)	–
Signs of post thrombotic syndrome (HER)	–	Yes (1 point)	–
Site of first VTE	Proximal DVT or PE	–	–
1st VTE associated with hormonal trigger	–	–	Yes (−2 point)
Suggested cut-off score for low risk recurrent VTE	<180	≤1	≤1
Recurrent VTE rate for low score	4.4%/year over 5 years	1.6%/year over 4 years	3.1%/year over 7 years

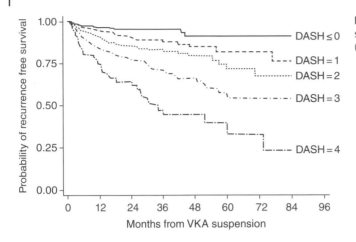

Figure 27.2 Cumulative rates of VTE recurrence-free survival according to DASH score. *Source*: Tosetto *et al.* (2012). Reproduced with permission of Wiley.

In each case, the aim was to identify a subgroup of patients with unprovoked VTE that had a low risk of rVTE (e.g. ≤ 20% at five years), such that long-term anticoagulant therapy was not indicated. In the Canadian HERDOO2, study no such group could be identified for men, although females with a low HERDOO score had a very low risk of rVTE. The Vienna study of unprovoked VTE patients, which did not include women with oral oestrogen-related VTE, identified site of initial VTE, male sex and D-dimer level three weeks following anticoagulant cessation as independent risk factors for rVTE.

Using D-dimer as a continuous variable, the Vienna Prediction Model nomogram was developed, allowing estimation of an individual's cumulative risk of rVTE at five years. This model has subsequently been updated to allow re-calculation of rVTE risk with D-dimer levels assessed at different time points, up to 15 months after anticoagulation cessation. The DASH model was derived from an IPD cohort of over 1800 patients with unprovoked VTE from seven separate, mainly observational, studies. This data set included oral oestrogen-related VTE as unprovoked, and weighted the independent risk factors according to their strength: 1 point for male sex and for age ≤ 50 years, 2 points for elevated D-dimer four weeks after anticoagulant cessation, and −2 points if initial VTE was oestrogen-related. An increasing DASH score was associated with an increasing risk of rVTE (Figure 27.2). In both the HERDOO and DASH cohorts, around 50% of patients had low scores with predicted rVTE rates < 4%/year.

Only the DASH score has been validated in separate patient cohorts with similar results. Using data from the MEGA follow-up study, consisting of more than 1000 patients with initial unprovoked VTE, a Dutch group confirmed the discriminative ability of the DASH score, with a *c*-statistic of 0.64. Interestingly, the *c*-statistic could be slightly improved to 0.67–0.68 by adding Factor VIII level to the model, or replacing D-dimer with Factor VIII.

Irrespective of their CPR score, it is clear that men suffering unprovoked VTE appear to have a particularly high risk of rVTE. Therefore, a valid question is whether they should ever stop anticoagulant therapy. Indeed, in a recent management study, those men ($n = 180$ aged ≤ 75 years) who had a normal D-dimer level following anticoagulant cessation, and did not restart anticoagulation, had a rVTE rate of 9.7%/year over an average follow-up period of 2.2 years. In the same study, women who had a normal D-dimer after stopping anticoagulation had an annual rVTE rate of 0% after an oestrogen therapy-related VTE, or 5.4% after an otherwise unprovoked VTE.

Conclusions

Decisions regarding the need for extended or indefinite anticoagulation appear straightforward for patients suffering a provoked VTE. On the other hand, for the 50% of patients who suffer an unprovoked VTE, a careful risk: benefit assessment is required, taking account of the relevant risk factors for rVTE, the potential consequences of rVTE, and also the risk of major bleeding should anticoagulation be continued. To aide this process, a variety of clinical prediction rules have been generated, although these remain imperfect – only applicable following DVT or pulmonary embolism and, in the most part, unvalidated.

Where the predicted risk of rVTE is around 20% at five years, there remains significant clinical uncertainty and, in these situations, patient perspectives (as regards their fears of rVTE or of bleeding complications of anticoagulant therapy) are paramount. It is possible that anticoagulation with one of the direct oral anticoagulants may confer a lower risk of major and fatal bleeding than with a vitamin K antagonist. If this is borne out from 'real life' experience with these agents, then the rVTE threshold for deciding upon indefinite anticoagulation may in the future be lowered.

Key Points

- Recurrent VTE is common, on average occurring in 40% patients over ten years following initial VTE.
- Following a VTE associated with a major permanent or persisting risk factor (e.g. cancer), long-term anticoagulation is indicated with reassessment if the risk factor is removed.
- Long-term anticoagulation is rarely, if ever, indicated following a VTE associated with a transient risk factor (e.g. surgery, pregnancy).
- Patients who suffer an unprovoked VTE require an individualised risk assessment for rVTE and its consequences, compared to their risk of bleeding, before deciding on the need for long-term anticoagulation.
- In general, following an unprovoked proximal DVT or pulmonary embolism, long-term anticoagulation is unlikely to be of net clinical benefit if the predicted risk of rVTE is ≤ 5% at one year or ≤ 15–20% at five years.
- Following unprovoked proximal DVT or pulmonary embolism, male sex and D-dimer level after anticoagulant cessation appear to be the most important and reproducible risk factors for rVTE.
- Clinical prediction scores for rVTE are still imperfect, and patients with low risk scores should be reminded that this does not mean 'no risk' of rVTE.

Further Reading

Ageno W, Dentali F, Donadini MP, Squizzato A (2013). Optimal treatment duration of venous thrombosis. *Journal of Thrombosis and Haemostasis* **11**(Suppl 1): 151–60.

Carrier M, Le Gal G, Wells PS, Rodger MA (2010). Systematic review: case-fatality rates of recurrent venous thromboembolism and major bleeding events among patients treated for venous thromboembolism. *Annals of Internal Medicine* **152**(9): 578–89.

de Jong PG, Coppens M, Middeldorp S (2012). Duration of anticoagulant therapy for venous thromboembolism: balancing benefits and harms on the long term. *British Journal of Haematology* **158**(4): 433–41.

Kearon C, Stevens SM, Julian JA (2015). D-Dimer Testing in Patients With a First Unprovoked Venous Thromboembolism. *Annals of Internal Medicine* **162**(9): 671.

Kearon C, Akl EA, Ornelas J, Blaivas A, Jimenez D, Bounameaux H, et al. (2016). Antithrombotic Therapy for VTE Disease: CHEST Guideline and Expert Panel Report. *Chest* **149**(2): 315–52.

Kearon C, Ageno W, Cannegieter SC, Cosmi B, Geersing GJ, Kyrle PA (2016). Categorization of patients as having provoked or unprovoked venous thromboembolism: guidance from the SSC of ISTH. *Journal of Thrombosis and Haemostasis* **14**(7): 1480–3.

Iorio A, Kearon C, Filippucci E, Marcucci M, Macura A, Pengo V, et al. (2010). Risk of recurrence after a first episode of symptomatic venous thromboembolism provoked by a transient risk factor: a systematic review. *Archives of Internal Medicine* **170**(19): 1710–6.

Prandoni P, Noventa F, Ghirarduzzi A, Pengo V, Bernardi E, Pesavento R, et al. (2007). The risk of recurrent venous thromboembolism after discontinuing anticoagulation in patients with acute proximal deep vein thrombosis or pulmonary embolism. A prospective cohort study in 1,626 patients. *Haematologica* **92**(2): 199–205.

Tosetto A, Iorio A, Marcucci M, Baglin T, Cushman M, *et al.* (2012). Predicting disease recurrence in patients with previous unprovoked venous thromboembolism: a proposed prediction score (DASH). *Journal of Thrombosis and Haemostasis* **10**(6): 1019–5.

Section VII

Controversies

28

Cancer Screening in Unprovoked Venous Thromboembolism
David Keeling

Consultant Haematologist, Oxford Haemophilia and Thrombosis Centre, Oxford University Hospitals, Oxford, UK

The association of cancer and venous thromboembolism (VTE) is well recognised. A number of mechanisms have been proposed, including release of inflammatory cytokines and pro-angiogenic factors by an underlying tumour, interaction between tumour cells and vascular endothelium leading to endothelial damage and platelet activation, and mass effect causing impaired venous return. On the basis of this association, it has become controversial as to how far to investigate someone presenting with unprovoked venous thromboembolism for possible underlying cancer, and whether computerised tomography (CT) screening for occult malignancy in asymptomatic patients is of clinical benefit.

A systematic review of 14 studies and an additional abstract (Carrier *et al.*, 2008) reported the prevalence of undiagnosed cancer in patients with unprovoked VTE as 6.1% (95% CI 5.0–7.1) at presentation, increasing to 10.0% (CI 8.6–11.3) at 12 months. Approximately 50% of these occult malignancies are picked up by standard clinical assessment, including history and examination, full blood count, urea and electrolytes, liver function tests, calcium, urinalysis and chest radiograph. However, screening with CT of the abdomen and pelvis (CT AP) and mammography may increase this detection rate by a further 13–20% (Carrier *et al.*, 2008; Piccioli *et al.*, 2004).

It is, however, incorrect to assume that earlier cancer detection automatically results in improved clinical outcomes. The negative consequences for the patient as a result of an equivocal or false positive scan result also need to be taken into account. These include patient anxiety and exposure to further high radiation doses (a CT of the abdomen is the equivalent of 400 chest radiographs) or other invasive investigations. Extended screening with CT and mammography also imposes a considerable burden on hospital economic and time resources.

The number of equivocal or false positive scans was very different in two influential studies in this area – the SOMIT study and the Trousseau study (Piccioli *et al.*, 2004; Van Doormaal *et al.*, 2011). These two studies, and a more recent larger randomised trial (Carrier *et al.*, 2015), are discussed below and summarised in Table 28.1.

In the SOMIT study, patients without cancer detected by standard care were randomised to extensive screening for occult cancer (*n* = 99) or to no further testing (*n* = 102) (Piccioli *et al.*, 2004). In 13 (13.1%) patients, extensive screening identified occult cancer, with a single (1.0%) further malignancy becoming apparent during two-year follow-up. In the control group, a total of 10 (9.8%) malignancies became apparent during two-year follow-up. Mean delay to diagnosis was reduced from 11.6 months to 1.0 month (*p* < 0.001). Cancer-related mortality during the two years follow-up period occurred in two (2.0%) of the 99 patients in the extensive screening group, versus four (3.9%) of the 102 control patients (non-significant absolute difference 1.9% (95% CI −5.5 to 10.9)).

Handbook of Venous Thromboembolism, First Edition. Edited by Jecko Thachil and Catherine Bagot.
© 2018 John Wiley & Sons Ltd. Published 2018 by John Wiley & Sons Ltd.

Table 28.1 Summary of key trials. See text for details.

	Number of patients	Cancer detected at baseline (%)	Additional cancers during follow-up (%)	Statistical differences in additional cancers during follow-up	Cancer deaths (%)	Statistical differences in cancer deaths
Piccioli *et al.*, 2004. Prospective randomised controlled study (patients with cancer detected at baseline with standard care excluded).						
SC	102	0 (0)	10/102 (9.8)	95% CI 1.3–36.8; $p < 0.01$	4 (3.9)	95% CI −5.5 to 10.9 $p = $ N/S
SC + ES	99	13 (13.1)	1/86 (1.2)		2 (1.9)	
Van Doormaal *et al.*, 2011. Not randomised (see text).						
SC	288	7 (2.4)	14/281 (5)	Adjusted HR 0.86 (95% CI 0.38–1.96)	8 (2.8)	Adjusted HR 1.79 (95% CI 0.74–4.35)
SC + ES	342	18 (5.3)	12/324 (3.7)		17 (5)	
Carrier *et al.*, 2015. Prospective randomised controlled study.						
SC	431	10 (2.3)	4/421 (0.9)	$P = 1.0$	6 (1.4)	$P = 0.28$
SC + ES	423	14 (3.3)	5/409 (1.2)		4 (0.9)	

SC – standard care; ES – extensive screening. CI –confidence intervals; HR – hazard ratio; OR – odds ratio; N/S – non-significant.

A year after publication, the data from the SOMIT trial were used to perform a decision analysis (Di Nisio *et al.*, 2005). The screening tests were divided into several possible strategies and the number of detected cancers, and the number of patients investigated further for what eventually turned out to be a benign condition, were calculated for each strategy. As an example, CT of the abdomen and pelvis detected ten of the 14 patients with occult cancer and had only one false-positive result. The authors concluded that screening for cancer with a strategy including abdominal/pelvic CT appears potentially useful, although its cost-effectiveness needs confirmation in a large trial.

The Trousseau study was a larger, prospective cohort study which compared limited and extensive cancer screening strategies (Van Doormaal *et al.*, 2011). All patients underwent baseline screening, consisting of history, physical examination, basic laboratory tests and chest X-ray. Of the 630 patients studied, 342 were seen in hospitals that performed additional extensive screening with CT chest/abdomen and mammography, and 288 in hospitals that did not. The initial limited screening detected malignancy in 12 out of 342 (3.5%) and seven out of 288 (2.4%), respectively.

In hospitals performing extensive screening 302 of the 330 remaining patients underwent screening, and suspicion of cancer was raised in 91 (30% of 302) and confirmed in six (2.0% of the 302), of which three were potentially curable. During a median 2.5 years of follow-up, cancer was diagnosed in an additional 12 patients in the extensive screening group, and an additional 14 patients in the limited screening group. In the extensive screening group, 26 patients (7.6%) died compared, with 24 (8.3%) in the limited screening group; adjusted hazard ratio 1.22 (95% CI 0.69–2.22). Of these deaths, 17 (5.0%) in the extensive screening group and eight (2.8%) in the limited screening group were cancer-related; adjusted hazard ratio 1.79 (95% CI 0.74–4.35). The study was designed to have cancer-related mortality as an end-point but, although recruitment was stopped when the numbers required were judged unobtainable, the authors nevertheless concluded that the low yield of extensive screening and lack of survival benefit did not support routine screening for cancer with abdominal and chest CT scan and mammography in patients with a first episode of unprovoked VTE.

In the United Kingdom, the National Institute for Health and Care Excellence (NICE) examined this issue for their June 2012 clinical guideline 'Venous thromboembolic diseases: the management of venous thromboembolic diseases and the role of thrombophilia testing' (NICE, 2012). Their rules for guideline production meant that they only considered the SOMIT study, as it was the only randomised controlled trial available. NICE recommended: 'Consider further investigations for cancer with an abdomino-pelvic CT scan (and a mammogram for women) in all patients aged over 40 years with a first unprovoked DVT or PE who do not have signs or symptoms of cancer based on initial investigation'.

NICE use the word 'consider' when they are confident that an intervention will do more good than harm for most patients, and be cost-effective, but other options may be similarly cost-effective. They accept that the choice of intervention, and whether or not to have the intervention at all, is more likely to depend on the patient's values and preferences than for a strong recommendation, so the healthcare professional should spend more time considering and discussing the options with the patient.

Whether to offer CT scanning remained controversial and, after the publication of the NICE guideline, practice varied considerably across the United Kingdom.

A large, multi-centre, open-label, randomised, controlled trial in Canada has now provided the best data to date (Carrier *et al.*, 2015). In this study, patients were randomly assigned to undergo limited occult-cancer screening (basic blood testing, chest radiography, and screening for breast, cervical, and prostate cancer) or limited occult-cancer screening in combination with CT abdomen and pelvis. The primary outcome measure was confirmed cancer that was missed by the screening strategy and detected by the end of the one-year follow-up period. Of the 854 patients who underwent randomisation, 33 (3.9%) had a new diagnosis of occult cancer between randomisation and the one-year follow-up: 14 of the 431 patients (3.2%) in the limited-screening group and 19 of the 423 patients (4.5%) in the limited-screening-plus-CT group ($P = 0.28$).

In the primary outcome analysis, four occult cancers (29%) were missed by the limited screening strategy, whereas five (26%) were missed by the strategy of limited screening plus CT ($P = 1.0$). There was no significant difference between the two study groups in the mean time to a cancer diagnosis (4.2 months in the limited-screening group and 4.0 months in the limited-screening-plus-CT group, $P = 0.88$) or in cancer-related mortality (1.4% and 0.9%, $P = 0.75$).

The authors concluded that the prevalence of occult cancer was low among patients with a first unprovoked venous thromboembolism, and routine screening with CT of the abdomen and pelvis did not provide a clinically significant benefit. All patients had sex-specific screening for breast, cervical and prostate cancer, if it had not been performed in the previous year. A breast examination, mammography or both were performed in women older than 50 years of age, and Papanicolaou (Pap) testing and a pelvic examination were performed in women 18–70 years old who had ever been sexually active. A prostate examination, prostate-specific antigen (PSA) test or both were performed in men older than 40.

Following this pivotal study, and taking all the evidence into account, the view of the author is that patients over 40 years old with an unprovoked VTE should have a full history and examination, a full blood count, urea and electrolytes (including calcium), liver function tests, dip-stick urinalysis, chest X-ray and, if not performed in the past year, mammography and a cervical smear, or a PSA. They should not then have a CT abdomen and pelvis as a routine investigation.

Key Points

- Cancer increases the risk of venous thromboembolism (VTE).
- Whether to investigate patients presenting with VTE for occult malignancy has been controversial.
- Screening has not been shown to reduce mortality.
- A small randomised trial in 2004 found a significant number of additional cancers with extensive screening. Although this was not duplicated in a non-randomised study, it caused the National Institute for Care and Health Excellence (NICE) in England to recommend screening be considered in patients with unprovoked VTE.

- A more recent, larger, randomised controlled trial found that the prevalence of occult cancer was low among patients with a first unprovoked venous thromboembolism, and routine screening with CT of the abdomen and pelvis did not provide a clinically significant benefit.
- The opinion of the author is that patients over 40 years with an unprovoked VTE should have a full history and examination, a full blood count, urea and electrolytes (including calcium), liver function tests, dip-stick urinalysis, chest X-ray and, if not performed in the past year, mammography and a cervical smear, or a prostate-specific antigen (PSA). They should not then have a CT abdomen and pelvis as a routine investigation.

Further Reading

Carrier M, Lazo-Langner A, Shivakumar S, Tagalakis V, Zarychanski R, Solymoss S, Routhier N, Douketis J, Danovitch K, Lee AY, Le Gal G, Wells PS, Corsi DJ, Ramsay T, Coyle D, Chagnon I, Kassam Z, Tao H, Rodger MA (2015). Screening for Occult Cancer in Unprovoked Venous Thromboembolism. *New England Journal of Medicine* **373**: 697–704.

Carrier M, Le Gal G, Wells PS, Fergusson D, Ramsay T, Rodger MA (2008) Systematic review: the Trousseau syndrome revisited: should we screen extensively for cancer in patients with venous thromboembolism? *Annals of Internal Medicine* **149**: 323–333.

Di Nisio M, Otten HM, Piccioli A, Lensing AW, Prandoni P, Buller HR, Prins MH (2005) Decision analysis for cancer screening in idiopathic venous thromboembolism. *Journal of Thrombosis and Haemostasis* **3**: 2391–2396.

NICE (2012). *Venous thromboembolic diseases: the management of venous thromboembolic diseases and the role of thrombophilia testing.* http://guidance.nice.org.uk/cg144.

Piccioli A, Lensing AW, Prins MH, Falanga A, Scannapieco GL, Ieran M, Cigolini M, Ambrosio GB, Monreal M, Girolami A, Prandoni P (2004) Extensive screening for occult malignant disease in idiopathic venous thromboembolism: a prospective randomized clinical trial. *Journal of Thrombosis and Haemostasis* **2**: 884–889.

Van Doormaal FF, Terpstra W, Van Der Griend R, Prins MH, Nijziel MR, Van De Ree MA, Buller HR, Dutilh JC, ten Cate-Hoek A, Van Den Heiligenberg SM, Van Der Meer J, Otten JM (2011) Is extensive screening for cancer in idiopathic venous thromboembolism warranted? *Journal of Thrombosis and Haemostasis* **9**: 79–84.

29

Sub-segmental and Incidental PE – to Treat or Not?

Jecko Thachil

Department of Haematology, Manchester Royal Infirmary, Manchester, UK

Introduction

Pulmonary embolism (PE) is associated with high mortality. In an increasingly medico-legal world, there are major concerns about missing a diagnosis like that of a PE, which has serious consequences, including fatality. This has translated to larger number of investigations for any symptom which may be loosely related to a PE. The easier availability of D-dimer testing is one of the commonest 'tests' in this context. Despite clear evidence to state that D-dimers are indicated in individuals in whom the diagnosis of a thromboembolism like PE is unlikely, most often these tests are performed to rule in a PE.

In addition, there is also an increasing trend towards radiological imaging for ruling out cancers and other diagnoses which have led to the identification of incidental findings, including a PE. Staging CT scans are one of the commonest radiological investigations in the current era, where the treatment of cancers has improved drastically and requires confirmation of the treatment success. Besides all of these, anxiety about missing a PE diagnosis also means there is an increased number of requests for computed tomography pulmonary angiography (CTPA), with less than 20% being identified to be positive. On the other hand, increased use of D-dimers and CT imaging means more PE are likely to be diagnosed, including incidental and sub-segmental PE.

Definitions

Incidental PE is defined as PE identified on radiological imaging performed for indications other than for the identification of thromboembolism. Although the terms 'silent PE' and 'unsuspected PE' have been used in publications, the current accepted terminology is 'incidental PE', probably because reports have concluded that many such patients may actually have symptoms suggestive of PE which are overlooked, and thus are not unsuspected or silent. The definition of sub-segmental PE is the presence of filling defects in the smaller branches of the pulmonary vasculature or the sub-segmental vessels.

Who Gets Incidental/Subsegmental PE?

The probability of finding a PE is higher in patients who have inherent risk factors for developing such thrombo-embolic problems. These groups of patients most commonly include those with an underlying malignancy. Cancer is one of the most thrombogenic conditions, and there are several publications which confirm the very strong association between thrombosis and malignancies, including treatment-resistant thrombosis. PE in these patients may be picked in the absence of definitive symptoms of breathlessness, chest pain or haemoptysis, because of radiological imaging done for staging of the cancer or confirming remission. In this context, we should consider fatigue as a 'symptom' of an underlying PE in the cancer setting. A retrospective case-control analysis of nearly 60 patients noted that 40% had signs or symptoms commonly associated with PE but, when the additional symptom of fatigue was included, 75% were symptomatic. This study showed that, in comparison with control patients, incidental PE was more common if there was a prior history of venous thromboembolism.

Another cohort of patients where incidental PE is likely to be identified is hospital in-patients. These individuals are, for obvious reasons, more likely to have scans and blood tests performed, which can pick up a PE. Also, the very fact that such patients may be less mobile, and have underlying disease states and co-morbidities which can increase the risk of thromboembolism, means they are more likely to get a PE. It may be argued that widespread use of prophylactic anticoagulation decreases the risk of hospital-acquired thrombosis, but it needs to be borne in mind that pharmacological thromboprophylaxis is not 100% effective. Added to this, there is the problem of under-dosing the prophylactic dose when prescription of the drug is not accurately based on the patient's weight.

The third group of patients who are more likely to be diagnosed with incidental PE is the group with high body mass index (BMI). Increased BMI and obesity is considered to be the new epidemic. Similar to cancer, there are several publications confirming the link between obesity and thrombosis. These patients very often have several co-morbidities, which require hospital admission and investigations which can pick up an incidental PE. This provides a dilemma when several symptoms of venous thromboembolism, including shortness of breath, palpitations, leg swelling and pain may have been attributed to being obese. It also opens up the conundrum of how to manage these cases, since there is no detailed literature about which is the best anticoagulant in this cohort of patients.

The Issue of Sub-segmental PE

The diagnosis of PE has become very streamlined in the current era. However, one of the big changes which has been noted in the diagnostic pathway for PE is that ventilation-perfusion (VQ) scanning, which was often the first-line imaging for PE, is rarely performed these days. These may be due to various reasons, including the high incidence of inconclusive results, easy availability out of hours of CT scanning, and the ability to diagnose conditions other than PE with a CT. Another sobering fact is that the widespread availability of CTPA has probably persuaded healthcare professionals to have a very low threshold for using the test to exclude PE.

The downside of this change in practice is the higher incidence of sub-segmental PE being diagnosed. Unlike the older single-slice CT scanners, the multi-detector CTPA has translated to more sub-segmental PE being diagnosed. This is evident from a systematic review and meta-analysis which noted the incidence of sub-segmental PE diagnosis with multiple-detectors being nearly 10%, compared with just below 5% with single detector CTPA. Another interesting aspect in this context is that, if V/Q scans were considered for the diagnosis of PE, the pivotal Prospective Investigation of Pulmonary Embolism Diagnosis (PIOPED) study showed that patients who had PE limited to sub-segmental branches of the pulmonary artery tend always to have low-probability V/Q scans, in the absence of prior cardiopulmonary disease. This would pull up the debate that, if a patient were suspected to have PE has a normal chest radiograph, shouldn't VQ scans be the next line of investigation, rather than CTPA? Also, with the arrival of the SPECT VQ sans, which are more sensitive and likely to have fewer intermediate-probability scans, this should certainly be the case.

Management Approach to Incidental/Sub-segmental PE

This is an area which has lot of prospective studies being undertaken at the current time. Hence, the landscape may change drastically in the near future. However, based on the current literature, the following approach may be followed:

1. Is it Really a PE?

The groups of patients who are diagnosed with incidental/sub-segmental PE are likely to have an increased baseline risk of PE, due to their co-existing illnesses or reduced mobility. But what needs to be certain is whether the abnormality on the CT scan really represents a PE. In other words, are the filling defects on the CT imaging representative of a clot? There is controversy among the experts about the correct diagnosis of a sub-segmental PE. An analysis of nearly one-third of sub-segmental PE on expert review was deemed indeterminate, and approximately one-fifth were considered false positive. The likelihood of false-positive interpretation is higher if the PE was located more peripherally, and was of a very small size. One additional practical issue in this regard is the respiratory motion artefacts, which is a significant contributor to false-positive results.

2. If a True PE, Do They Need Anticoagulation? If So, Whom?

The best answer to this dilemma comes from the study by den Exter and colleagues. When they analysed over 3700 patients with clinically suspected PE, of whom 16% had a sub-segmental PE, they found no differences in the risk of recurrent thrombosis or mortality between these patients and those with more proximal PE. This study would clarify any doubts on whether sub-segmental PE needs anticoagulation – the simple answer is 'yes'. However, expert recommendations have made a two-tier approach in this clinical area. All patients with sub-segmental PE should have bilateral lower limb Doppler examination, to exclude a deep vein thrombosis. If a clot is present, then it is logical to think that it could have embolised to cause the sub-segmental PE, and can be dangerous if left untreated.

3. Does the Patient Have Cardio-respiratory Symptoms?

If the patient does have a true PE but no associated DVT, can such patients be followed up without anticoagulation? This would be based pretty much on the patient's cardio-respiratory reserve. If the patient does have pre-existing cardio-respiratory problems, such as chronic obstructive airways disease or congestive cardiac failure, then even a minor decrease in pulmonary perfusion may be considered to be detrimental and, as such, even a sub-segmental PE should be considered for anticoagulation. On the other hand, if the patient is otherwise fit and well, close follow-up may be reasonable. Once again, in the oncology patients, the symptom of fatigue should not be overlooked as being due to a PE. In those for whom no anticoagulation route is chosen, detailed explanation is given, with advice to contact the emergency department if any features of clot develop.

Conclusion

In summary, incidental and sub-segmental PEs are an increasing problem in the current era. Patients with these diagnoses require anticoagulation if they have co-existing lower limb thrombosis, associated thrombotic risk factors or cardio-respiratory diseases, in the absence of any contraindications (increased bleeding risk). Those patients who do not fall into any of these categories may not require anticoagulation, but should have a close follow-up arranged.

Further Reading

Carrier M, Righini M, Le Gal G (2012). Symptomatic subsegmental pulmonary embolism: what is the next step? *Journal of Thrombosis and Haemostasis* **10**: 1486–90.

Carrier M, Righini M, Wells PS *et al.* (2010). Subsegmental pulmonary embolism diagnosed by computed tomography: incidence and clinical implications. A systematic review and meta-analysis of the management outcome studies. *Journal of Thrombosis and Haemostasis* **8**: 1716–22.

den Exter PL, van Es J, Klok FA *et al.* (2013). Risk profile and clinical outcome of symptomatic subsegmental acute pulmonary embolism. *Blood* **122**(7): 1144–1149.

Khorana AA, O'Connell C, Agnelli G, Liebman HA, Lee AYY, on Behalf of the Subcommittee on Hemostasis and Malignancy of the SSC of the ISTH (2012). Incidental venous thromboembolism in oncology patients. *Journal of Thrombosis and Haemostasis* **10**: 2602–4.

Miller WT Jr, Marinari LA, Barbosa E Jr. *et al.* (2015). Small pulmonary artery defects are not reliable indicators of pulmonary embolism. *Annals of the. American Thoracic Society* **12**: 1022–9.

O'Connell C (2015). How I treat incidental pulmonary embolism. *Blood* **125**(12): 1877–82.

O'Connell CL, Boswell WD, Duddalwar V *et al.* (2006). Unsuspected pulmonary emboli in cancer patients: clinical correlates and relevance. *Journal of Clinical Oncology* **24**(30): 4928–32.

Stein PD, Goodman LR, Hull RD, Dalen JE, Matta F (2012). Diagnosis and management of isolated subsegmental pulmonary embolism: review and assessment of the options. *Clinical and Applied Thrombosis/Hemostasis* **18**(1): 20–26.

Stein PD, Henry JW (1997). Prevalence of acute pulmonary embolism in central and subsegmental pulmonary arteries and relation to probability interpretation of ventilation/perfusion lung scans. *Chest* **111**: 1246–8.

Wiener RS, Schwartz LM, Woloshin S (2013). When a test is too good: how CT pulmonary angiograms find pulmonary emboli that do not need to be found. *BMJ* **347**: f3368.

30

Management of Distal Vein Thrombosis

Giuseppe Camporese[1] and Enrico Bernardi[2]

[1] Unit of Angiology, Department of Cardiac-Thoracic-Vascular Sciences, University Hospital of Padua, Italy
[2] Department of Emergency and Accident Medicine, Hospital of Conegliano, Italy

Diagnosis of Distal Deep-vein Thrombosis

Distal deep-vein thrombosis (DVT) involves the paired deep veins (i.e. the anterior tibial, the posterior tibial, and the peroneal veins), and the muscular veins (i.e. the gastrocnemius, and the soleal veins) of the calf. Distal DVT accounts for between 20% and 60% of all DVTs, in studies using venography or ultrasonography as the reference standard, respectively. When compared with proximal DVT, isolated distal DVT (IDDVT) is more frequently associated with transient risk factors (such as recent surgery, plaster-cast immobilisation, air travel, etc.), and carries an overall halved risk of death, pulmonary embolism – either symptomatic or asymptomatic – and recurrent venous thromboembolic events (VTE).

Ultrasonography of the whole-leg venous system (WLUS) is currently the first-line test for patients with suspected distal DVT. The proximal-vein system is examined first, with the patient supine, starting from the femoral veins (common, superficial and deep), and the proximal part of the great saphenous vein; then, with the patient sitting, the popliteal vein down to the trifurcation, and the proximal part of the small saphenous vein, are scanned. Only if proximal DVT is ruled out are the distal veins (see above) evaluated. The only validated diagnostic criterion is vein compressibility, although a lack of spontaneous or reverse-flow intraluminal colour-filling after augmentation manoeuvres may represent an adjunctive abnormal finding, limited to the muscular veins.

According to a meta-analysis of validation studies of WLUS versus venography, the sensitivity of WLUS is suboptimal, with a false-negative rate of up to 30% in symptomatic patients, reaching 60% in asymptomatic patients (Table 30.1). Nonetheless, a recent meta-analysis, pooling seven cohort studies of symptomatic patients managed with WLUS, reported a < 2% upper confidence limit of the three-month pooled incidence of VTE in untreated symptomatic patients, indicating that WLUS can safely rule out distal DVT in *unselected* patients. It is noteworthy that the corresponding figure in patients with a high pre-test probability for DVT (i.e. those with 'likely' or 'high' Wells score, or positive D-dimer) ranges between 3–6%, suggesting that WLUS may not be as efficient at ruling out DVT in that population.

By contrast, the specificity of WLUS is adequate in both symptomatic and asymptomatic patients (see Table 30.1), with a low probability of false-positive results in unselected patients. However, some authors claim that its indiscriminate use in low-risk patients may produce a number of false-positive results, resulting in potential overtreatment. Accordingly, the latest ACCP Guidelines do not recommend WLUS in these patients. Indeed, in the only two randomised studies comparing two-point US (i.e. limited to the proximal veins) with

Table 30.1 Performance of diagnostic test in patients with suspected distal DVT.

Test	Population	Sensitivity	Specificity	Reference
Whole-leg US	Symptomatic	75 (68–82)	94 (93–96)	Venography
Whole-leg US	Asymptomatic	39 (35–44)	97 (96–98)	Venography
D-dimer (ELISA)	Symptomatic	86 (84–88)	–	Mixed
D-dimer (Latex)	Symptomatic	79 (75–83)	–	Mixed
D-dimer (whole-blood)	Symptomatic	64 (55–73)	–	Mixed
Wells' score	Symptomatic	47 (36–57)	74 (70–77)	US
CT-venography	Symptomatic *	95 (91–97)	97 (95–98)	Mixed
MR-venography	Symptomatic	92 (88–95)	95 (93–97)	Venography

Data are reported as percentage (95% confidence interval)
US: ultrasonography; –: not reported; H: high; I: intermediate; L: low; Mixed: venography + US.
* Most studies included patients with suspected symptomatic PE.

WLUS in symptomatic patients, the 6–15% excess DVT recorded at baseline in the WLUS arm, solely due to the detection of IDDVT, did not result in a lower incidence of VTE during follow-up.

In addition, WLUS is time-consuming, requires expertise and dedicated equipment, and is only available during working hours, so alternative, readily available, low-cost non-invasive strategies would be desirable. In this respect, the sequential use of the Wells rule and D-dimer may be adequate. Indeed, although pooled data suggest that both are more accurate for proximal DVT than distal DVT, several randomised and cohort studies have demonstrated that it is safe to withhold anticoagulation in patients with suspected DVT with both a low pre-test probability and a normal D-dimer, irrespective of the location of symptoms (i.e., proximal versus distal deep-vein system).

Furthermore, a recent prospective study of patients with suspected IDDVT reported that, in patients with a low pre-test clinical probability, the negative predictive value of D-dimer is as high as 99% (95% CI 95–100%). Another possible approach, tested in a single randomised study, is to spare distal-vein testing in patients with normal two-point US who do not complain of calf symptoms or signs (so-called 'selective WLUS'). Such an approach has proved to be both safe, as the three-month pooled incidence of VTE in untreated symptomatic patients randomised to selective WLUS was 0.8%, and effective, as more than 40% of the patients in the selective WLUS arm were spared distal-vein testing.

Finally, CT- and MR-venography, two potential alternative diagnostic strategies, both possess adequate accuracy for IDDVT (Table 30.1). Unfortunately, no management studies with these techniques are available to date, so the consequences of basing treatment decisions on the results of CT- or MR-venography are still unknown. Furthermore, both techniques are invasive, and require sophisticated, costly equipment and high technical skills.

Conclusion

In conclusion, WLUS is the preferred approach to rule out and rule in distal DVT in symptomatic, unselected patients. Patients with suspected isolated DVT and either a low pre-test probability and a normal D-dimer, or without calf signs/symptoms and a normal proximal-vein ultrasonography, can be spared further testing. The safety of withholding treatment in high-risk patients with normal WLUS findings should be further investigated.

Treatment of Isolated Distal Deep-vein Thrombosis

Anticoagulant therapy is the mainstay for the treatment of proximal DVT and PE. However, whether anticoagulation for IDDVT is mandatory is still controversial.

To Treat or Not to Treat?

The suspicion rate for VTE has dramatically increased during the last 20 years, and IDDVT, as diagnosed by WLUS, accounts for roughly half of all DVTs. Despite the increasing frequency of IDDVT, there is ongoing debate in the literature regarding systematically searching for and treating IDDVT. This uncertainty is reflected in international guidelines and national policies.

Interestingly, the 10th edition of the ACCP guidelines for VTE treatment suggest serial imaging surveillance for two weeks, instead of anticoagulation in patients with acute symptomatic IDDVT without either severe symptoms, or risk factors for thrombus extension (Table 30.2) (grade 2C). Conversely, in patients with these features, anticoagulation is suggested (grade 2C), using the same therapeutic approach adopted for proximal DVT (grade 1B).

Indeed, ultrasonographic surveillance and compression therapy remain the commonly used approaches in patients with IDDVT in the USA, Canada and the Netherlands. In contrast, mandatory anticoagulation for IDDVT is recommended by the Australasian Society of Thrombosis and Haemostasis, by the British DVT

Table 30.2 Major and minor risk factors for IDDVT extension or recurrence.

Factors thought to be strongly associated with a higher risk of extension or recurrence
Previous VTE events
Unprovoked events
Secondary events but with persistently incomplete mobilization
VTE during pregnancy or puerperium
Multiple calf vein involvement with or without involvement of the venous tibio-peroneal trunk
Bilateral leg distal DVT
Active cancer with or without chemotherapy
Concomitant predisposing diseases (e.g. inflammatory bowel disease)
Known thrombophilia
Permanent risk factors
In-patient status
Initial calf vein diameter > 7 mm and/or thrombus length > 5 cm
Positive D-Dimer
Residual thrombus on ultrasonography > 4 mm
Presence of severe symptoms in the affected leg
Factors thought to be moderately associated with a higher risk of extension or recurrence
First thrombotic event secondary to surgery or other removable risk factors (e.g. plaster cast, immobilization, trauma, travel DVT)
Oral contraceptives or hormonal replacement treatment (treatment must be interrupted)
Patients able to recover an immediate full mobilization

Modified from Palareti (2014).

Consensus Group (2012), and by the International Consensus Statement on Prevention and Treatment of Venous Thromboembolism (2013). Accordingly, anticoagulation is prescribed to all symptomatic patients with IDDVT in some European countries, such as France, Spain, Italy and Germany.

Such heterogeneity is due to two main reasons. On one side, guidelines for IDDVT management do not provide a common management strategy or highlight a clear decision-making process, due to the scarce and conflicting evidence available. On the other side, cost-effectiveness or cost-minimisation are major issues for most healthcare services, and local reimbursement policies strongly influence treatment choice. Thus, it is conceivable that treatment costs may be felt to be potentially unnecessary by some health authorities, given that IDDVT is considered low-risk for life-threatening complications.

In our opinion, when a patient attends medical services with symptoms in his/her calf, he/she wants to know what is happening to his/her leg. From a practical point of view, it seems quite unfair to avoid investigating a symptomatic patient and, when a IDDVT is diagnosed, not to treat it. In this respect, the position paper by Palareti clearly states that diagnosing a calf DVT without giving any treatment causes anxiety in the patient, and disappointment in the physician concerning the management of the disease. Moreover, even if IDDVT is ruled out, the ultrasonographic investigation of the calf may be able to establish a differential diagnosis in up to 70% of patients with suspected IDDVT, frequently providing a conclusive answer to the patients' complaints.

Generally, we believe that when considering whether to treat or not to treat IDDVT, one must consider the following criteria: VTE complication rate (including extension to either the distal or the proximal-vein systems, fatal/symptomatic non-fatal PE); axial (tibial or peroneal veins) or muscular (gastrocnemial or soleal) involvement; risk of bleeding; late sequelae and VTE recurrence.

VTE Complication Rate

Some authors affirm that a systematic search for calf DVTs and their subsequent treatment appear to be at least debatable, due to the low VTE complication rate occurring in 15–25% of untreated patients. Also, three recent prospective trials investigating the natural history and treatment of IDDVT reported conflicting results. Palareti (2014) showed a cumulative 8% complication rate in 65 patients with objectively confirmed IDDVT who were left untreated, and monitored by means of serial WLUS. Horner *et al.* (2015) randomly assigned 70 patients to receive low molecular weight heparin (LMWH) and vitamin K antagonists (VKA) or no treatment for three months. In untreated patients, the complication rate was 11%, compared with 0% in patients receiving anticoagulation.

Conversely, Righini *et al.* (2006) randomised 259 patients with symptomatic IDDVT to receive LMWH plus graduated compression stockings, or placebo plus graduated compression stockings for six weeks. At the end of the three-month follow-up, the complication rate was not statistically different in the two randomisation groups (3.3% vs. 6.1%, $p = 0.51$); instead, the bleeding rate (major and clinically relevant non-major bleeding) was significantly higher in the LMWH group (4% vs. 0%, $p = 0.03$).

The major issue when considering VTE complications in patients with untreated IDDVT is the risk of PE and/or PE-related death. Obviously, PE may be caused either by partial dislodgement of a proximal-vein clot, leaving a residual thrombus in the calf-veins, or by IDDVT. Unfortunately, there is currently no way to distinguish if a PE is provoked by an IDDVT or by a proximal DVT; hence, it is almost impossible to estimate the real IDDVT-associated PE-risk. Nonetheless, an older study by Moreno-Cabral *et al.* (1976) reported a 33% incidence of asymptomatic PE at presentation in patients with IDDVT, while the corresponding figure in a more recent review was 13%. Finally, the incidence of non-fatal PE (mostly asymptomatic) in patients with objectively documented IDDVT undergoing WLUS surveillance is about 3.5%.

Axial or Muscular Involvement

Based on anatomical considerations, axial IDDVT might display a different clinical course compared to muscular-vein thrombosis (MVT). However, no randomised clinical trials are available on this issue. Several cohort studies have reported conflicting results, in terms of extension and need for anticoagulation. A small cohort study suggested that a short ten-day course of anticoagulation may reduce the extension of MVT to the axial calf veins or to the popliteal vein, while other studies reported no differences in prognosis at three months between muscular and axial IDDVT. Summarising, the currently available evidence does not support different treatment regimens for axial IDDVT, compared with MVT.

Bleeding Risk

The bleeding risk is higher in patients treated for proximal DVT and PE than in those with IDDVT, probably because patients with proximal DVT are treated for a longer time, and with higher doses of anticoagulants, compared with IDDVT patients. The risk of major and fatal bleeding is reported to be approximately 0.6–2.0% and 0.1–0.5%, respectively. This risk must be balanced against some 10% cumulative risk of local and proximal extension, PE and VTE-related death associated with IDDVT.

Recurrences and Late Sequelae

The risk of recurrence is reported to be higher in patients presenting with a proximal DVT or PE, compared with patients with IDDVT. A recent meta-analysis by Baglin *et al.* (2010) confirmed these data, showing that the cumulative five-year recurrence rate is five times higher in patients with proximal DVT than in patients with IDDVT (HR 4.76, 95% CI 2.06–10.98). Some risk factors have been identified that increase the risk of recurrence (Table 30.2), prompting treatment, while serial ultrasound testing is the suggested approach in patients without these risk factors.

In the long term, IDDVT may lead to post-thrombotic syndrome (PTS). In a mean five-year follow-up period, the incidence of PTS, as assessed by both the CEAP classification or Villalta Score, was reported to be as high as 11%. However, with a lack of prospective, blinded and well-designed randomised trials in this setting, no conclusive results can be drawn about the incidence and severity of PTS and its prevention with the use of prompt treatment for IDDVT.

Which Drug for Treatment of IDDVT?

The 10th edition of the ACCP guidelines suggest the use of standard anticoagulation (LMWH, fondaparinux, VKAs) for the treatment of IDDVT, but not the direct oral anticoagulants (DOACs), because IDDVT was excluded from all the phase III clinical trials involving DOACs. However, in all countries where DOACs are registered, approved and reimbursed for VTE treatment, their use for the treatment of IDDVT is not considered off-label, being not formally excluded by the package leaflet.

It is possible that the bleeding risk could be reduced with the use of DOACs, and a recent meta-analysis reported a risk ratio of 0.60 (95% CI 0.46–0.77) for fatal bleeding and 0.80 (95%CI 0.63–1.01) for major bleeding when DOACs are compared to warfarin. Interestingly, the few available data on the use of DOACs for treatment of IDDVT are safety data (major and fatal bleeding events) coming from prospective international registries (such as the RIETE and the PREFER-VTE, the latter still not published). For instance, the RIETE registry reported no major bleeding events in 163 patients with IDDVT treated with rivaroxaban. Similarly, in our personal experience at the Unit of Angiology of the University Hospital of Padua, only one major bleeding event was observed in 85 patients with IDDVT treated with rivaroxaban.

Duration of Treatment

The 10th edition of the ACCP guidelines suggested anticoagulant treatment for three months over a shorter time-period (grade 2C), and recommended anticoagulant treatment for three months over 6–24 months (grade 1B), or indefinite duration (grade 1B) in all patients with an IDDVT of the leg provoked by surgery or by a non-surgical transient risk factor. In patients with unprovoked IDDVT, anticoagulant therapy is recommended for at least three months over either a shorter period or longer time period (both grade 1B), but a new evaluation of patients for the risk-benefit ratio of the therapy is recommended at the end of the first three-month course of treatment.

Conclusion

The current body of literature does not provide conclusive recommendations on the treatment of IDDVT. Currently, two management strategies are available for patients with objectively documented symptomatic IDDVT:

1) anticoagulation for a period ranging from six weeks to three months, and a subsequent evaluation for treatment extension in patients with an unprovoked presentation; or
2) serial imaging surveillance to intercept local or proximal extension leading to mandatory anticoagulant treatment.

While awaiting properly, well-designed, rigorous, and adequately powered randomised clinical trials, we believe that all patients with an objectively documented IDDVT should be preferentially treated with DOACs for at least three months, depending on the nature of the presentation (i.e. provoked versus unprovoked).

Key Points

- Isolated distal DVT (IDDVT), as diagnosed by WLUS, accounts for roughly half of all DVTs.
- Compared to proximal DVT, IDDVT is more frequently associated with transient risk factors.
- Compared to proximal DVT, IDDVT is associated with significantly less risk of death, pulmonary embolism and recurrent venous thromboembolism.
- Whole-leg ultrasonography (WLUS) is the preferred approach to rule out and rule in distal DVT in symptomatic, unselected patients. Low-risk patients with suspected isolated DVT and a normal proximal-vein ultrasonography can be spared further testing.
- The safety of withholding treatment in high-risk patients with normal WLUS findings requires further investigation.
- The incidence and severity of PTS associated with IDDVT is unclear.
- The use of anticoagulation to treat IDDVT is controversial.
- Current evidence does not support different treatment regimens for axial IDDVT, compared with muscular vein IDDVT.
- Although IDDVT was excluded from all phase III clinical trials involving DOACs, their use for the treatment of IDDVT is not considered off-label.

References

Baglin T, Douketis J, Tosetto A, Marcucci M, Cushman M, Kyrle P, Palareti G, Poli D, Tait RC, Iorio A (2010). Does the clinical presentation and extent of venous thrombosis predict likelihood and type of recurrence? A patient-level meta-analysis. *Journal of Thrombosis and Haemostasis* **8**(11): 2436–42.

Bernardi E, Camporese G, Büller HR, Siragusa S, Imberti D, Berchio A, Ghirarduzzi A, Verlato F, Anastasio R, Prati C, Piccioli A, Pesavento R, Bova C, Maltempi P, Zanatta N, Cogo A, Cappelli R, Bucherini E, Cuppini S, Noventa F, Prandoni P; Erasmus Study Group (2008). Serial 2-point ultrasonography plus D-dimer vs whole-leg color-coded Doppler ultrasonography for diagnosing suspected symptomatic deep vein thrombosis: a randomized controlled trial. *JAMA* **300**(14): 1653–9.

Galanaud JP, Quenet S, Rivron-Guillot K *et al.*; Riete Investigators (2009). Comparison of the clinical history of symptomatic isolated distal deep-vein thrombosis vs. proximal deep-vein thrombosis in 11086 patients. *Journal of Thrombosis and Haemostasis* **7**(12): 2028–2034.

Galanaud JP, Sevestre MA, Genty C, Kahn SR, Pernod G, Rolland C, Diard A, Dupas S, Jurus C, Diamand JM, Quere I, Bosson JL; OPTIMEV-SFMV investigators (2014). Incidence and predictors of venous thromboembolism recurrence after a first isolated distal deep vein thrombosis. *Journal of Thrombosis and Haemostasis* **12**(4): 436–43.

Horner D, Hogg K, Body R, Nash MJ, Baglin T, Mackway-Jones K (2014). The Anticoagulation of Calf Thrombosis (ACT) Project. Results from the randomized controlled external pilot trial. *Chest* **146**(6): 1468–1477.

Horner D, Hogg K, Body R (2015). Should we be looking for and treating isolated calf vein thrombosis? *Emergency Medicine Journal* **33**(6): 431–7.

Hughes MJ, Stein PD, Matta F (2014). Silent pulmonary embolism in patients with distal deep venous thrombosis: systematic review. *Thrombosis Research* **134**(6): 1182–5.

Moreno-Cabral R, Kistner RL, Nordyke RA (1976). Importance of calf vein thrombophlebitis. *Surgery* **80**(6): 735–42.

Palareti G (2014). How I treat isolated distal deep vein thrombosis (IDDVT). *Blood* **123**: 1802–1809.

Righini M, Paris S, Le Gal G, Laroche JP, Perrier A, Bounameaux H (2006). Clinical relevance of distal deep vein thrombosis. Review of literature data. *Thrombosis and Haemostasis* **95**(1): 56–64.

Sartori M, Cosmi B, Legnani C, Favaretto E, Valdré L, Guazzaloca G, Rodorigo G, Cini M, Palareti G (2012). The Wells rule and D-dimer for the diagnosis of isolated distal deep vein thrombosis. *Journal of Thrombosis and Haemostasis* **10**(20): 2264–9.

Section VIII

Prevention

31

A Summary of the Evidence for VTE Prevention, with a Focus on the Controversies

Catherine Bagot

Consultant Haematologist, Department of Haematology, Glasgow Royal Infirmary, Glasgow, UK

Introduction

Venous thromboembolism (VTE) is a common problem with an incidence of approximately one per 1000 in the general population and associated sequelae of post-thrombotic syndrome, pulmonary hypertension, VTE recurrence and death. Strategies that can reduce this incidence and its associated morbidity and mortality should, therefore, be employed.

Over the years, a significant amount of evidence has accumulated regarding which measures may be effective at reducing the risk of VTE. This chapter provides a summary of the strategies that have been demonstrated to be effective in reducing VTE risk, and also those where perhaps more evidence is still required, and where their use remains controversial.

One major issue in the more controversial areas of this topic is the gap in evidence regarding an absence of significant decreases in symptomatic VTE with the use of prevention strategies – particularly LMWH. This lack of evidence often deters clinicians from exposing their patients to anticoagulation when the risk of bleeding is perceived as being higher than the risk of a clinically significant VTE. To detect a beneficial effect with LMWH use, patient groups need to be very large, as PE and symptomatic DVT are uncommon, so recruiting large patient numbers to randomised, controlled trials can be challenging and, therefore, often unable to be achieved. Studies will usually justify using the surrogate markers of asymptomatic and distal DVT, as there is a correlation between these and symptomatic DVT and PE. An assumption is made that if a significant reduction is seen in asymptomatic and/or distal DVT then, in a larger group, a reduction in the more significant VTE events would be shown.

This chapter is divided into strategies for reducing VTE risk in hospitalised patients, a group with a significantly increased VTE risk, followed by approaches for reducing risk in the general population outside of the hospital setting.

Hospitalised Patients

What is the Level of Risk?

Patients admitted to hospital are at significantly increased risk of VTE compared with those in the community. This risk is increased in all patient groups: In patients admitted to hospital with acute medical conditions, the risk increases at least eight-fold; for patients who undergo surgical procedures, the level of risk is affected by the surgical procedure being undertaken, and also the patient's associated co-morbidities (Sweetland *et al.*, 2009). For example, orthopaedic surgery (particularly joint arthroplasty) and cancer surgery are associated with a very high thrombotic risk that may be as high as 100-fold compared with the general population.

Risk Assessment Tools

Various risk assessment tools (RATs) for different patient groups are now being applied, based on variable levels of evidence. Their aim is to allow healthcare workers to make an easy, efficient, yet effective assessment of a patient's risk of VTE. RATs are most commonly used for patients admitted to hospital. Usually, risk factors are listed with associated tick boxes, to allow an easy assessment as to whether a particular patient would benefit from intervention to reduce their VTE risk. These risk factors will include risks inherent to the patient (e.g. age, weight), but also temporary risk factors associated with the inpatient stay (e.g. stroke, heart failure, surgical procedures).

Risk assessment tools usually also contain contraindications to prevention strategies. These can include an increased bleeding risk, such as thrombocytopaenia, haemophilia or renal failure, preventing safe use of low molecular weight heparin (LMWH). Contraindications to anti-embolism stockings (AES) are also usually listed (e.g. peripheral vascular disease or significant peripheral oedema). An example of the RAT used in Glasgow Royal Infirmary, Scotland, for most groups of medical and surgical patients, is shown in Figure 31.1.

Medical

There is now significant evidence that, if a patient is admitted to hospital with an acute medical illness and has at least one additional risk factor for VTE, their relative risk of VTE while in hospital will be reduced by approximately 60% with the daily use of prophylactic dose LMWH (Kahn *et al.*, 2012). Large international trials performed in the 1990s examined the effect on VTE risk of different forms of LMWH, and all demonstrated effectiveness in reducing the risk of VTE. The Medenox (enoxaparin) and Prevent (dalteparin) studies demonstrated a significant decrease in proximal DVT risk, the effect of which continued beyond the course of the LMWH treatment. The Artemis (fondaparinux) study reported a significant decrease only in the rate of asymptomatic distal DVT events, likely due to a very low rate of symptomatic events in either the treatment or placebo arms of the study. This study did not report on events beyond the period of treatment.

There is no evidence that antiembolism stockings (AES) are an effective strategy for reducing VTE risk in medical inpatients. Indeed, in patients admitted to hospital with acute stroke, the use of AES may be detrimental to patient outcomes. However, the recent CLOTS3 study demonstrated that, in this group of patients, who are both at high risk of bleeding during the first days following stroke, and also at very high risk of VTE, can have their risk of proximal DVT significantly reduced with the use of intermittent pneumatic compression (IPC) devices ($p = 0.001$). Furthermore, the probability of death at six months was significantly reduced in the IPC group ($p = 0.042$), suggesting that the use of IPC may improve overall mortality in this patient group. There was a significant increase in the prevalence of skin ulcers in patients using IPC, but the absolute incidence in both groups was low. The installation of IPC on stroke wards does have significant resource implications, but this study indicates that a safe method of VTE risk reduction in this high-risk patient group is available.

Surgical

General

Over many years, a significant amount of evidence has accumulated which indicates that unfractionated heparin (UFH) significantly reduces the risk of VTE in general surgical patients, including fatal PE and overall mortality. When LMWHs became available in the 1990s, they were compared to UFH, and were shown to

NHS GG&C Adult Risk Assessment for Venous Thromboembolism (VTE)

[excluding orthopaedics, obstetrics & ENT who have specialty-specific policies]

NHS
Greater Glasgow
and Clyde

- **Risk Assessment must be completed for all patients within 24 hours of admission to hospital**
- **Patients must be reassessed every 48-72 hours or sooner if condition changes**
- **Reassessment must be documented in Kardex**
- **Please complete risk assessment and then sign and date Risk Assessment Result box at bottom of page.**

Pt Addressograph

Operative patients	Non-operative patients

Is the patient bed-bound or expected to have reduced mobility relative to normal state for ≥ 2 days?

Yes ☐   No ☐

Does the patient have any risk factors for thrombosis? (tick √ all that apply)

Age >60	☐	Use of oestrogen-containing contraceptive therapy	☐
Active cancer or cancer treatment	☐	Use of hormone replacement therapy or tamoxifen	☐
Dehydration	☐	Pregnancy or < 6 weeks post partum	☐
Known thrombophilias	☐	Critical care admission eg HDU/ITU	☐
Obesity (BMI>30)	☐	Surgical procedure with total anaesthetic/surgical time >90 min, or >60 min if surgery on lower limb or pelvis	☐
Current significant medical condition e.g. Serious infection, Heart failure, Respiratory disease or Inflammatory disease	☐	Acute surgical admission with inflammatory or intra-abdominal condition including Pelvic Inflammatory Disease	☐
Personal history or first degree relative with a history of VTE	☐	Hip fracture	☐
Varicose veins with phlebitis	☐	All gynaecological surgery except uncomplicated gynaecological diagnostic day case procedures	☐

- No thromboprophylaxis required.
- Continue to reassess every 48-72 hours or sooner if condition changes.
- Document all reassessments in drug kardex.
- **Complete Risk Assessment Result Box.**

Yes, 1 or more risk factors identified ☐   No risk factors identified ☐

Indicators of high risk bleeding (tick √ all that apply)

Active bleeding	☐	Lumbar puncture, epidural/spinal anaesthesia • Expected within the next 12 hours • Within the previous 4 hours	☐
Acquired bleeding disorders (e.g. liver failure)	☐		
Concurrent use of other anticoagulants (e.g. warfarin, rivaroxaban, apixaban, edoxaban) is a contra-indication to additional phamacological thromboprophylaxis	☐	Other procedure with high bleeding risk – discuss with senior if unsure	☐
Acute stroke (within 14 days)	☐	Acute bacterial endocarditis	☐
Persistent uncontrolled hypertension (BP > 230/120 mmHg)	☐	Surgery expected within the next 12 hours	☐
Thrombocytopenia (<75 x 10⁹/l)	☐	Trauma with high bleeding risk e.g. Head Injury	☐
Untreated inherited bleeding disorders (e.g. haemophilia or von Willebrands)	☐	eGFR <30ml/minute/1.73m²: Dose reduction required	☐
High risk of peri- or post-procedural bleeding, e.g. neurosurgery , spinal, posterior eye surgery and thyroid surgery	☐	Heparin induced Thrombocytopenia	☐

- **Discuss with senior clinical staff before deciding to prescribe pharmacological prophylaxis**
- Consider mechanical prophylaxis e.g. AES unless contra-indicated.
- Reassess patient every 48-72 hours or sooner if condition changes.

No contraindications to pharmacological prophylaxis identified ☐   Contraindications to pharmacological prophylaxis identified ☐

Operative patients – Enoxaparin 40mg + AES ☐*
*prior to application of AES, please check contraindications to AES
Non-operative patients – Enoxaparin 40mg ☐
Prescribe Enoxaparin at 6pm
[on day of surgery, at the later of either 4h post-op or 6pm]
Reduce Enoxaparin to 20mg if <50Kg or eGFR <30ml/minute/1.73m² ☐
If weight> 120kg, consider Enoxaparin 40mg bd (see StaffNet Guideline).
Discontinue at discharge or when returned to pre-morbid mobility.

Contraindications to anti-embolism stockings (AES)   Y ☐   N ☐

Peripheral neuropathy	☐
Peripheral arterial disease	☐
Cellulitis or Gross oedema	☐
Leg deformity or Fragile skin	☐
Leg / foot ulcers	☐
Allergy	☐
Unusual leg size/shape	☐

Risk assessment result – please tick √ all that apply

VTE risk factors: YES ☐ NO ☐   Indicators of high risk bleeding: YES ☐ NO ☐   Prescribed: LMWH ☐ AES ☐ NONE ☐

Patient informed of VTE risks and benefits of thromboprophylaxis YES ☐ NO ☐ N/A ☐   Information leaflet provided YES ☐ NO ☐

Print Assessor's Name: _____   Signature: _____   Date: _____

RAT Medicine & Surgery – TEST OF CHANGE 09   Copyright © NHS Greater Glasgow and Clyde, 2016   **mi** • 250744 Version 9_0 • GGC0015

Figure 31.1 VTE risk assessment tool for medical and surgical inpatients (excluding orthopaedics, obstetrics and gynaecology) (reproduced with kind permission from NHSGGC Health Board).

have comparable efficacy. Given the favourable safety profile of LMWHs compared to UFH, LMWH is now the pharmacological prophylaxis of choice in general surgical patients (Gould *et al.*, 2012). In contrast to patients admitted with medical conditions, in surgical patients there is an additive benefit from the concurrent use of LMWH with AES and/or IPC. However, such studies have only indicated an improvement in the rate of asymptomatic DVT when pharmacological and mechanical methods are used concurrently.

AES can also reduce VTE risk when used alone in surgical patients, if the patient is unable to receive LMWH safely, due to the presence of additional bleeding risks. This benefit applies to general, gynaecological and orthopaedic surgery.

Orthopaedic

LMWH and mechanical thromboprophylaxis have similar rates of effectiveness in orthopaedic patients in reducing the incidence of VTE. Orthopaedic patients undergoing hip or knee arthroplasty also experience a reduction in VTE risk with the use of the recently introduced oral anticoagulants (either dabigatran, rivaroxaban or apixaban), which is comparable to that obtained with the use of prophylactic dose LMWH. The effectiveness of the new oral anticoagulants in reducing VTE risk is yet to be demonstrated in other surgical (or medical) patient groups.

Immobilisation of Lower Limb (Plaster Casts)

Patients who are immobile are at increased risk of VTE, probably resulting from stasis in the lower limb deep veins. This is particularly applicable to patients who have minimal calf muscle contractions when immobilised in a lower limb plaster cast. Reported VTE incidence varies widely, between 4–40% when patients do not receive thromboprophylaxis, with incidence rates likely being dependent on the severity of the underlying injury. and associated surgery.

Studies to date have been inconclusive as to whether LMWH is effective at reducing the rate of VTE in such patients. Furthermore, the duration of anticoagulation that may be appropriate is also not clear. Reasons for these results include the low rate of symptomatic events, heterogeneous groups included in each study, which likely had different levels of VTE risk, and the exclusion of high-risk VTE patients from the studies. A Cochrane review of the data involving immobilisation following fracture indicated a decreased risk of VTE with the use of LMWH, but highlighted the fact that the patient groups included were heterogeneous.

Guidelines vary in their recommendations, with NICE stating that pharmacological thromboprophylaxis can be considered in this patient group, but the ACCP stating that LMWH is not indicated. This conflicting guidance likely results from the fact that LMWH has only been shown to reduce asymptomatic VTE, and a reduction in symptomatic DVT and PE has not been demonstrated, the latter likely due to the fact that rates of PE in this patient group are very low.

Obstetrics

Pregnant women have a significantly increased risk of venous thrombosis of approximately one per 1000 pregnancies. Furthermore, VTE is one of the commonest causes of maternal mortality in the Western world. For this reason, there has been a significant drive, in recent years, to accurately assess a pregnant woman's risk of VTE during her pregnancy, and use pharmacological thromboprophylaxis if it is thought to be indicated.

The Royal College of Obstetricians and Gynaecologists (RCOG) provide guidelines for the prevention of VTE in pregnant women and when specific preventative measures should be used. The Royal College of Obstetricians and Gynaecologists (RCOG) have been providing comprehensive risk assessment tools to assess pregnant women and women in the post-partum period for a number of years. The most recent guidelines were released in April 2015, and recommend that all women should be risk-assessed during the antenatal period and post-natal period, and considered eligible for prophylactic dose LMWH if they have a significant number of risk factors for VTE (RCOG, 2015).

One method of risk assessment recommended in the guidelines uses a point system, awarding a greater number of points to the factors carrying the greatest VTE risk, and the number of points awarded determines the time point during the pregnancy at which thromboprophylaxis with LMWH should commence. For example, patients with a previous VTE, unprovoked, or provoked by anything other than surgery, gain four points, and are recommended to receive prophylactic dose LMWH from early in pregnancy until six weeks post-partum; women with a previous VTE in association with surgery gain three points when LMWH is recommended from 28 weeks gestation (Figure 31.2; RCOG, 2015).

Every woman who is recommended to receive LMWH during the antenatal period should receive six weeks post-partum LMWH, as the latter is the time of highest risk. Admission to hospital is considered a significant risk factor for VTE in all pregnant women, and all pregnant women admitted to hospital should receive LMWH, unless there is a contraindication such as an increased bleeding risk.

All evidence for the effectiveness of LMWH during pregnancy is extrapolated from other patient groups, and LMWH remains unlicensed for use during pregnancy. However, given the high risk of VTE during pregnancy, particularly in the post-partum period, and also the demonstrable low risk associated with LMWH use during pregnancy, it has gained an entrenched role in VTE prevention in pregnancy.

Cancer

Patients with cancer have a very high risk of VTE, and are known to benefit from LMWH during hospital admissions, whether for surgical or medical reasons (Lyman *et al.*, 2015). The VTE risk in cancer patients remains high while they are out of hospital, particularly during treatment with chemotherapy or radiotherapy.

A risk assessment tool has recently been produced for patients with myeloma, a malignant haematological condition, associated with a particularly high risk of VTE. The International Myeloma Working Group (IMWG) has produced a risk assessment tool categorising patients into low- and high-risk groups, depending on concurrent risk factors. Low-risk groups have been shown to benefit from aspirin alone, whereas high-risk patients have been shown to benefit from LMWH. High-risk patients include those who are receiving chemotherapy, or who have two additional risk factors for VTE, such as obesity, diabetes or previous VTE.

A risk assessment tool for outpatient cancer patients has been produced, using a points system which allocates points to markers of known thrombosis risk. Although this has been shown to demonstrate which outpatient cancer patients are at the greatest VTE risk, it has not yet been demonstrated that LMWH or another anticoagulant will safely reduce the VTE risk in outpatients shown to be at the greatest risk using this system. Trials in this area are ongoing (Di Nisio *et al.*, 2012).

Central Venous Catheters

Central venous catheters (CVCs) are associated with an increased risk of VTE, and the risk is known to be particularly high in patients with either a previous CVC thrombosis, previous PE or previous upper limb DVT.

A significant number of trials have been performed, including a meta-analysis, and these have shown that neither LMWH nor warfarin reduce the risk of VTE in such patients (Akl *et al.*, 2014), compared with placebo. Therefore, despite the high risk of VTE in this patient group, the use of pharmacological prophylaxis is currently not recommended.

Aspirin

Aspirin is now rarely used for VTE prevention. Although it may reduce the risk of VTE, compared with placebo, in some surgical patients, there is now a significant amount of evidence that UFH, LMWH and the new oral anticoagulants are highly effective at VTE prevention in some or all patient groups, and are likely to be far more effective than aspirin. The PEP study indicated that the use of aspirin for 35 days post-operatively

Appendix III: Risk assessment for venous thrombeoembolism (VTE)

- If total score ≥ 4 antenatally, consider thromboprophylaxis from the first trimester.
- If total score 3 antenatally, consider thromboprophylaxis from 28 weeks.
- If total score ≥ 2 postnatally, consider thromboprophylaxis for at least 10 days.
- If admitted to hospital antenatally consider thromboprophylaxis.
- If prolonged admission (≥ 3 days) or readmission to hospital within the puerperium consider thromboprophylaxis.

For patients with an identified bleeding risk, the balance of risks of bleeding and thrombosis should be discussed in consultation with a haematologist with expertise in thrombosis and bleeding in pregnancy.

Risk factors for VTE

Pre-existing risk factors	Tick	Score
Previous VTE (except a single event related to major surgery)		4
Previous VTE provoked by major surgery		3
Known high-risk thrombophilia		3
Medical comorbidities e.g. cancer, heart failure; active systemic lupus erythematosus, inflammatory polyarthropathy or inflammatory bowel disease; nephrotic syndrome; type I diabetes mellitus with nephropathy; sickle cell disease; current intravenous drug user		3
Family history of unprovoked or estrogen-related VTE in first-degree relative		1
Known low-risk thrombophilia (no VTE)		1[a]
Age (> 35 years)		1
Obesity		1 or 2[b]
Parity ≥ 3		1
Smoker		1
Gross varicose veins		1
Obstetric risk factors		
Pre-eclampsia in current pregnancy		1
ART/IVF (antenatal only)		1
Multiple pregnancy		1
Caesarean section in labour		2
Elective caesarean section		1
Mid-cavity or rotational operative delivery		1
Prolonged labour (> 24 hours)		1
PPH (> 1 litre or transfusion)		1
Preterm birth < 37^{+0} weeks in current pregnancy		1
Stillbirth in current pregnancy		1
Transient risk factors		
Any surgical procedure in pregnancy or puerperium except immediate repair of the perineum, e.g. appendicectomy, postpartum sterilisation		3
Hyperemesis		3
OHSS (first trimester only)		4
Current systemic infection		1
Immobility, dehydration		1
TOTAL		

Abbreviations: ART assisted reproductive technology; IVF in vitro fertilisation; OHSS ovarian hyperstimulation syndrome; VTE venous thromboembolism.

[a]If the known low-risk thrombophilia is in a woman with a family history of VTE in a first-degree relative postpartum thromboprophylaxis should be continued for 6 weeks.

[b]BMI ≥ 30 = 1; BMI ≥ 40 = 2

Figure 31.2 VTE risk assessment for obstetric patients, using a points system. Reproduced with kind permission from RCOG (2015).

reduced the risk of VTE in patients with arthroplasty, irrespective of whether other thromboprophylaxis was used concurrently. A similar reduction in risk was not seen for hemiarthroplasty. All reported VTE were symptomatic, with half being distal DVT.

Aspirin, however, did not have a significant effect when used alongside LMWH, and the use of aspirin resulted in a significant increased risk of bleeding, which was comparable to the reduction in symptomatic VTE risk. For this reason, although this study is often quoted as justification for the use of aspirin in thromboprophylaxis, the confounding effect of concurrent LMWH use, the increased bleeding risk, and the more recent accumulated evidence of better overall effectiveness of LMWH and the new oral anticoagulants, makes aspirin the less favourable option.

Mechanical Methods of Thromboprophylaxis

Anti-embolism Stockings

Anti-embolism stockings (AES) apply compression to the lower limb, resulting in increased venous flow in patients with reduced mobility. Their effectiveness in VTE prevention requires appropriate measurement of the patient's legs and the appropriate stocking pressure profile: 18 mm Hg at the ankle, 14 mm Hg at the mid-calf and 8 mm Hg at the upper thigh. Knee-length stockings, however, have been found to be as effective as thigh-length, and therefore either can be used. Both are commercially available at the appropriate pressures described. This has an additive effect on VTE prevention in surgical patients when used in addition to LMWH.

There are a number of contraindications to their use, including the following;

- Severe peripheral neuropathy.
- Severe peripheral arterial disease
- Diabetes.
- Severe peripheral oedema.
- Pulmonary oedema secondary to congestive cardiac failure.
- Severe leg deformity.
- Leg ulceration.

Intermittent Pneumatic Compression (IPC) Devices

IPC devices intermittently compress the leg, usually at the level of the calf, at a pressure of 35–40 mm Hg for approximately ten seconds every minute. They consist of a pump usually attached to the end of the patient's bed, with an attached sleeve placed around each calf. These are usually used peri- and post-operatively. They have recently been shown to also be effective in stroke patients, as described earlier.

The IPC devices reduce the risk of asymptomatic DVT in patients undergoing general surgery by over 60%, and significant reduce the risk of symptomatic DVT in patients undergoing hip arthroplasty. Therefore, there remains a need to accept the validity of extrapolation of distal/asymptomatic VTE to symptomatic/proximal DVT and PE events when using these devices.

What is the Most Appropriate Duration of Thromboprophylaxis?

Patients who are admitted to hospital for surgical procedures remain at increased risk of thrombosis for up to 90 days following discharge, with the duration in risk being shorter in patients who undergo day surgery procedures. What is unclear is whether such patients would benefit from extended thromboprophylaxis to reduce that risk. There is good evidence in patients undergoing knee and hip arthroplasty that a duration of thromboprophylaxis to ten days and 35–42 days, respectively, with either LMWH or a new oral anticoagulant, is beneficial in reducing risk. However, in other surgical and medical inpatients, there is no evidence, to date, that extended thromboprophylaxis beyond hospital discharge is beneficial.

In light of the lack of evidence in this area, clinicians will often consider extending thromboprophylaxis if they consider that they have a patient who is at particularly high risk of VTE (such as surgical cancer patients). National and international guidelines also recommend such a policy.

Prevention Strategies in the General Population

Body Weight

There is an increase in the risk of VTE that correlates not only with Body Mass Index (BMI), but also with waist circumference. These correlations apply equally to both DVT and PE.

The effect of losing weight translates into a decreased risk of VTE. Therefore, all patients with an increased BMI should be encouraged to lose weight, particularly if they have previously experienced a VTE, in order to reduce their thrombotic risk.

COCP/HRT

Medication containing estrogenic compounds increases the risk of VTE. These include the combined oral contraceptive pill (COCP) and Hormone Replacement Therapy (HRT). The risk is affected by the type of oestrogen and progestogen and the route of administration used. Tamoxifen, used for its anti-oestrogen effect in women with oestrogen receptor-positive breast cancer, also imparts an increased risk of VTE, due to its concurrent oestrogen agonist effect.

The use of the COCP, HRT or tamoxifen is contraindicated in women with a previous VTE. Such women should be advised to use alternative forms of contraception that do not contain oestrogen. Epidemiological and laboratory data suggests that the risk of VTE is very low in women who use transdermal HRT, although this reduced risk does not translate to transdermal contraception, probably due to the different formulation of oestrogen used in the latter group.

Despite the decreased VTE risk with transdermal HRT, it remains unclear whether this can be used safely in a woman with a previous VTE. In women for whom oestrogen-containing medications cannot be avoided, concurrent use of anticoagulation can be considered. Anastrozole can be considered as an alternative anti-cancer therapy to tamoxifen in post-menopausal women with oestrogen receptor positive breast cancer, and is not associated with an increased VTE risk.

Smoking

There appears to be a small increased risk of VTE of around 1.5 fold for smokers, compared to non-smokers, which does not completely return to baseline following discontinuation of smoking. The higher quantity of cigarettes smoked per day, alongside the younger age at which smoking starts, increases the risk further.

However, although smoking in itself may increase the risk of VTE, there is a significant possibility that there are confounders affecting the data, including obesity and other health problems associated with smoking, that also impart an increase VTE risk (e.g. heart failure, respiratory impairment).

Discontinuing smoking will, therefore, likely decrease the risk of subsequent VTE, either as a direct effect or via other health benefits associated with stopping smoking.

Travel

Travel is often promoted in the media as being associated with a high risk of VTE. However, the increased VTE risk associated with travel is much lower than that associated with other risk factors for VTE, which people might encounter during their lives.

The evidence as to how this risk can be decreased with interventions is very limited (Watson and Baglin, 2011). Clinicians will often recommend good hydration and frequent mobilisation. However, an association between dehydration and increased VTE risk has not been demonstrated. Given that immobility is likely to be one of the drivers for increased thrombotic risk in travellers, it seems reasonable to suggest frequent mobilisation, but this has not been demonstrated to reduce VTE risk in this cohort.

There are no studies indicating that LMWH, or any other form of anticoagulation, decreases the risk of travel related VTE in travellers at high VTE risk, and its use in this population can only be based on indirect evidence that anticoagulation such as LMWH is effective in other groups at high VTE risk. Travellers at high risk of VTE could be considered to be either those who have undergone recent surgery, or who have active cancer.

Only one trial of acceptable quality has investigated the effectiveness of compression stockings in travellers considered to be at low risk of VTE. Two hundred and thirty-one air travellers considered to be at low risk of VTE were randomised to wear either Class 1 compression stockings or no stockings. Twelve travellers developed asymptomatic distal DVT, none of whom wore stockings. This was a small trial, where asymptomatic distal DVT had to be considered a surrogate marker for clinical relevant VTE.

Lifestyle Advice

Some risk factors for VTE are modifiable, and therefore patients can be given advice on measures they can take to reduce the risk of VTE. These include maintaining a normal body weight, such that BMI remains between 20 and 25. Smoking increases the risk of VTE, either directly or indirectly and should, therefore be avoided for this, as well as for other, health reasons. Patients who have had a previous VTE should avoid oestrogen-containing medications, including the COCP, HRT and tamoxifen. However, progesterone-only contraception can be used safely.

While on long journeys, whether by car, train or plane, mobilising every two hours, remaining well-hydrated and performing ankle flexion and extension exercises while seated, is pragmatic advice, with minimal evidence being available on this topic. Compression stockings and prophylactic doses of anticoagulation, such as LMWH or the direct oral anticoagulants, can be considered for high-risk travellers, but the evidence for their effectiveness in this group is minimal (Figure 31.3; Watson and Baglin (2011)).

Figure 31.3 Proposed risk assessment and preventative measures in travellers. *Source*: Watson and Baglin (2011). Reproduced with permission of Blackwell Publishing Ltd.

Duration of travel	<3 h	3–8 h	>8 h
Risk group			
Low	Nil	Nil	Nil
Intermediate	Nil	Nil or stockings	Stockings
High	Nil	Stockings	Stockings ± anticoagulant

Risk group	Examples of risk factors for VTE
Low	None
Intermediate	All others e.g. Up to 6 weeks post-partum. Previous unprovoked VTE no longer on anticoagulants Previous travel-related VTE Combinations of risk factors
High	Major surgery in previous 4 weeks Active cancer undergoing chemo-radiotherapy in the previous 6 months, awaiting surgery or chemo-radiotherapy or in palliative phase

Key Points

1) LMWH reduces VTE risk in hospitalised medical patients with at least one additional risk factor.
2) LMWH reduces VTE risk in hospitalised surgical patients.
3) Risk reduction must always be balanced against risk of bleeding when anticoagulation is used.
4) Obstetric patients are at increased risk of thrombosis, and evidence for the effectiveness of LMWH in pregnant women is extrapolated from other patient groups.
5) The direct oral anticoagulants are as effective as LMWH in reducing VTE risk in patients undergoing either hip or knee arthroplasty.
6) No pharmacological intervention can reduce risk of VTE associated with central venous catheter use, although risk factors are known.
7) Cancer patients are at very high VTE risk, particularly in hospital but, to date, effectiveness of LMWH in ambulatory cancer patients has only been demonstrated in myeloma.
8) Oestrogen-containing medications should be avoided in women with previous VTE. Transdermal HRT is associated with the lowest VTE risk.
9) A healthy lifestyle of normal weight and non-smoking should be promoted for VTE risk reduction.

Further Reading

Akl EA, Ramly EP, Kahale LA, Yosuico VED, Barba M, Sperati F, Cook D, Schünemann H (2014). Anticoagulation for people with cancer and central venous catheters. *Cochrane Database of Systematic Reviews* **10**. Art. No.: CD006468. doi: 10.1002/14651858.CD006468.pub5.

Di Nisio M, Peinemann F, Porreca E, Rutjes AWS (2012). Primary prophylaxis for venous thromboembolism in ambulatory cancer patients receiving chemotherapy. *Cochrane Database of Systematic Reviews* **2**. Art. No.: CD008500. doi: 10.1002/14651858.CD008500.pub2.

Gould MK, Garcia DA, Wren SM, Karanicolas PJ, Arcelus JI, Heit JA, Samama CM; American College of Chest Physicians (2012). Prevention of VTE in nonorthopedic surgical patients: Antithrombotic Therapy and Prevention of Thrombosis, 9th ed: American College of Chest Physicians Evidence-Based Clinical Practice Guidelines. *Chest* **141**: e227S-e277S.

Kahn SR, Lim W, Dunn AS, Cushman M, Dentali F, Akl EA, Cook DJ, Balekian AA, Klein RC, Le H, Schulman S, Murad MH; American College of Chest Physicians (2012). Prevention of VTE in non-surgical patients. *Chest* **141**: e195S–e226S.

Lyman GH, Bohlke K, Khorana AA, *et al.* (2015). Venous thromboembolism prophylaxis and treatment in patients with cancer: American Society of Clinical Oncology clinical practice guideline update 2014. *Journal of Clinical Oncology* **33**: 654–656.

Royal College of Obstetricians and Gynaecologists (2015). *Reducing the Risk of Venous Thromboembolism during Pregnancy and the Puerperium* (Appendix 3). Green-top Guideline No. 37a, April 2015.

Sweetland S, Green J, Liu B, Berrington de González A, Canonico M, Reeves G, Beral V (2009). Million Women Study collaborators. Duration and magnitude of the postoperative risk of venous thromboembolism in middle aged women: prospective cohort study. *BMJ* **339**: 4583.

Watson HG, Baglin TP (2011). Guidelines on travel-related venous thrombosis. *British Journal of Haematology* **152**: 31–34.

32

VTE Prevention: Real World Practice

Emma Gee

Nurse Consultant, Thrombosis and Anticoagulation, King's College Hospital NHS Foundation Trust, London, UK

This chapter will discuss real-world experiences of implementing venous thromboembolism (VTE) prevention strategies, and ways to overcome common challenges. The broad structure of a successful VTE prevention strategy will be examined, followed by discussion of two fundamental elements of VTE prevention; risk assessment and appropriate thromboprophylaxis.

The Strategy

The Thrombosis Team

The Agency for Healthcare Research and Quality (AHRQ; Maynard and Stein, 2008) in the USA recommends 'assembling an effective team' as an essential first step in ensuring success in VTE prevention. In England, multi-disciplinary thrombosis teams, comprising of specialist doctors, nurses, pharmacists and diagnostic technicians are common. Their role is to work collaboratively, to ensure an effective and sustainable systems-based approach to VTE prevention.

A thrombosis committee, made up of stakeholders involved in VTE, oversee the work of the thrombosis team. Their remit encompasses the writing and implementation of local protocols, leading audit, delivering an education and support programme for clinical staff, working with patient representative groups, and developing VTE governance structures. In practice, the combined efforts of the thrombosis teams and committees have expedited and maintained change that has directly improved patient outcomes (Roberts *et al.*, 2013). The thrombosis committee has an essential role in creating the VTE prevention vision for an organisation, and engaging and empowering staff to deliver that vision. They are also a great source of support and advice to the organisation, and their expertise enables them to influence national and international practice by contributing to the existing evidence base.

Best Practice

The definition of best practice will dictate the standards an organisation should strive for. National and international peer-reviewed VTE prevention guidelines are available which set out these standards. In England, as part of the National VTE Prevention Programme, the National Institute for Health and Care Excellence (NICE) have published guidelines and quality standards (NICE, 2010a, 2010b). The quality standards cover aspects of care such as risk assessment, appropriate thromboprophylaxis and patient information (https://www.nice.org.uk/Guidance/QS3). The American College of Chest Physicians (ACCP) (Holbrook *et al.*, 2012) has also published evidence-based practice guidelines.

The challenges for health care providers often involve the implementation of guidance, assessment of outcomes and decisions in areas that lack a scientific evidence base. Thrombosis committees are, therefore, tasked with the development of local guidelines that are clear and accessible, to ensure standardised high-quality practice throughout the organisation. The challenge here is providing clarity that can result in consistent practice, while allowing for clinical judgement to be applied to individualised care. For example, at King's College Hospital, London, the stroke and thrombosis teams worked closely to develop guidelines that were practical and also addressed the risk benefit dilemma appropriately. This was necessary, because the interpretation of the recommendation from NICE – to consider chemical thromboprophylaxis if risk of bleeding is deemed to be low in stroke victims – is subjective, potentially leading to variation in practice.

Once best practice has been defined and agreed, it is necessary to gain an understanding of the baseline – that is, how guidelines are currently implemented. This could be in the form of an audit and discussion with key members of the organisation to discover what current practice, perceptions and cultures are like. From this baseline, goals and timelines can be formed as part of the quality improvement strategy.

Support

The AHRQ (Maynard and Stein, 2008) suggest that gaining support from the institution is another essential first step. Practice experience has shown that support from key leaders in an organisation is vital in enabling meaningful changes to practice to be embedded. It aids access to financial and knowledge resources, provides senior leadership, and allows for alignment of goals within an organisation.

Another integral part of the VTE prevention programme in England was the establishment of a National VTE Exemplar Centres Network tasked with improving patient outcomes through sharing best practice and resources. Exemplar centres are required to demonstrate excellence in the field of VTE prevention and an ongoing commitment to quality improvement. The broad aims of the VTE Exemplar Centres are summarised in Figure 32.1.

In practice, the network is an active community that shares guidelines, materials, effective strategies and innovative solutions. They are a form of support to each other, and also to other organisations wishing to benefit from the resources, experience and expertise of these centres. Essential criteria for centres applying for exemplar status are shown in Figure 32.2.

Education

A quality education programme is an important part of achieving engagement with the VTE prevention pathway. For individuals to commit to an organisation's VTE prevention strategy, understanding of its vision, its necessity and how it can be achieved needs to be communicated.

- To support implementation of the National VTE Prevention Programme in England, ensuring VTE risk assessment and appropriate thromboprophylaxis for all adult patients admitted to hospital.
- To develop a holistic approach to VTE prevention.
- To ensure that VTE prevention is fully integrated into NHS systems.
- To ensure that the three dimensions of quality: clinical effectiveness; patient safety; and patient experience, are met in regard to VTE prevention.

Figure 32.1 Aims of National VTE Exemplar Centres in England.

Criteria	Assessment
1. VTE strategy	• Chief executive agreement • Thrombosis committee / VTE implementation group established • VTE guidance and protocol in place
2. Compliance and processes	Satisfactory performance: • VTE risk assessment • Root cause analysis • Audit of VTE prevention pathway • Reporting within Trust and to commissioners
3. Training and education	• Appropriate thromboprophylaxis training • Mandatory induction programmes on VTE • E-learning modules • National and regional learning events and forums
4. Communications	• Staff VTE communication strategies in place • Use of social media, newsletters, intranet, league tables • Patient information leaflets and verbal explanation • Hospital patient groups are informed about VTE
5. Implementation	• VTE process diagram and protocol • VTE champions • Innovations around care, education, audit
6. Patient and community	• Patient care plans • Protocols for transition to the community • Education for self-injection with low molecular weight heparin or regarding adherence to oral agents

Figure 32.2 Essential criteria for VTE Exemplar Centres.

In practice, decisions need to be made regarding delivery of the education programme, the format and content. In small healthcare settings, this may be achievable through face-to-face teaching. Larger organisations can benefit from the use of e-learning, e-assessment and use of local champions to disseminate information. There is a portfolio of national e-learning modules available in England, targeting a range of different healthcare professionals. These are listed in Figure 32.3.

'Reaching' staff is another challenge, particularly in a large institution. Liaising with education departments to ensure VTE features in induction and mandatory update programmes is effective in reaching the majority. It is important that the VTE messages delivered in such programmes are easily retained and are likely to translate into positive changes to practice. Some hospitals have developed mnemonics, stickers, pocket cards and mobile device apps to facilitate access to information when it is most needed.

While planned education programmes will address what best practice should look like in an organisation, another, more responsive, education system needs to be in place to deal with issues as they arise, such as learning from adverse incidents. The multi-professional thrombosis team is well placed to undertake this reactive teaching, in collaboration with risk, governance and clinical teams. In reality, this approach can translate into changes in practice more effectively than formal programmes. There is also an opportunity to learn from examples of best practice.

VTE prevention e-learning course
http://www.vteprevention-nhsengland.org.uk/resources/e-learning

This e-Learning resource, updated in May 2013, is designed to help nurses, pharmacists and junior doctors understand quickly the concept of hospital-associated venous thromboembolism, how to prevent it and to identify which steps of the prevention pathway are necessary to audit.

Developed by the King's Thrombosis Centre and VTE Prevention England
Published Oct 2010
Updated May 2013 (3rd edition)

E-learning for Healthcare
http://www.e-lfh.org.uk/programmes/vte-%28public-access%29/how-to-access/

These resources have been developed in partnership with the NHS England National VTE Prevention Programme, these modules were developed in 2014:
VTE prevention in primary care
VTE prevention: A Guide for Commissioners
VTE prevention for Healthcare Undergraduate Students

Members of the Royal College of Midwives can access an e learning module developed specifically for midwives:
https://www.rcm.org.uk/user/login?destination=node/13942

The Royal College of Nursing have developed a freely accessible module aimed at nurses.
http://www.rcn.org.uk/development/practice/cpd_online_learning/nice_care_preventing_venousthromboembolism/understanding_v

Figure 32.3 e-learning modules available in England.

Risk Assessment

The implementation of VTE risk assessment for all patients admitted into an acute setting is aimed at more accurately identifying patients at risk of VTE, and enabling better decisions to be made in relation to appropriate thromboprophylaxis. It can potentially provide a tool for collecting valuable data concerning risk factors and their relationship with VTE.

In the absence of a validated risk assessment tool, decisions need to be made regarding which tool to use, and whether local adaptations need to be made to better reflect the needs of areas such as stroke and critical care. These decisions need to be balanced against complicating the risk assessment, as they could potentially hinder its accurate use. In England, the Department of Health has created a national risk assessment tool, based on the available evidence; this has enabled standardised use of one tool nationally (Gee and Bonner, 2012).

Clarity around when, and by whom, the risk assessment will be completed is important to aid adherence. This may call for intra-hospital variation, which can be successful, provided that lines of responsibility are clear. For example, the admitting doctor may be best placed to complete the risk assessment in most areas but, in obstetrics, midwives may be more suitable – or, in critical care, it may be nurses.

Measuring Risk Assessment Performance

Collection of performance data has been one of the major challenges of the VTE Prevention Programme nationally. 'Census' data collection has been mandatory in England since 2010, and it is aimed at ensuring that every patient receives a risk assessment on admission to trigger appropriate thromboprophylaxis prescription. Data from each organisation is published, and financial incentives were in place for the first four years as a very effective driver to expedite change.

In 2010, few hospitals had electronic systems able to support risk assessment and data collection, so many employed an innovative approach, adapting existing resources where possible. Some centres incorporated the risk assessment into the medication prescription chart, to encourage prescription of thromboprophylaxis following risk assessment. Other areas incorporated the risk assessment into existing care pathways, or into admission documentation. Electronic systems have the advantage of allowing easy data collection and the use of prompts and prospective surveillance. Conversely, manual data collection can be time consuming, expensive and subject to human error. Electronic systems are at risk of IT errors and crashes, so contingency systems need to be in place to cope in these situations.

Good communication with information technology and business departments are essential to facilitate the process of obtaining good quality data. The manner in which data is then used should be carefully planned; it is a good tool to measure the quality of VTE prevention practice, and enable easy identification of areas that are performing well and those that require further improvement.

For areas in which census data is not mandatory, decisions regarding the nature of snapshot audits need to be made, such as how and when the patients will be selected, who will perform the audit, and what number of patients will give sufficient representation of the patient population.

Reassessment

Thrombosis and bleeding risks can fluctuate throughout a patient's admission, making reassessment necessary whenever the clinical condition changes, to ensure that thromboprophylaxis remains appropriate. In practice, this has the scope to directly impact patient outcomes, since reassessment may prompt a change in thromboprophylaxis, but achieving this can be challenging. Education can be effective in reinforcing the importance of reassessment, but mandating daily consideration of thrombosis and bleeding risk factors may be necessary. The right approach may vary from area to area. Sharing of relevant clinical case scenarios can be a useful tool in achieving adherence with reassessment.

Implementation

For risk assessment to be completed accurately and to be valued as a tool to inform prophylaxis, clinicians need to understand the problem of hospital-associated thrombosis, and how risk assessment can reduce the risk.

In practice, this requires clear articulation of the vision and strategy at all levels within the organisation, and access to necessary resources. There are several strategies that can be employed to help achieve engagement. A link or champion network has worked well in many health care settings. This is where a clinician with a particular interest in VTE prevention will be appointed as a local source of information and guardian of best practice. They should have support from a VTE specialist to ensure their knowledge is up to date, and to coordinate efforts for maximum gain.

The use of appreciative enquiry – that is, creating a culture of affirmation and positivity by celebrating and sharing ideas and strategies, is effective at achieving engagement with VTE prevention (Gee and Bonner, 2012). Good work is recognised and celebrated, and others are inspired to strive to achieve similar high standards. Dissemination of performance and audit findings can be a valuable driver in raising standards, and all available formats should be utilised to distribute this information, including newsletters (electronic and paper versions), email, posters and face-to-face meetings. Obtaining support from senior members of the leadership team adds credibility to this information. Using national outcome data to support the benefits of a VTE Prevention Programme may also be an effective driver.

Solutions to promote VTE risk assessment that have been used with success in practice include a VTE column on the ward patient board (to be ticked when risk assessment is completed), incorporation of risk assessment into nursing and medical handover sheets, and electronic departmental summaries of risk assessment rates to enable prospective surveillance and electronic alerts.

Appropriate Thromboprophylaxis (TP)

This is clearly the vital link in the chain in protecting patients from VTE, but perhaps the hardest to achieve in practice. Interpretation of what constitutes appropriate TP can vary widely, calling for clear local guidelines to aid decisions. For example, clarity is needed around the platelet count cut-off at which chemical prophylaxis is deemed a contraindication, the weight adjustment criteria for LMWH, the unit and level of renal impairment required for LMWH to be contraindicated, and so on.

Mechanical Thromboprophylaxis

The paucity of clinical outcome evidence for mechanical TP sets a challenge to achieving implementation. As before, it is important that national guidelines are used to aid local decisions, to guide clinicians in making consistent choices. Clinicians need to work with procurement teams to ensure that products selected for use have good clinical outcome data wherever possible. Other decisions, such as the length of stockings to be used (thigh or knee length) and duration of use need to be clear.

With all modes of mechanical TP, good quality basic care is required to ensure risks outweigh the potential to cause harm (Gee and Doyle, 2015). For example, in practice, skin damage can result from fitting the wrong size of anti-embolism stockings, or incorrectly positioning intermittent pneumatic compression (IPC) device tubing. This highlights the need for clinicians to receive training on all devices used, and for guidelines to promote their proper use. Documentation of device applied, size of stocking or IPC sleeve, limb measurements and observations from daily skin checks, are essential.

Errors commonly observed with the use of anti-embolism stockings are: failure to measure legs; failure to re-measure in the presence of swelling or weight loss; and failure to comply with recommended skin checks. These can be overcome by ensuring that proper training is given, and that regular audit against local standards takes place as part of continuous quality improvement and is fed back to the appropriate clinical team.

Implementation

Education, audit and feedback are key to achieving success with appropriate TP. Easy access to guidelines and specialist advice may also help implementation.

Logistical considerations may need to be made to optimise appropriate TP, such as ensuring easy access to all modalities. Clinical areas should have easy access to all sizes of anti-embolism stockings and intermittent pneumatic compression device sleeves that may be required, as inadequate stock levels can be a barrier to the correct TP being offered.

A consistent approach to interpretation of appropriate TP should be employed when auditing, in order to optimise the validity of results. For example, one auditor may deem it appropriate to withhold LMWH on the evening after surgery, while another may not. Link staff and champions are well placed to help collect audit data, and this can encourage ownership of the results and increase motivation to implement necessary changes. Investigation into underperforming areas may reveal barriers (such as having insufficient space to store stockings, or having an influx of new staff without training) that, once identified, can be easily remedied.

Patient Empowerment

Empowering patients by educating and supporting them to be involved in thromboprophylaxis decisions is another key part of any VTE prevention programme. An awareness campaign incorporating World Thrombosis Day, and other national and local awareness events, can have a positive impact on the knowledge patients bring to such decisions. NICE promotes the delivery of providing patients with written and verbal information on admission and discharge, and this should include involving patients in their care, and ensuring signs and symptoms of VTE are recognised and acted upon by patients.

Providing this information in a format that is well understood by a diverse patient population can be a significant challenge. It calls for written information to be available in multiple languages, and in versions suitable for patients with impaired cognition and senses. Giving information via a multi-disciplinary approach, and using relevant opportunities (such as during risk assessment) when giving anticoagulants or fitting stockings, may help patients to apply and retain the information.

Conclusion

Outcome evidence exists to support the implementation of a comprehensive VTE prevention programme in acute care organisations, and this chapter has highlighted some of the complexities involved in achieving this. The key factors to success are having a strong team with support at all levels within an organisation, having and articulating clear goals, and having access to adequate resources. Above all else, good quality VTE prevention relies on engagement from all clinical staff. Therefore, having strategies to achieve engagement from staff within the organisation to work towards delivering its goals is vital, and requires commitment, enthusiasm and creativity from the thrombosis team. Having clear guidelines, and empowering patients to be involved in their care, are also important elements in ensuring the success of a programme.

Key Points

1) A multi-disciplinary team of key VTE stakeholders with support from senior leadership is an essential component of a VTE prevention programme.
2) Best practice should be clearly defined, based on national guidelines, and should be easily accessible to clinical staff.
3) An education programme based on local needs is an effective way of improving knowledge and awareness around VTE prevention in an organisation.
4) Risk assessment, and ensuring appropriate thromboprophylaxis through education and audit, requires a multi-faceted approach that can positively impact on patient outcomes.
5) Maximising patient empowerment through information-giving and patient involvement in TP decisions is vital.

Further Reading

Gee E, Bonner L (2012). Collaborative working to reduce VTE. *Nursing Times* **108**(36): 24–6.

Gee E, Doyle C (2015). Best practice in the use of VTE prevention methods. *Nursing Times* **111**(16): 12–14.

Holbrook A, Schulman S, Witt DM, American College of Chest Physicians (2012). Evidence-based management of anticoagulant therapy: Antithrombotic Therapy and Prevention of Thrombosis, 9th ed: American College of Chest Physicians Evidence-Based Clinical Practice Guidelines. *Chest* **141**(2 Suppl): e152S–e184S.

Maynard G, Stein J (2008). *Preventing Hospital-Acquired Venous Thromboembolism: A Guide for Effective Quality Improvement. Prepared by the Society of Hospital Medicine.* AHRQ Publication No. 08-0075. Rockville, MD: Agency for Healthcare Research and Quality. http://www.ahrq.gov/qual/vtguide/.

National Institute for Health and Care Excellence (2010a). Clinical Guideline 92: *Venous thromboembolism in adults admitted to hospital: reducing the risk.* https://www.nice.org.uk/guidance/cg92.

National Institute for Health and Care Excellence (2010b). *Venous thromboembolism prevention quality standard.* NICE Quality Standard 3: http://guidance.nice.org.uk/QS3.

Roberts L, Porter G, Barker R, MD, Yorke R, Bonner L, Patel R, Arya R (2013). Comprehensive VTE Prevention Program Incorporating Mandatory Risk Assessment Reduces the Incidence of Hospital-Associated Thrombosis. *Chest* **140**(4) **144**(4): 1276–1281.

33

VTE Root Cause Analysis – How To Do It

Alison Moughton,[1] Francesca Jones[2] and Will Lester[1]

[1] Department of Haematology, University Hospital Birmingham NHS Foundation Trust
[2] Department of Haematology, University Hospital Coventry and Warwick, NHS Foundation Trust, UK

Background

Root Cause Analysis (RCA) is a structured approach of identifying the underlying cause of a problem. From its inception in the engineering and aviation industries in the 1950s, it has become a key component of health care systems over the past two decades. RCA is now a well recognised process for identifying how and why patient safety incidents have occurred. More importantly, the analysis can be used to identify areas requiring change, and to develop recommendations in order to deliver safer care for patients.

Root cause analysis can provide a methodical system of identifying factors leading to the development of venous thromboembolism (VTE) in a patient, with the aim of enabling learning from these episodes, promoting better practice, improve patient safety and reducing the incidence of hospital-acquired thrombosis (HAT). HAT is commonly defined as any new episode of VTE diagnosed during hospitalisation or within 90 days of discharge following an inpatient stay of at least twenty four hours, or following a surgical procedure under general or regional anaesthesia (NHS England, 2016).

Proven beneficial outcomes of RCA in monitoring of HAT include identification of troublesome areas in VTE prevention and increased awareness by clinicians of VTE. Implementation of standards incorporating RCA has led to a reduction in numbers of episodes of HAT by as much as 20% (Roberts *et al.*, 2013; Rowswell and Nokes, 2013).

RCA Goes Political; the English Experience

In 2005, a Health Committee report highlighted the high number of deaths relating to venous thromboembolism (VTE) acquired in hospital, emphasising the preventable nature of many of these deaths (House of Commons Health Select Committee, 2005). This report generated considerable interest in HAT. In 2010, the NHS Contract for Acute Services in England endorsed a requirement to investigate all episodes of HAT and, in the same year, the move to reduce deaths associated with HAT gained further momentum by the introduction of financial implications linked to performance measures in this field by the

Department of Health framework, Commissioning for Quality and Innovations (CQUIN) (Department of Health, 2010). This financial incentive initially included the undertaking of risk assessment for VTE for all hospital admissions, but was subsequently expanded to incorporate RCA for all cases of HAT. Within the national VTE CQUIN goal for 2013/14, health care providers were given quarterly targets for completion of HAT RCA.

Aims

With any type of root cause analysis, it is key to establish what you are aiming to achieve. Below are some aims to consider when performing HAT RCA at a local level:

- To enable monitoring of HAT and identify cases of potentially preventable events.
- To facilitate learning from individual episodes of HAT within each organisation.
- To identify common themes and facilitate wider learning by reviewing accumulated data locally and, ideally, at a national level.
- To identify and promote local and national solutions from this learning, to consistently reduce the incidence of VTE.

The following steps will assist in the successful identification of HAT and enable data to be extracted through effective RCA:

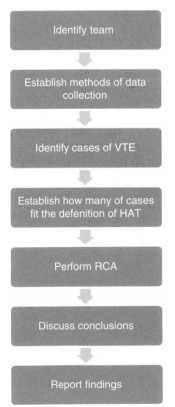

Figure 33.1 An effective path to follow when planning an RCA.

Process

Figure 33.1 identifies an effective path to follow when planning to carry out an RCA.

It is important to give each of the stages in Figure 33.1 careful consideration, as the process of capturing data and successfully performing RCA on such a large group of patients can be very challenging. Systematic methods should ensure effective data capture, and enable the necessary information as to the root cause of an event to be extracted, in order to understand why the VTE event happened and the lessons that can be learned. The data collection tool should be designed so that it is simple to use and gives clear themes on which to assess patient care. It is recommended that the process of data collection should be carried out regularly (at least monthly), to ensure timely identification of potential HAT.

Identify your Team

Firstly, identify the team structure (see Figure 33.2).

It is necessary to engage a gatekeeper, such as a lead consultant. The gatekeeper plays a crucial role in ensuring the process is seen through to completion, as demonstrated above. The team involved must be established at the outset of the process, in order to coordinate data and feedback effectively and should be incorporated into their clinical governance/clinical risk departments, so that findings can be escalated appropriately and dealt with through recognised channels. The process can be lengthy, from the start of a RCA to achieving closure as to the actual root cause for an event; hence, the need for a well-informed team who are all aware of their own and others' roles throughout the process, in order to achieve targets. A key role for specialist thrombosis nurses in this process has been recognised (Rowswell and Law, 2011).

Establish Methods of Data Collection

It is vital to establish whether there are sufficiently robust methods in place to identify all cases of HAT. The most effective method may vary, depending on a hospital's organisational structure. Data can be collected through a variety of methods, including radiology reports, anticoagulant clinic referrals, mortuary/bereavement data and hospital coding (e.g. hospital episode statistics). If available, it can be useful to utilise a computerised patient care system to extract data on discharge, and health insurance data is commonly used in the United States. In the UK, the most robust methodology to capture VTE events appears to be interrogation of radiology reporting (Rowswell and Nokes, 2013).

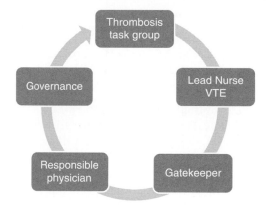

Figure 33.2 Team structure.

A significant challenge is establishing the correct questions to ask, in order to extract the most accurate data and to ensure that the process is repeatable. Hospital coding may be insufficiently sensitive or accurate for the purpose of identifying HAT, unless an effective electronic hospital patient record system is available from which to extract data. VTE deaths (where VTE is the primary cause of death on the death certificate) may be identified by liaison with the bereavement office and mortuary, if suitable. Once the method of data capture has been formalised, it is then possible to begin to derive the number of HATs.

Identify Cases of VTE

At this point, a medical professional with knowledge of VTE – for example, a lead thrombosis nurse can examine the data captured. VTE cases identified using the chosen methodologies need to be cross-checked with admission records, to identify cases that satisfy the definition of HAT (NHS England, 2013) and, therefore, require RCA. This process should ideally be performed at regular intervals, to allow for data to be dealt with in a timely fashion. It is recommended to perform this task at least monthly, and to use a secure electronic database from the outset.

Performing RCA

Although time-consuming, it is essential to ensure that all identified cases of HAT are subject to RCA and, moreover, that there are systems in place to consider the results of RCAs and to take appropriate action. Analysis of circumstances pertaining to the HAT should ideally be reviewed by the designated VTE lead and the lead clinician responsible for the patient's admission. In the author's experience, engagement from the clinicians involved in patient care at the time of HAT can be very difficult to achieve, and requires considerable effort. It is essential to utilise an agreed RCA tool, and it may be prudent to make use of an existing tool to correlate data in line with other centres. A tool is available from the National VTE Prevention Programme website for use in paper or electronic format.

The use of local and national VTE registries could prove invaluable in the future to facilitate sharing of data and to learn from other centres, analogous to haemovigilance schemes such as SHOT. It is recommended that data collection be standardised and electronically stored, so that a hospital can participate actively in wider learning about the nature of HAT. A lead nurse for VTE can ensure thorough record-keeping at all stages of the process, utilising an electronic version of the tool and capturing data regarding HAT themes for feedback purposes.

Discuss Conclusions

Discussion with a lead clinician for thrombosis, and feedback from the physician responsible for the patient's care, will help determine the root cause of the HAT, and can prove an invaluable exercise in establishing the facts surrounding the event. When collating the data, it is useful to identify themes, in order to target areas for improvement in patient care. Some potential common themes are listed below:

- **Thromboprophylaxis (TP) Failure** – patient with high VTE risk who was prescribed and administered chemical prophylaxis as indicated, but still went on to have a VTE event. TP failure is one of the most common findings (Nieto *et al.*, 2014) and is to be expected, as current pharmacological thromboprophylaxis regimens (commonly LMWH) in medical and surgical inpatients are only associated with an approximate 50% and 70% risk reduction, respectively (Turpie and Norris,2004; Collins *et al.*, 1988). Risk factors for thromboprophylaxis failure include increased BMI and a history of VTE (Lim *et al.*, 2015).
- **Inadequate Thromboprophylaxis (TP)** – patient with high VTE risk with an unjustified omission or inadequate dose of chemical or mechanical prophylaxis during their index admission.
- **Contraindication to Thromboprophylaxis (TP)** – patient with bleeding risk factors, such as thrombocytopenia, may not be suitable for LMWH, and patients with acute stroke are not suitable for passive mechanical TP.

Report Findings

Throughout the RCA process, the aim is to establish whether the VTE event was hospital-associated, whether that event could potentially have been prevented, and what can be learned to reduce the risk of HAT in future. As part of the review process, it is necessary to report these findings. Conclusions from the RCA process should be shared with relevant frontline clinicians, managers and overseeing bodies responsible for patient safety and care quality. Root causes should be specific enough that precise action can be taken on the basis of their identification, and recommendations made regarding specific solutions. This should demonstrably reduce the likelihood of recurrence.

If the reason why the event happened is still unclear, then the root cause has not yet been reached, and the process should continue until this is resolved. Duty of candour should also be considered, in terms of informing patients when care has been sub-standard. Ideally, on a larger scale, consistent evidence of thromboprophylaxis failure in specific patient groups should be a catalyst to develop more effective thromboprophylaxis regimens in future.

Key Points

- Hospital-acquired venous thromboembolism (HAT) is a recognised cause of significant morbidity and mortality.
- The preventable nature of HAT has been acknowledged as a key patient safety issue.
- Root Cause Analysis (RCA) is a systematic approach which can be used to reduce the risk of future HAT events.
- The RCA of individual HAT episodes can identify underlying contributing factors with the opportunity for subsequent implementation of changes to clinical practice, in order to reduce the occurrence of HAT.
- RCAs are undertaken by a designated investigating team, using an agreed methodology and RCA tool, in close collaboration with the health care professionals responsible for the patient's care. They should be incorporated into the existing clinical governance infrastructure of each organisation.

- The dissemination of review findings and recommendations, both at a local, and ideally at national/international level, are key to improving quality of patient care.
- The identification of recurring themes, such as thromboprophylaxis failure, are important in guiding future developments/research in this area.
- Duty of candour should always be considered in circumstances where patients have received sub-optimal care.

References

Collins R, Scrimgeour A, Yusuf S, Peto R (1988). Reduction in fatal pulmonary embolism and venous thrombosis by perioperative administration of subcutaneous heparin. Overview of results of randomized trials in general, orthopedic, and urologic surgery. *New England Journal of Medicine* **318**: 1162–73.

Department of Health (2010). *The standard NHS contracts for acute hospital, mental health, community and ambulance services and supporting guidance.* Available at: http://www.dh.gov.uk/en/Publicationsandstatistics/Publications/PublicationsPolicyAndGuidance/DH_111203.

House of Commons Health Select Committee (2005). *The Prevention of venous thromboembolism in hospitalised patients.* The Stationary Office, London. Available at: www.publications.parliament.uk/pa/cm200405/cmselect/cmhealth/99/99.pdf.

Lim W, Meade M, Lauzier F, Zarychanski R, Mehta S, Lamontagne F, Dodek P, McIntyre L, Hall R, Heels-Ansdell D, Fowler R, Pai M, Guyatt G, Crowther MA, Warkentin TE, Devereaux PJ, Walter SD, Muscedere J, Herridge M, Turgeon AF, Geerts W, Finfer S, Jacka M, Berwanger O, Ostermann M, Qushmaq I, Friedrich JO, Cook DJ; PROphylaxis for ThromboEmbolism in Critical Care Trial Investigators (2015). Failure of anticoagulant thromboprophylaxis: risk factors in medical-surgical critically ill patients. *Critical Care Medicine* **43**: 401–10.

NHS England (2013). *VTE Prevention England; The Website of the National VTE Prevention Programme.* Available at: https://www.england.nhs.uk/blog/prevent-venous-thromboembolism/.

Nieto JA, Cámara T, Camacho I; MEDITROM Investigators (2014). Venous thromboembolism prophylaxis in acutely ill hospitalized medical patients. A retrospective multicenter study. *Eur J Intern Med.*;**25**:717–23.

Roberts LN, Porter G *et al.* (2013). Comprehensive VTE Prevention Program Incorporating Mandatory Risk Assessment Reduces the Incidence of Hospital-Associated Thrombosis. *Chest* **144**(4): 1276–1281.

Rowswell H, Law C (2011). Reducing patients risk of venous thromboembolism. *Nursing Times* **107**: 12–4.

Rowswell H, Nokes TJC (2013). *Real Time Radiological Data for Hospital Acquired Thrombosis associated with improved outcomes for Patients.* Plymouth Hospitals NHS Trust. (http://www.vteprevention-nhsengland.org.uk/nnmnweb/index.php/component/k2/item/download/145_0bb2884ecc30f2da65ba7e112b91ae98).

Turpie AG, Norris TM (2004). Thromboprophylaxis in medical patients: the role of low-molecular-weight heparin. *Thrombosis and Haemostasis* **92**: 3–12.

Index